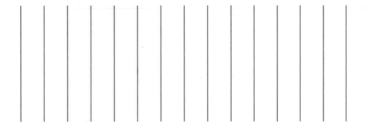

CURRENT TECHNIQUES IN
Laparoscopy

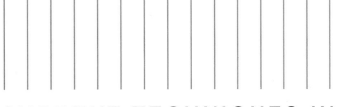

CURRENT TECHNIQUES IN
Laparoscopy

DAVID C. BROOKS, MD, FACS

Harvard Medical School
Brigham and Women's Hospital
Boston, Massachusetts

1 9 9 4

CM

CURRENT ■
MEDICINE

Philadelphia

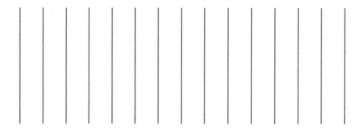

Current Medicine

20 NORTH THIRD STREET
PHILADELPHIA, PA 19106

DEVELOPMENTAL EDITOR:................Bonnie R. Meyers

ILLUSTRATION DIRECTOR:...........................Larry Ward

ART DIRECTOR:.......................................Paul Fennessy

DESIGNER: ....Maria Sarli

MANAGING EDITOR: ....Navasha Barman-Roy

PRODUCTION MANAGER:...........................David Myers

TYPESETTING DIRECTOR:...........................Bill Donnelly

Printed in Hong Kong
by Paramount Printing Group Limited

5 4 3 2 1

ISBN: 1-878132-05-9
ISSN: 1068-4123

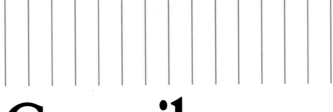

Contributors

RICCARDO ANNABALI, MD
Laparoscopic Research Fellow
Department of Surgery
Creighton University School of Medicine
Omaha, Nebraska

KEITH N. APELGREN, MD
Associate Professor
Department of Surgery
College of Human Medicine
East Lansing, Michigan

DAVID C. BROOKS, MD, FACS
Assistant Professor
Department of Surgery
Harvard Medical School
Attending Surgeon
Brigham and Women's Hospital
Boston, Massachusetts

DOUGLAS BROWN, MD
Fellow, Critical Care Anesthesia
Division of Anesthesiology and
Critical Care Anesthesia
Johns Hopkins Medical School
Baltimore, Maryland

BERNARD DALLEMAGNE, MD
Department of Surgery
Centre Hospitalier Saint Joseph-Esperance
Liege, Belgium

DOUGLAS DORSAY, MD
Department of Surgery
University of South Carolina
School of Medicine
Columbia, South Carolina

ROBERT FITZGIBBONS, JR., FARS
Associate Professor
Department of Surgery
Creighton University School of Medicine
Omaha, Nebraska

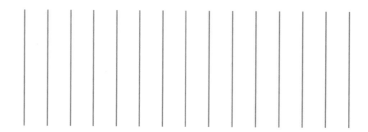

DAVID R. FLETCHER, MBBS, MD, FRACS
Associate Professor
University of Melbourne
Director, Minimal Access Surgery
Austin Hospital
Melbourne, Australia

MORRIS E. FRANKLIN, JR., MD, FACS
Clinical Professor of Surgery
University of Texas Health Science Center
Director, Texas Endosurgery Institute
San Antonio, Texas

FREDERICK L. GREENE, MD
Department of Surgery
University of South Carolina
School of Medicine
Columbia, South Carolina

JOHN G. HUNTER, MD, FACS
Associate Professor of Surgery
Department of Surgery
Emory University School of Medicine
Atlanta, Georgia

CONSTANT JEHAES, MD
Department of Surgery
Centre Hospitalier Saint Joseph-Esperance
Liege, Belgium

NAMIR KATKHOUDA, MD
Chief, Division of Laparoscopic Surgery
Hospital Saint Roch
University of Nice School of Medicine
Nice, France

STEPHEN M. KURTZER, DVM
Medical Concepts Incorporated
Goleta, California

KEVIN R. LOUGHLIN, MD
Associate Professor of Surgery
Brigham and Women's Hospital
Boston, Massachusetts

SERGE MARKIEWICZ, MD
Department of Surgery
Centre Hospitalier Saint Joseph-Esperance
Liege, Belgium

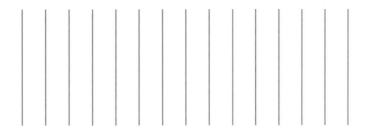

STEVEN J. MENTZER, MD
Division of Thoracic Surgery
Brigham and Women's Hospital
Harvard Medical School
Boston, Massachusetts

JEAN MOUIEL, MD
Chief, Department of Surgery
Hospital Saint Roch
University of Nice School of Medicine
Nice, France

ADRIAN E. ORTEGA, MD
Assistant Professor of Surgery
University of Southern California
Healthcare Consultation Center
Los Angeles, California

JOSEPH B. PETELIN, MD, FACS
Clinical Assistant Professor
Department of Surgery
University of Kansas School of Medicine
Kansas City, Kansas

JEFFREY H. PETERS, MD
Assistant Professor of Surgery
Chief, Division of General Surgery
USC University Hospital
University of Southern California
Healthcare Consultation Center
Los Angeles, California

ELIZABETH J. REDMOND, FRCS
Research Fellow, Department of Surgery
Creighton University School of Medicine
Omaha, Nebraska

PETER ROCK, MD
Associate Professor, Anesthesiology
and Critical Care Medicine
Director, Division of Critical Care Anesthesia
Johns Hopkins Medical School
Baltimore, Maryland

JONATHAN M. SACKIER, MB, FRCS
Associate Professor of Surgery
Department of Surgery
University of California, San Diego, Medical Center
San Diego, California

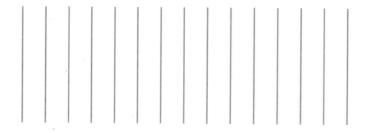

GIOVANNI M. SALERNO, MD
Laparoscopic Research Fellow
Department of Surgery
Creighton University School of Medicine
Omaha, Nebraska

BRUCE D. SCHIRMER, MD
Associate Professor
Department of Surgery
University of Virginia Health Sciences Center
Charlottesville, Virginia

NATHANIEL J. SOPER, MD, FACS
Associate Professor of Surgery
Department of Surgery
Washington University
School of Medicine
St. Louis, Missouri

DAVID J. SUGARBAKER, MD
Chief, Division of Thoracic Surgery
Brigham and Women's Hospital
Harvard Medical School
Boston, Massachusetts

ROBERT D. TUCKER, PHD, MD
Associate Professor
Department of Pathology
University of Iowa
Iowa City, Iowa

STEPHEN WISE UNGER, MD, FACS
Director, Surgical Endoscopy
and Laparoscopy
Mount Sinai Medical Center
of Greater Miami
Miami Beach, Florida

C. RANDLE VOYLES, MD, MS
Associate Clinical Professor
Department of Surgery
University of Mississippi
Jackson, Mississippi

JOSEPH M. WEERTS, MD
Department of Surgery
Centre Hospitalier Saint Joseph-Esperance
Liege, Belgium

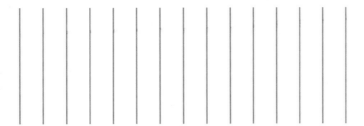

Contents

Chapter 1

Techniques in Laparoscopy: Training, Credentialing, and Socioeconomic Considerations

David C. Brooks

It is difficult to appreciate fully the changes that have occurred in surgery in the 4 years since laparoscopic cholecystectomy was introduced and popularized and an entirely new field entered the realm of general surgery. In the interim the vast majority of general surgeons performing gallbladder surgery in the United States have been taught the technique, and fully 85% of the cholecystectomies performed in the United States are performed laparoscopically [1]. This volume examines available laparoscopic techniques in light of current knowledge and future directions in the field. The emphasis is technical, but the authors have also included important review information reflecting a wide diversity of opinion.

Laparoscopic surgery and its offspring, such as laparoscopic urology and thoracoscopy, have responded to a growing consumer demand to minimize iatrogenic trauma, as well as a socioeconomic demand to decrease hospital stays and return patients to the workplace sooner. Laparoscopic surgery, however, is only the most visible technique in a growing trend toward minimally invasive therapies.

Few events in the history of surgery have had the impact of laparoscopic cholecystectomy. Wickham [2] noted that three seminal events have indelibly altered surgery: the introduction of anesthesia, the development of antisepsis, and endoscopy, a general term that includes both endoluminal and endosurgical procedures. Although many would add organ transplantation to that list, it is hard to differ with Wickham's assessment. Since the first laparoscopic cholecystectomy was performed in the late 1980s, the field of laparoscopic surgery, minimally invasive surgery, endosurgery, or whatever one chooses to call it, has been embraced with a fervor that defies description.

It is both fitting and timely that this first edition of *Current Techniques in Laparoscopy* be published now. The past 4 years have witnessed the introduction, acceptance, and expansion of a dramatically new way to perceive and perform surgery. The authors assembled here represent the pioneers in this new field. Each is an expert in the field, with broad experience. Moreover, these authors have all pushed the technologic envelope as leaders in advancing minimally invasive surgery. This volume provides an overview of the currently available techniques for laparoscopic general, thoracic, and urologic surgery.

The tremendous growth of laparoscopic surgery has raised a number of important sociologic, legal, and ethical issues that continue to fuel debate and controversy within both medicine and the lay public. It is difficult to comprehend the magnitude of changes that have occurred within surgery as a result of this controversy. The consensus panel convened by the National Institutes of Health (NIH) [3] on laparoscopic cholecystectomy in 1992 has placed its imprimatur on the procedure, and although that clears the way for an increasing acceptance of the operation, it would be naive to think that surgeons and the public had waited for the NIH seal of approval before thoroughly using the technique. With the controversy surrounding laparoscopic cholecystectomy somewhat diminished and with the growth curve nearing the shoulder, it is useful to look at the sociologic, legal, and ethical issues that affect the medical establishment, the payers, and the public.

TRAINING

The introduction of laparoscopic cholecystectomy in 1987 required the vast majority of general surgeons in the United States, some of whom had had only a small amount of laparoscopic training during their residencies, to acquire an entirely new set of skills. Because of the eminent popularity of this procedure among both patients and insurers, most surgeons in the United States felt the need to acquire these skills rapidly. During 1989 and 1990, 2- and 3-day courses in laparoscopic cholecystectomy sprang up across the country [4]. These courses were sponsored by individual surgeons, academic institutions, and manufacturing companies. By the end of 1991, nearly all the surgeons interested in gallbladder disease had acquired the basic skills to perform the operation through these courses.

Although none of the courses were regulated or officially accredited at the outset, they had a number of

unifying attributes. The courses could be divided into three different segments. The first involved *didactic* teaching related to laparoscopy, the videoendoscopic imaging systems, and the laparoscopic instruments. Some courses also involved basic laser instruction. During the early part of the laparoscopic cholecystectomy experience, the laser was thought to facilitate this procedure. Laser training, which accompanied courses in laparoscopic surgery, was inadequate to meet most hospital laser credentialing criteria but offered the enterprising surgeons an easy introduction to the field. (Subsequent experience has shown that there is no advantage to using lasers.) The didactic portion of these courses generally lasted from 4 to 6 hours, during which the faculty outlined the basics of laparoscopic surgery and described their personal experiences with laparoscopic cholecystectomy.

The second portion of the training courses consisted of *inanimate* training to acclimate the surgeon to a two-dimensional world in which tactile feedback and proximity are lost. Using what are referred to as *pelvic trainers* (black boxes in which a video camera had been inserted), surgeons were able to practice basic procedures such as trocar insertion, tissue dissection, and vascular clipping. A number of cleverly chosen objects were used to simulate "real life," such as grapes, beans, and balloons. None of these had the normal consistency of human tissue, but at least they allowed the operator to practice in this new two-dimensional world with slippery and often awkward items. The inanimate practice generally lasted 4 to 6 hours, and by the end students were familiar with cannulas and trocars, operating instruments, the basic operation of videoendoscopic equipment, and operative strategies for dissection. Importantly, these sessions allowed the surgeons to become accustomed to working from a television screen, and to the unequivocally distracting phenomenon of looking away from the operative field and watching one's hands on a television.

The final and most satisfying portion of most laparoscopic courses dealt with a hands-on animal laboratory using, most commonly, the small domestic swine. These animals, weighing between 30 and 40 pounds, allowed the student surgeons to practice the skills they had learned in the pelvic trainers and to finally appreciate the sense of operating on living tissue. Skill stations for these procedures involved three people. One student functioned as the camera operator, one as the first assistant, and one as the operating surgeon. Roles were rotated through these various positions until everyone had had an opportunity to appreciate the difficulties and obstacles involved in each position. The biliary tree of the swine is quite similar to gross human anatomy, although the size and delicacy of the structures does not correspond to those of diseased human gallbladders. Nonetheless students soon became aware of the need for meticulous dissection, the difficulty of controlling bleeding, and the strength and weaknesses of both electrocautery and laser dissection.

Although many of these courses were given under the auspices of individual surgeons or academic institutions, all were supported by generous donations from manufacturing companies. These companies often provided all the cannulas and trocars, video equipment, and instruments necessary to complete these procedures. The donations obviously did not represent an altruistic effort on the part of the companies, but rather an opportunity to highlight their merchandise and introduce surgeons to their products in the burgeoning marketplace.

These courses also offered an opportunity for the entrepreneurial surgeon to enter the educational marketplace. During 1989, 1990, and 1991, surgeons with familiarity in laparoscopic cholecystectomy were generously rewarded for their teaching skills. This policy was viewed as a disturbing trend because of the historical willingness of surgeons to share their expertise and skills with others and to encourage the free flow of ideas and experience. Nonetheless, the cost of organizing the courses, securing manufacturing sponsorship, and reimbursing faculty surgeons who took time away from their practices necessitated a hefty tuition for some of these courses, often in the range of $2500 to $3000. For the student, however, this investment was well worth the future benefits. The public demanded this new technology and surgeons who did not learn it were left in the dust. By the end of 1991, virtually all interested surgeons had completed courses, and that fact alone led to the estimation that 85% of all cholecystectomies were performed laparoscopically during 1992.

Training for resident physicians has taken on a slightly different form. As laparoscopic cholecystectomy has been introduced successfully into academic institutions, attending surgeons have gradually involved house officers in the procedure. At our institution, fifth-year residents were initially taught laparoscopic cholecystectomy. Since then the procedure has gradually evolved downward in the residency, so that now second-year residents typically perform the case. In the more than 1200 procedures performed at our institution since 1990, residents have been the operating surgeons in all but the first 20 cases. Many academic programs have used formal courses to demonstrate these techniques. Residents are required to attend didactic lessons, practice on pelvic trainers, and demonstrate skills on living swine. Others, such as ours, have opted to introduce resident surgeons to laparoscopic procedures in much the same way we do to other procedures. In other words, the house staff assists in the first six to 10 cases and gradually assumes more and more responsibility after demonstrating their understanding of the anatomy, the instrumentation, and the necessary skills. Resident interest and skill are variable and unpredictable. We have noted that certain residents require a longer training period to acclimate themselves to a two-dimensional world and to become comfortable with a dissecting technique that does not involve tactile feedback. Others rapidly assimilate the surgical skills necessary and show an impressive aptitude for two-dimensional surgery.

The future of training in laparoscopic surgery will eventually become a nonissue as more and more residents are exposed to a greater variety of advanced laparoscopic procedures during their training and translate these skills into practical experience when they join attending staffs. In the meantime, however, questions still persist as to the utility of training courses for the more advanced procedures. Many institutions have been ambivalent in their credentialing and have not required specific courses for each individual procedure. On the other hand, surgeons with only a limited laparoscopic experience feel more comfortable taking advanced courses to learn the strategies involved in dealing with complex procedures such as herniorrhaphy, colon resection, and gastroesophageal surgery. Most people acknowledge that the transition from laparoscopic cholecystectomy to laparoscopic appendectomy is sufficiently straightforward and easy to not require additional advanced training. As a general rule, laparoscopic procedures that are more destructive than reconstructive are easier to do and require less facility with the more advanced techniques, such as knot tying and intracorporeal anastomoses. It seems clear, however, that there will be a place for advanced training courses in the foreseeable future and until a larger portion of the operating surgeons in the country become familiar with other aspects of laparoscopic surgery.

The training of surgeons in advanced laparoscopic procedures will also depend largely on future trends in laparoscopic surgery. The most optimistic prognosticators expect that 60% to 70% of general surgical procedures will be conducted laparoscopically within the next decade. Others believe that this approach may be too optimistic and that once the initial wave of enthusiasm for laparoscopic cholecystectomy has passed, a more rigorous examination of advanced laparoscopic procedures will need to be undertaken before they are wholeheartedly embraced by the surgical community in the United States.

CREDENTIALING

A general surgeon who completes 5 years in an accredited residency currently applies for operating room privileges and admitting privileges at the hospital in which he or she practices. Credentialing committees have generally assumed that a surgeon completing a fully accredited training program is capable of performing those operations considered within the purview of general surgery. There has never been a requirement to demonstrate technical competence, nor has there been any mechanism to observe a surgeon at work. The introduction of laparoscopic surgery has altered our philosophy toward credentialing at a time when there is a greater concern for liability and culpability issues within the medical profession. As a result laparoscopic credentialing committees have sprung up in most hospitals where this new technology is available. Various national organizations, such as the Society for Surgery of the Alimentary Tract and the Society of American Gastrointestinal Endoscopic Surgeons, have delineated general credentialing criteria despite the fact that there is no uniform state or federal legal requirement [5]. Nonetheless, the litigious atmosphere surrounding surgery in the 1990s has prudently dictated that hospitals assume the responsibility of oversight. In the last 2 years, a general consensus has been built across the country to define the requirements for laparoscopic credentialing. These requirements comprise, at a minimum, a) a course that includes didactic, inanimate, and live operating experience; b) a preceptorship as an assistant surgeon of no fewer than five cases; and c) a preceptorship of no fewer than five cases as the operating surgeon under the guidance of an experienced laparoscopic surgeon. Many institutions have requested that surgeons applying for laparoscopy credentials also submit tapes of their work.

Residents who have completed the majority of their training during the postlaparoscopy, postpelviscopy period should not require attendance at a formal course, although it is still considered prudent for them to undergo a five-case preceptorship. Many surgeons view these credentialing criteria as odious; however, surgery in general has been sadly remiss in regulating the types of work performed by surgeons. It is also important for credentialing committees to maintain longitudinal records concerning morbidity and mortality. This ensures appropriate ongoing credentialing.

State review of credentialing criteria has been sporadic. The most notable case is New York, which has aggressively pursued the rate of laparoscopic complications in a number of hospitals and has issued disciplinary notices based on the findings [6]. It is incumbent on organized surgery to anticipate these issues and to adequately police and monitor the performance of laparoscopic surgery from within the profession.

THE RISING INCIDENCE OF LAPAROSCOPIC SURGERY

Not only are the types of laparoscopic procedures increasing, as can be seen from the topics included in this volume, but the total number of cases done in a particular area also appears to be increasing. This has been documented in both Connecticut and California. During the calendar year 1991, Orlando reported that the state of Connecticut showed an increase of approximately 25% in the number of cholecystectomies done as compared with the prior 2 to 3 years [7]. In California, Blue Cross–Blue Shield reported that laparoscopic cholecystectomies increased from approximately 140 to 155 per 100,000 [8]. Because there is no reason to believe that the pathophysiology of symptomatic cholelithiasis is changing, two possible explanations remain. The first is that there is a large backlog of symptomatic gallbladder patients who had postponed recommended surgery. With the advent of laparoscopic cholecystectomy and the promise of diminished pain and rapid return to the normal activities of daily living, these patients opted to undergo surgery at an earlier date than they might otherwise have done. This explanation undoubtedly holds true in a large percentage of patients. Symptomatic cholelithiasis affects a young, otherwise healthy female population, many of whom are active in the workforce or pursuing busy schedules as homemakers. In the past, this patient cohort could often control their symptoms by strict dietary manipulation and would expect only occasional episodes of biliary colic when they were indiscreet with their diets. Because active professional women with responsibilities at home can anticipate surgical care with a maximum of 24 hours' hospitalization and 1 week of convalescence, early acceptance of laparoscopic surgery allows minimal interruption in their lifestyle.

A more troubling explanation, however, is that surgeons are no longer offering the procedure simply to patients who have moderate to severe symptomatic cholelithiasis. In other words, the mere presence of gallstones associated with dyspepsia and mild upper abdominal discomfort is being invoked as reason to undergo surgery. Although there are no data to support this explanation, I suspect that it accounts for a proportion of the increased number of cholecystectomies performed in the United States today.

There are major implications in pursuing a policy of early cholecystectomy. Although the procedure is safe and has acceptable associated morbidity and mortality rates, as suggested by the NIH consensus conference, complications and death will continue to occur. No useful service is provided if cholecystectomy is performed with questionable indications and an untoward outcome ensues. Furthermore, the financial savings to the American health system, which surgeons were quick to understand in the case of laparoscopic cholecystectomy, will not be fully realized if cholecystectomy is performed for marginal indications. Surgeons must continue to offer laparoscopic cholecystectomy only to symptomatic patients. There is no role, with a few minor exceptions, for prophylactic cholecystectomy. Likewise, other, newer procedures should be performed with the same indications as traditional procedures and only if a comparable procedure can be completed with at least similar morbidity and mortality rates.

SURGEONS AND INDUSTRY

In addition to the many issues surrounding training, credentialing, and regulation, the relationship between surgeons and industry has changed dramatically in the last 4 years. The sudden emergence of laparoscopic surgery as an alternative to painful, debilitating, and morbid open surgical procedures has brought together two groups who would not otherwise have been in close contact. Prior to the advent of laparoscopic surgery, a surgeons' contact with industry was limited, desultory, and minimal. Drug representatives have always been present, touting new antibiotics and so forth, but device manufacturers have not had large dealings with individual surgeons. Certainly the advent of stapling devices in the late 1960s and early 1970s brought manufacturers' representatives in close contact with surgeons, but eventually acquisition decisions were largely taken over by hospital purchasing departments, with the advice and consent of the operating surgeon.

Laparoscopic surgery, on the other hand, has required an entirely new armamentarium and this has brought the device manufacturers ever closer to the surgeons. These devices include video systems, insufflators, cannulas and trocars, and instruments. For the surgeon, this relationship has been necessary both to enhance training and as an introduction to the procedures; for industry it has been an opportune time to both sell devices and garner ideas for new and innovative instruments. This symbiotic relationship has had the potential for great advances in a new and emerging field, but also the potential for collusive and venal motives. For surgeons unaccustomed to the entrepreneurial side of industry, this relationship has been fraught with potential conflicts of interest. Fortunately the mood within the profession demands ethical conduct at all costs. Surgeons who present data in national forums must now acknowledge any and all relationships with industry. It remains incumbent on surgeons to acknowledge these relationships and to remember that the patient is truly our only customer. Unfortunately, from the standpoint of the industry, the profits to be made are too large to allow the marketing of these instruments to proceed solely on the basis of product merit. Whereas surgeons may find minimal and unimportant differences in competing equipment, to industry, two similar products are as different as night and day. Surgeons by nature are adaptable and generally achieve their operative results in spite of their instruments. It is difficult to take seriously the competing claims of manufacturers. Surgeons must bargain on behalf of the patient and the hospital, not their own gain. We will certainly lose what little trust is invested in us if we are seen as being stooges of industry.

THE FUTURE

The procedures outlined and presented in this volume are only the beginning of a true revolution in surgery and medicine, a revolution that will accompany our government's hopes and plans for a major change in the way health care is delivered. Surgeons have taken the forefront of this revolution, bringing to fruition a vision of safe, effective, and minimally invasive therapy. There seems little doubt that we will continue to advance the science of surgery toward the least morbid, least invasive, and most acceptable therapy.

Not mentioned in this volume is the tremendously exciting area of robotics and virtual reality, pursuits that are only a short way from the clinic and that will further refine and alter the way medicine is practiced. The promise of ever newer techniques and ever less traumatic therapies challenges and emboldens us to imagine ways of treating disease never before considered. This is an exciting time to be a surgeon. We have it within our power to push forward the confines of traditional surgery while remaining true to the precepts of care, such as gentleness of tissue handling, asepsis, and hemostasis, that are central to all surgical procedures.

REFERENCES

1. Invisible mending. *Economist*, April 10, 1993:93.

2. Wickham JEA: *Editorial. J Minimally Invasive Surg* 1991, 1:1–5.

3. National Institutes of Health NIH Consensus Development Panel on Gallstones and Laparoscopic Cholecystectomy. *JAMA* 1993, 269:1018–1024.

4. Zucker KA, Bailey RW, Graham SM, Scovil W, Imbembo AL. Training for Laparoscopic Surgery. *World J Surg* 1993, 17:3–7.

5. Hershman MJ, Turner G, Drew P, Rosin RD: Laparoscopic Cholecystectomy: Views of a Surgeon in Training. *J Minimally Invasive Surg* 1992, 1:267–271.

6. *Gen Surg Laparoscopy News* 1992, 13:1.

7. Russel JC, Orlando R, Cahow CE, Laffaye HA: Laparoscopic Cholecystectomy: A Statewide Experience. *Arch Surg* (in press).

8. *Am Med News*, May 4, 1992:9.

Chapter 2

Laparoendoscopic Imaging Equipment and Devices

Stephen M. Kurtzer

Medical imaging has been around for many years in several different modalities. Roentgenography, fluoroscopy, ultrasound, computed tomography (CT), magnetic resonance imaging (MRI), and more recently endoscopic video systems have provided medical professionals with a means of "seeing" internal structures of the human body. Before these inventions, the human eye was the physician's only tool for seeing, and although limited, the eye is still a major factor in all imaging systems.

TODAY'S ENDOSCOPIC SURGICAL SUITE

Today's endoscopic surgical suite includes an endoscope, high-resolution video camera, high-resolution video monitors, high-intensity light source, insufflator, irrigator, electrocautery or laser unit, and possibly other means of visualization [1•].

In Figure 1A, the most important part of the system is missing—the viewer (Fig. 1B). The surgeon's eyes are the basic image processor for the entire system. No matter how "high tech" the endoscopic suite becomes, endoscopic procedures always require a surgeon, who stands next to the patient or works from a console in a different area. We cannot overlook the human aspect of the surgeon as an important, unpredictable part of the system. The unpredictability stems from the fact that no two people perceive the same thing when viewing the same scene. This disparity creates an enormous challenge for people in the business of manufacturing imaging systems.

Before we discuss current laparoendoscopic technology, we should explain the evolution of endoscopy and what prompted the recent acceptance of laparoscopic procedures by general surgeons.

HISTORICAL OVERVIEW

Endoscopy (visualization of the interior of a living organism) began in the early 1800s when an obstetrician by the name of Philipp Bozzini realized his dream of constructing a device that could be used to look into the human body. Bozzini constructed this first endoscope, called the *Lichtleiter*, in 1806. Although the original Lichtleiter was never used on a patient, Bozzini is credited with inventing the first endoscope. Bozzini's principles of light, reflection of light, and light conduction are still applicable today.

Expanding on Bozzini's principles, Antonin Jean Desormeaux, a French surgeon, was the first to use an endoscope on a patient (1853). He is considered the father of endoscopy. Desormeaux's endoscope used a concave reflector and plane mirror with central aperture and spirit lamp flame. The instrument was clumsy and had to be used with great care so as not to burn the patient's legs. Although the light source was weak, Desormeaux was able to visualize disease in the urethra and stones in the bladder [2].

Thomas Edison's invention of the light bulb in the late 1800s provided the early endoscopists with an important answer to the illumination question. Maximillian Nitze, a German physician, took Edison's concept of electrical illumination and produced a tiny light bulb for placement at the distal end of the cystoscope. He also recognized the importance of an optical system. Nitze invented the first optical endoscope using electrical incandescent light (1876). This breakthrough is considered the birth of modern urology [2]. Nitze and Josef Leiter, a Viennese instrument maker, went on to produce the first set of electroendoscopic instruments.

In the early 1900s gynecologists, otorhinolaryngologists, and urologists around the world began using endoscopes first for diagnosis then later for therapeutic procedures. The physician viewed inside the body directly through the endoscope, which was placed through a naturally occurring orifice. This technique was not practical for general surgeons, however, because the abdomen is a closed structure, and most procedures require a second surgeon who must also be able to view the operative area with uncompromising accuracy.

Only after many years did general surgeons embrace the idea of laparoscopy, even though a few physicians and gastrointestinal surgeons (*eg*, Charles Lightdale, MD, George Berci, MD, Barry Salky, MD, H. Juergen Nord, MD, Worth Boyce Jr., MD) had performed abdominal laparoscopy for decades [3•].

PENETRATING THE GENERAL SURGERY MARKET

In the 1970s, the emphasis in laparoscopy was on diagnostic, not therapeutic, procedures other than in gynecology. According to Dr. Charles Lightdale, the CT scan became the preferred method in the mid-1970s for diagnostic use and biopsy collection because it was less invasive than surgery and provided additional information to laparoscopy.

The lack of long-handled instruments similar to those recently introduced to laparoscopists and high-resolu-

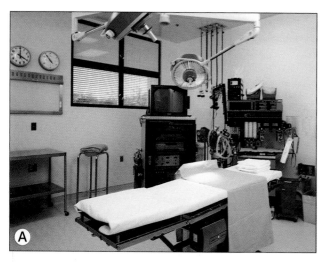
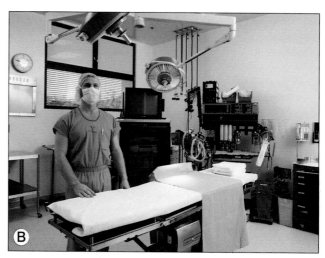

Figure 1. **A,** What's missing? **B,** The surgeon is the most important part of the imaging system.

tion video systems precluded the use of laparoscopes for operative therapeutic procedures.

Another factor was the general surgeon's resistance to the ideas of the early laparoscopists [8]. The concept of moving away from traditional open procedures to the less-known, minimally invasive methods was initially met with doubt and skepticism. Some general surgeons clung to the adage of "why look through the keyhole when you can open the door?"

Kurt Semm, MD, of Kiel, Germany, a world-renowned pioneer of intra-abdominal laparoscopy, developed an automatic insufflation device in 1964 that monitored abdominal pressure and gas flow. This device, along with safer insufflation needles, greatly reduced the potential risk of injury to patients, but the timing was not right for what was still considered a "blind" procedure [4].

Gynecologists moved the cause forward by recognizing the possibilities of endoscopic sterilization. In 1970, Jordan Phillips, MD, of Santa Fe Springs, CA, and other leading gynecologists founded the American Association for Gynecological Laparoscopists. As a result of this organization, endoscopic sterilization became widely discussed and accepted in the gynecologic field. Gynecologists (eg, Jaroslav Hulka, MD, developer of the Hulka clip, Inbae Yoon, MD, developer of the fallopian ring, Richard Soderstrom, MD, developer of the snare technique, Jacques Rioux, MD, Albert Yuzpe, MD, Franklin Loffer, MD, Richard Kleppinger, MD, and Stephen Corson, MD, leaders in the development of instruments for electrosurgical sterilization) pioneered modern laparoscopic instrumentation by creating and partially filling the need for long-handled instruments. The tools they required for sterilization were easily adapted in later years to general surgical procedures.

General surgeons continued to open the abdomen until the late 1980s, when the advantages of laparo-scopic cholecystectomy became well known throughout the medical community. Many leading surgeons (eg, Eddie Reddick, MD, Douglas Olsen, MD, George Berci, MD, and Ed Phillips, MD) shared their video-documentation and laparoscopic successes with their colleagues.

Douglas Olsen, MD, of Nashville, TN, attributes the sudden interest in laparoscopic surgery to the introduction of high-resolution video cameras. Although physicians in many other specialties had been using endoscopes and cameras, not until the late 1980s had the technology addressed the unique needs of the laparoscopic general surgeon.

MEDICAL VIDEO CAMERAS

Photographic endoscopy was first attempted by Nitze in 1890. A long time passed without any significant advances relative to the endoscope or endoscopic documentation. In the 1960s, British physicist Harold H. Hopkins perfected the use of glass fibers as well as the rod lens system for endoscopy. The Hopkins rod lens optical system dramatically improved the quality of endoscopic images. It offered surgeons very high quality endoscopic views worth documenting.

The evolution of photography for endoscopy was slow to progress until the development of fully automatic exposure flash systems that enabled surgeons to document their findings using 35-mm film cameras [5]. In the early 1970s, a handful of surgeons adapted large, broadcast-type video cameras for use with endoscopes and microscopes, but not until 1973 did a US company introduce a video camera specifically designed for use in endoscopic procedures. The camera used a single 2.5-cm (one inch) tube and produced full-color images. Weighing 1.7 kg (3.8 lbs), it was far too cumbersome for the average surgeon (Fig. 2). During the next several years, innovations were made that resulted in smaller tube cameras that were soakable.

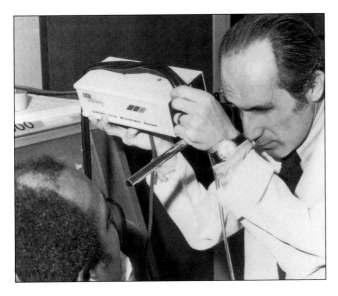

Figure 2. Dr. George Berci, video endoscopy pioneer, using one of the earliest video cameras designed specifically for endoscopy.

Soakability enhanced and increased the camera's usability, because the cumbersome use of sterile towels or drapes was no longer necessary.

In 1982, the first solid-state camera was introduced. "Chip" technology greatly reduced the size and weight of cameras to well under one quarter kilogram (one-half pound). This introduction was, perhaps, the most interest-generating technologic advance in the endoscopic evolution since the introduction of the Hopkins rod lens system. Now, high-resolution video cameras could be designed in small, light-weight packages that appealed to the surgeon both technologically and ergonomically. Orthopedic surgeons, gynecologists, otorhinolaryngologists, and urologists, already accustomed to using endoscopes, welcomed this new video technology to their endoscopy suites.

For general surgeons, the laparoscope and video camera came not simply as an addition to existing equipment but as an essential part of the operating system. The availability of a high-resolution video camera freed the surgeons' hands and made coordinated viewing between surgeons possible. Today, more than 80% (480,000) of all cholecystectomies performed in the United States are done laparoscopically [6•], and all of them rely on the visual capabilities of medical video cameras.

Biomedical Business International (Santa Ana, CA), a medical market research firm, estimates the number of laparoscopic general surgery procedures to reach 1.7 million by the year 1997. In addition, an estimated 700,000 laparoscopic procedures will be performed in other specialties such as gynecology and thoracoscopy. A complete endoscopic surgical estimate would take into account all other specialties (excluding gastrointestinal and pulmonary endoscopy) that use rigid and flexible scopes (*eg*, urology, otorhinolaryngology, and orthopedic surgery). This number, in my opinion, would exceed 4 million by 1997.

UNDERSTANDING THE KEY SPECIFICATIONS

The excitement and possibilities surrounding laparoendoscopic surgery resulted in many new medical companies entering the video and instrumentation marketplace. The large number of competitive companies has inevitably created an overwhelming amount of conflicting information regarding what is good and what is not. To gain a better understanding of what you can expect from video technology and to ensure you reap the full benefits from a system, you must familiarize yourself with a few key specifications before making a purchase.

RESOLUTION

Resolution is probably the most commonly discussed camera specification, for good reason. It determines the clarity and detail of the video image.

Resolution is usually measured by scanning an Electronic Industries Association resolution chart (Fig. 3) that fills the monitor screen. Horizontal resolution is measured by the number of vertically oriented alternating black and white lines that appear on three fourths of the screen's width. Three fourths of the width is equal to the screen height, so one can measure both vertical and horizontal resolution to the same standard.

Vertical resolution is measured by the number of observable, horizontally oriented, alternating black and white lines and is a function of the scanning system. A scanning system, which can vary in different countries, is the system that television monitors rely on for creating the video image.

If we rely on the number of lines seen by an observer to arrive at the measurement of resolution, then the resolution can vary from observer to observer. Resolution is a subjective measurement within certain limits as set forth by the camera's pixel count.

The number of picture elements, or pixels, on a solid-state sensor directly correlates to its ability to visually resolve detail. The higher the number of pixels, the more capable the camera is of resolving picture detail. Vertical resolution is fixed by the scanning system and should remain constant regardless of camera manufacturer.

Although resolution is somewhat subjective, there is a mathematic formula that defines the maximum horizontal resolution a camera is capable of reaching. For example, a black-and-white charge coupled device (CCD) sen-

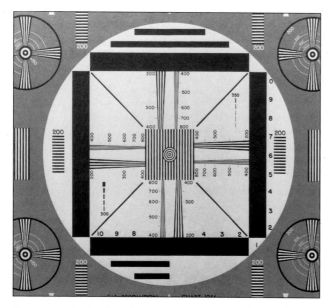

Figure 3. Electronic Industries Association resolution chart.

sor with 100 columns of pixels has one line of resolution for every row of vertical pixels. Because resolution is measured using only 75% of the screen, the maximum resolution this sensor could produce is 75 lines. For a color sensor, 20% (of the remaining 75%) of the pixels would be lost to reproducing color, *ie*, we would retain only 80% (of the remaining 75%) of the pixels for resolution, which in this example is 60 lines. (100%-25%)80% = 60% of total horizontal pixel count.

Therefore, a quick way to figure the maximum resolution of a single-chip color video camera is to take 60% of the total horizontal pixel count. This method works simply because it already takes into account the use of only 75% of the screen and the 20% demand for color. As the formula indicates, you cannot expect to find a resolution specification higher than or equal to the pixel count.

Unfortunately, no single measurement system is used consistently by video manufacturers. The industry standard is to measure horizontal resolution using 75% of the screen; however, some manufacturers have been known to use 100% of the screen and thus publish numbers much higher than their competitors' values. Be aware of such tactics, and arm yourself with the right questions.

LIGHT SENSITIVITY

Another important specification is light sensitivity. Light sensitivity refers to the minimum amount of light required by the camera to produce a usable image. This specification, too, is a subjective measurement that varies from observer to observer. Light sensitivity is the camera's ability to make a usable picture in low light conditions. Because lighting conditions vary during laparoscopic procedures, a camera's ability to respond to changing light is extremely important.

SIGNAL-TO-NOISE RATIO

The signal-to-noise ratio is a measurement that differentiates random video "noise" from useful video information. The specification is measured in decibels. A noise value is obtained by allowing no light to reach the sensor and measuring the signal generated by the system on an oscilloscope. In the absence of picture information, the signal contains only noise. A signal value is obtained by illuminating a scene as brightly as the sensor will allow and measuring the amplitude of the signal.

A larger ratio indicates that a picture is "cleaner," meaning it has less noise than a smaller ratio. A camera's signal-to-noise ratio is an indicator of how fine details will appear on the screen relative to background noise. This ability is most important for viewing scenes in low light levels.

These three specifications, resolution, light sensitivity, and signal-to-noise ratio, are, in my opinion, the most important specifications for a potential buyer to understand. Granted, we could discuss many other specifications, but if these three measurements do not meet your needs, then the myriad of other specifications is meaningless. The best way to determine whether a camera is appropriate for you is to arrange a live demonstration in your operating room or office. If you make an investment in a video system based solely on the specifications listed on promotional materials, you are robbing yourself of the chance to evaluate how the camera performs when viewed by you.

CURRENT IMAGING TECHNOLOGY

My intent here is to discuss current technology and available products. Although new imaging technology is always under research and development, this section focuses on technology commercially available at the time of this writing. All of the imaging systems discussed in this chapter were actively marketed at the 1992 American College of Surgeons meeting as well as other conventions and exhibitions around the world. Although some of the products were in prototype stages, they were all available for public viewing.

INTRAOPERATIVE ULTRASOUND

Intraoperative ultrasound (Fig. 4) is still in the early stages and is used mainly for the examination of the biliary tree. Although not yet widely embraced by laparoscopic surgeons, it seems to offer a reliable endoscopic method for diagnostic evaluation and identification of abdominal abnormalities. The ultrasonic images can be displayed in a picture-in-picture arrangement on the monitor screen with freeze frame and zoom capabilities. Intraoperative ultrasound will most likely find its niche

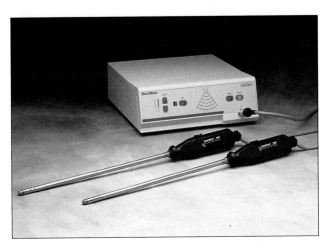

Figure 4. Recently introduced intraoperative ultrasound device.

as a complement to cholangiography as a screening procedure during laparoscopy prior to cholecystectomy, and as an evaluation tool in addition to the choledochoscope after the removal of the gallbladder near the end of the procedure.

MEDICAL VIDEO SYSTEMS

There are different styles of cameras on the market; some utilize one CCD sensor, others use three. Some are one-piece camera-lens designs, and others have detachable lenses. Some are specialty specific and are beneficial for purchase when other uses are not anticipated. Examples of specialized units are cameras with an integrated laparoscope (Fig. 5) designed specifically for laparoscopy and cameras with integral beamsplitters designed for urologic endoscopy. These types of cameras are not easily shared by other specialties within a hospital.

SINGLE-CHIP CAMERAS

Single-chip technology evolved from the first solid-state camera (1983) to the higher resolution systems of today. Several models are available that use a single CCD sensor; all offer approximately 300 to 450 lines of horizontal resolution. Single-chip cameras are generally small and compact and weigh approximately 42 to 84 g (1.5 to 3.0 ounces) (Fig. 6).

Most single-chip cameras reproduce color by using a mosaic filter pattern comprised of complementary (yellow, cyan, magenta) colors. Complementary color filters are placed precisely over the pixels in a pattern that resembles a mosaic. An electronic process is required to convert the complementary colors into primary colors (red, blue, green). Approximately 20% of the total number of pixels is lost in this reproduction process to produce color rather than used for resolution.

Image quality can vary greatly from manufacturer to manufacturer, so a personal demonstration is very useful. A variety of features are available, depending on the model you choose. Automatic exposure systems negate the need for automatic light sources. Zoom lenses (variable focal length) and focusing mechanisms facilitate the identification of anatomic features. Some cameras have control buttons on the camera head itself, and many offer a choice of focal lengths of endoscopic adaptors. One-piece camera-laparoscopes eliminate potential fogging at the junction of the endoscope and camera lenses. A camera has recently been introduced that incorporates not only a laparoscope but a built-in lens-washing and irrigation system (Fig. 7).

THREE-CHIP CAMERAS

At the heart of the three-chip camera is a prism that separates the light into the three primary colors of red, green, and blue (RGB) (Fig. 8). A sensor is mounted on each side of the prism. Each sensor "sees" one color and transmits the single color information to the video monitor.

A three-chip camera produces more accurate color than single-chip cameras because it has a true RGB prismatic color-separation system (Fig. 9). Since the system is RGB from beginning to end, no color accuracy is lost to electronic processing or encoding and decoding of the color signals. In non-RGB systems, all available color information is encoded into compatible formats (*eg*, NTSC, PAL, SECAM) and is then decoded by compatible video monitors to produce a final picture. Encoding and decoding of color information cause a loss of chromatic resolution.

In general, three-chip cameras available today have horizontal resolution counts of approximately 500 to 700 lines. Since no pixels are lost in color reproduction, the horizontal resolution of a three-chip camera can be computed by simply taking 75% of the total pixel count. The result of the high resolution is an extremely sharp image that captures fine detail. The resolution can be additionally increased by off-setting the green channel approximately one half pixel width. Pixels are

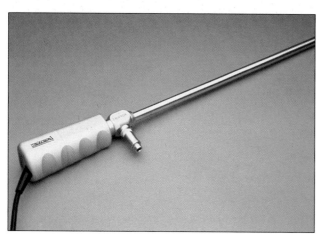

Figure 5. One-piece camera-laparoscope video system.

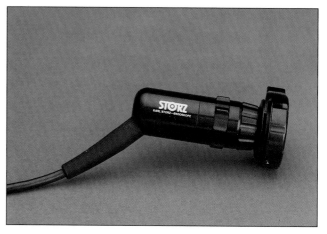

Figure 6. Single-chip camera with zoom lens and automatic exposure.

aligned in rows and columns and have small spaces between them. By filling some of the empty space, the horizontal resolution can be increased to approximately 90% of the camera's total pixel count. As this process is refined, you can expect to see three-chip cameras with horizontal resolution measurements as high as 725 lines (total horizontal pixel counts per CCD are approximately 800 pixels). (Remember, horizontal resolution cannot equal or exceed the total horizontal pixel count.) Three-chip cameras are more expensive than single-chip models and are usually larger; however, the improved picture quality often outweighs these drawbacks.

One piece of advice if you do use a three-chip camera: the monitor must equal or surpass the resolution of the video camera. Since a video system is only as strong as its weakest link, a 600-line camera connected to a 300-line monitor will produce a picture the quality of 300 lines. By making the extra investment in a good-quality, high-resolution monitor, you can truly benefit from the three-chip technology.

VIDEOENDOSCOPES

Several videoendoscopes, or "chips on sticks," have been introduced recently and seem to be a viable alternative to traditional add-on video systems. A videoendoscope is an endoscope with a camera sensor placed at the distal end (Fig. 10). The advantages of this type of configuration include reduced glass use by the manufacturer, lower cost, and an overall smaller package. Videoendoscopes are reported to be more durable and

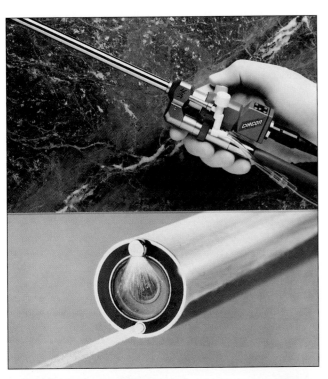

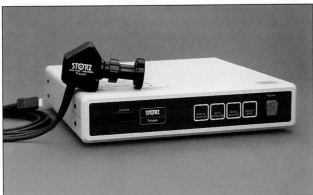

Figure 9. Three-chip cameras offer high resolution and true red-green-blue (RGB) color.

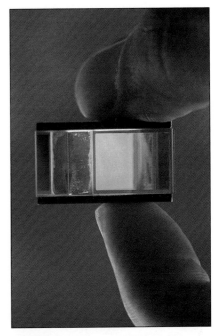

Figure 7. Laparoscopic video system (*top*) with built-in lens washing and irrigation system (*bottom*).

Figure 8. The three-chip prism separates light into red, green, and blue.

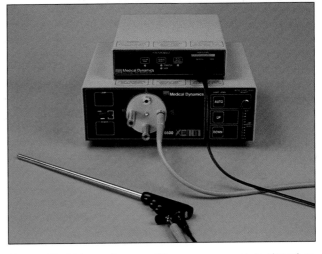

Figure 10. Videoendoscope. The camera sensor is placed at the distal end of the scope.

have less demand for light. The key disadvantage appears to be that when the system malfunctions, the scope cannot even be used for viewing by the naked eye. A surgeon will always need multiple backup systems.

Until recently, high-resolution sensors were not small enough to fit at the end of the scope, and there was no reason to trade resolution for the videoendoscope configuration. High-resolution sensors are now small enough for use in videoendoscope models without sacrificing image quality, and, therefore, their popularity should continue to grow.

THREE-DIMENSIONAL SYSTEMS

Three-dimensional imaging attempts to provide depth information not available with a monocular endoscopic video system. The increased depth perception enables surgeons to know where their instruments are in relation to tissues and organs. The dimension of depth is especially useful in laparoscopy, in which instruments enter the abdominal cavity from accessory portals.

Most three-dimensional systems require the use of some sort of eyewear (Fig. 11) so that the images in the left and right eyes are parallax to create depth. Our eyes are naturally separated, by an average of 63.5 mm (2.5 inches) in adults, which causes each eye to view the same object at a slightly different angle. The disparity is then processed by the brain into a single image [7]. Three-dimensional systems can recreate this phenomenon by utilizing eyewear that lets the left eye see only the left eye image and vice versa, or by using a binocular system.

There are two types of eyewear: active and inactive. As the names imply, in one instance the glasses continually adjust to the image, and in the other, the eyewear remains unchanged but the monitor or viewing instrument changes.

One manufacturer offers active eyewear with shuttering lenses. Each shutter is synchronized to occlude the unwanted image and transmit the wanted image. Thus each eye sees only its appropriate perspective view. The left eye sees only the left view, and the right eye only the right view. The eyewear receives a signal from an emitter placed in front of the monitor and synchronizes its shutters to the video field rate. If the images are alternated rapidly enough, the result is a flickerless image [7].

Inactive eyewear allows light to pass through the lenses in only one direction for each eye. If the lens over the left eye allows light to penetrate only on a horizontal plane, then the left eye will see only the alternating images that appear horizontally. Likewise, the right eye would be allowed to see only the vertical images. The screen, utilizing a liquid crystal display in front of the viewing monitor, alternately changes from horizontal to vertical images and allows only the correct perspective to be seen by the left and right eyes.

The disadvantages of three-dimensional systems with eyewear include a generally darker, lower-resolution image and potential eye strain from long-term use of an unnatural system. In the presence of highly concentrated, focused attention to the surgical procedure, a feeling of motion sickness may set in. In the 1950s

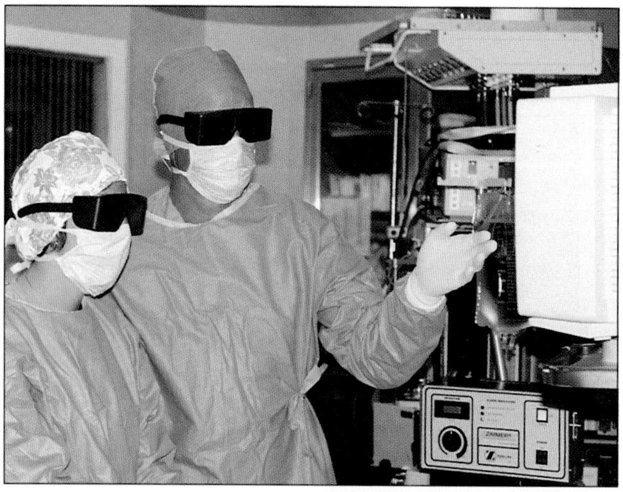

Figure 11. Three-dimensional systems require some form of eyewear. (Courtesy of Stereographics, San Rafael, CA.)

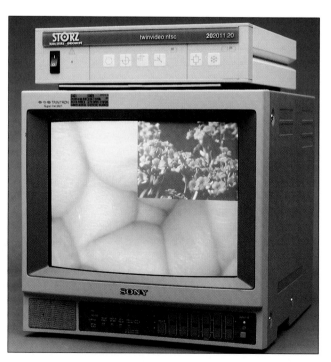

Figure 12. Picture-in-picture systems enable simultaneous viewing of two separate images. This photograph is an actual reproduction from the television monitor.

when three-dimensional movies were introduced to the public, similar reports were made by some viewers.

Binocular systems use completely separate viewing channels for each eye and, therefore, do not suffer from the disadvantages mentioned above. Binocular systems offer a brighter image and do not require eyewear. They are limited to one viewer at a time, however, and are fixed in space, so the surgeon is not able to move around.

These issues will undoubtedly be overcome as the technology matures. Mature three-dimensional technology can be defined as technology that does not compromise any existing benefits. The image will need to be as clear and bright as standard video cameras with at least the same resolution. The system should not sacrifice anything but should add depth without eye strain or nausea.

DIGITAL TECHNOLOGY

Digital technology has been around for many years; however, just recently, innovative uses have been developed. The word *digital* describes the type of technology employed in many camera systems today. Digital is not in itself a feature or benefit; it simply enables a manufacturer to build a wide variety of features into the system. Some of these features are long-term integration, picture-in-picture viewing, and image enhancement.

Long-term integration (long exposure or shutter times) greatly increases the camera's sensitivity to light but is not practical for real-time use during surgery. Picture-in-picture systems utilize digital technology to enable the viewer to see two live images simultaneously (Fig. 12). One image fills the monitor screen, while the secondary image appears as an inset in a portion of the screen. Picture-in-picture systems require two video

cameras and a picture-in-picture control box. Images can be frozen, printed, or videotaped as desired.

Image enhancement enables the viewer to accent structures that are difficult or impossible for the naked eye to see (Fig. 13). Small surface details can be enhanced in real time during endoscopic procedures. Digital image enhancement is a major breakthrough for purposes of further increasing the viability and efficacy of future video endoscopic imaging systems.

HIGH-DEFINITION TELEVISION

Although not practical for use in endoscopy at the time of this writing, high-definition television (HDTV) technology is being developed rapidly domestically and internationally. Several companies have made HDTV endoscopic systems and have demonstrated the system's capabilities at major medical conferences. HDTV is a system developed to create the picture and sound quality experienced in movie theaters. The interest in consumer and medical markets stems from the extremely high resolution capabilities. HDTV has the potential to offer 1150 lines of resolution.

The obvious disadvantages are the screen size and the large bulky cameras. The screen's aspect ratio [9], which has a horizontal dimension approximately twice the vertical dimension, is not ideally suited to endoscopic use. Another drawback is price: the cameras and monitors cost hundreds of thousands of dollars. The issue concerning screen size will most likely be overcome by using a portion of the screen for titling or monitoring vital signs or developing new HDTV cameras and monitors with 1:1 aspect ratios. The issue of price should be addressed as the technology becomes more widely available.

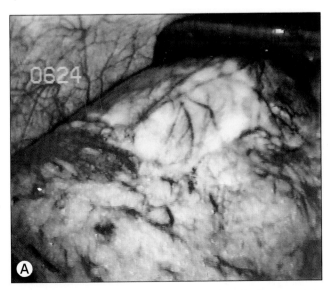 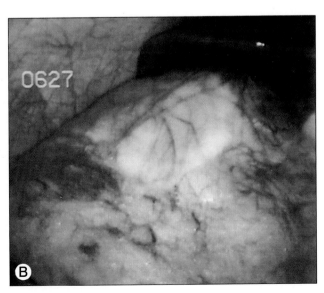

Figure 13. **A**, Digitally enhanced image. Note the improved clarity of the vascularity. Structures appear more obvious when enhanced. All differences noted are from the video monitor; no enhancements were made during film processing. **B**, Unenhanced, standard video image.

SUMMARY

The purpose of this brief overview of currently available laparoendoscopic imaging equipment and devices has been to increase your level of understanding and help you make a more informed buying decision when the opportunity presents itself.

Ultrasound, single-chip cameras, three-chip cameras, videoendoscopes, three-dimensional systems, digital technology, HDTV, and technology yet to come all have a place in today's evolving endoscopy market. There is not one system that fits every surgeon's needs; thus there is a need for variety in imaging systems, just as there is a need for variety in scopes and hand instruments, for example. Many factors will play a part in your decision-making process, and some of those factors may eliminate possible choices. For example, if you are performing laparoscopy and need to share your system with other departments, a one-piece camera/laparoscope is not the best choice. If you tend to get motion sickness, the current three-dimensional systems may make you uncomfortable; however, if your stomach can tolerate the environment, this is an exciting new technology worth exploring.

From a technical point of view, we know that certain systems are less advanced than others, but even this does not matter if the system meets your needs. The bottom line is that the quality of the image is in the eye of the beholder, regardless of technical specifications. Resolution, light sensitivity, and signal-to-noise ratio provide good guidelines for narrowing down the choices, but the true determining factor must be a personal demonstration. Do not underestimate the importance your eyes play in deciding what is good and what is not.

To date, imaging products have been driven by technologic advances instead of market needs. The reasons are twofold: first, technology has been advancing rapidly, quicker, in fact, than most individuals can keep up with, and second, most surgeons are not well versed in video technology and, therefore, are not able to communicate creative ideas to manufacturers. As time goes on and surgeons become more familiar with imaging technology and the language that surrounds it, a more productive relationship will ultimately develop between the users and manufacturers of the products. I believe that manufacturers and surgeons are looking forward to exchanging ideas and producing advanced imaging products that continue to benefit the medical field.

ACKNOWLEDGMENT

I express my sincere thanks to Bethany Rushing Thornton for her assistance in writing this chapter.

REFERENCES

Papers of particular interest, published within the period of review, have been highlighted as:
• Of special interest
•• Of outstanding interest

1.• Berci G, Cuschieri A, Sackier J: *Problems in General Surgery*, vol. 8. Lippincott; 1991.
A compilation of chapters written by leading laparoscopic surgeons. Contains descriptions of a variety of laparoscopic operations and several color photographs and illustrations for explanatory purposes.

2. Reuter HJ, Reuter MA: *Philipp Bozzini and Endoscopy in the 19th Century*. Stuttgart, Germany: Max Nitze Museum; 1988.

3.• Lightdale C: Diagnostic Laparoscopy in the Era of Minimally Invasive Surgery. *Gastrointest Endosc* 1992, 38:392–394.
Dr. Lightdale's review of the "Laparoscopy in Diagnosis and Therapy" conference held January 1992. The conference involved experts from the United States, Europe, and Japan.

4. Zucker KA: *Surgical Laparoscopy*. St. Louis: Quality Medical Publishing; 1991.

5. Kurtzer S: Automated Still Photography for Endoscopy. *Int J Fertil* 1981, 26.

6.• Biomedical Business International (BBI), Santa Ana, California.
Biomedical Business International (BBI) publishes detailed market analysis reports and a monthly newsletter containing medical market research. Trends and projections for endoscopic procedures are included in the newsletter on a regular basis.

7. Lipton L: *The Crystal Eyes Handbook*, San Rafael, CA: Stereographics Corporation; 1991.

8. Sackier J, Berci G: Diagnostic and Interventional Laparoscopy for the General Surgeon. *Contemp Surg* 1990, 37(4):14–26.

9. Kraszna-Krausz A, Mannheim LA, Buckmaster D, *et al.*: *The Focal Encyclopedia of Photography*. New York: McGraw-Hill-Focal Press Ltd.; 1969.

Chapter 3

Anesthetic Considerations for Endoscopic Surgery

Peter Rock
Douglas Brown

Although once considered a technique only for gynecologic surgery, laparoscopy is becoming increasingly popular for the performance of other abdominal procedures. These procedures include cholecystectomy, bowel resection, and inguinal hernia repair. Compared with open procedures, laparoscopy results in a shorter postoperative hospital stay, a reduced recovery period until full activity is resumed, reduced hospital costs, and an earlier return to the work force [1•]. Laparoscopic surgery avoids a large abdominal incision, thereby yielding an improved cosmetic result. The incidence of postoperative intra-abdominal adhesions is reduced by a laparoscopic approach to a procedure [2]. Another advantage of laparoscopic surgery over open procedures is that postoperative pain is generally considered less. Additionally, pulmonary function is less severely compromised after laparoscopic surgery than after open procedures.

Laparoscopic surgery uniquely involves intraoperative intraperitoneal gaseous insufflation. The induced pneumoperitoneum by itself affects respiratory and cardiac homeostasis and may lead to morbidity including cardiovascular compromise. Laparoscopic procedures are associated with an increased incidence of postoperative emesis. Mediastinoscopy and thoracoscopy are other endoscopic procedures that require special anesthetic consideration.

PREOPERATIVE ASSESSMENT

The preoperative assessment of the patient undergoing a laparoscopic procedure differs little from that required for a similar procedure performed by laparotomy. Because a wide range of procedures are now performed laparoscopically, patients may be varied in regard to age and general health. Many patients scheduled for laparoscopic surgery arrive in the preoperative area without first having been seen by an anesthesiologist, and a rapid but complete history and physical examination must be performed.

Pulmonary and cardiac disease are of particular importance because surgical conditions, anesthetic agents, and intraoperative abdominal gaseous insufflation affect pulmonary and cardiac physiology. Medications for chronic conditions are usually administered on the day of surgery. Insulin is administered at a reduced dose, as the lower caloric intake in the perioperative period necessitates less insulin for control of blood glucose. Diuretics are often omitted. Allergies are documented, and previous anesthetic exposure and difficulties ascertained. Of course, airway assessment is essential.

TECHNIQUE OF ANESTHESIA

Laparoscopic procedures can be performed using local, regional, or general anesthesia. Laparoscopy with local anesthesia requires a well-motivated patient. To enable a patient to tolerate the procedure, supplemental sedation to the point of obtundation may be required. Additionally, surgical conditions are not optimal [3]. Bridenbaugh and Soderstrom [4] describe 100 laparoscopic tubal ligations using epidural anesthesia. Patients and surgeons were satisfied with the technique, but the amount of sedation administered, level of sensory block, and percent of patients with intraoperative pain were not described. Ciofolo and coworkers [3] administered epidural anesthesia with sensory block between the second and fifth thoracic dermatome to seven patients, four of whom complained of shoulder pain with gaseous insufflation, but severity of pain, patient satisfaction, and surgical conditions were not addressed. Epidural anesthesia involving upper thoracic dermatomes results in profound sympathetic block. This procedure may be tolerated in healthy patients in the Trendelenburg position. Hemodynamic compromise, however, may result from a loss of sympathetic tone in the less healthy patient undergoing a laparoscopic cholecystectomy in the reverse Trendelenburg position. Additionally, epidural catheter placement and block onset require significantly more time than induction of general anesthesia and may delay a busy operating-room schedule unless the surgical suite has locations and personnel to allow preoperative placement of spinal axis anesthesia.

A general anesthetic is most commonly employed in laparoscopic procedures. Because regurgitation of gastric contents and subsequent pulmonary aspiration is a concern, the trachea is intubated. Increased intra-abdominal pressure with insufflation, surgical compression of the stomach, and the Trendelenburg position are factors that tend to increase gastric pressure and may precipitate regurgitation. Moreover, the outpatient population has larger gastric volumes than their inpatient counterparts [5]. A greater gastric volume increases the risk of regurgitation and the risk of a significant pneumonitis, should aspiration occur. Using an oral pH monitor, Duffy [6] found two of 93 patients undergoing laparoscopy with evidence of regurgitation. Emergency laparoscopic procedures have a 20% incidence of regurgitation [7]. Seed and coworkers [8] found two of 10 of his study patients regurgitated gastric contents. Scott [9], however, reports no cases of aspiration in 50,000 laparoscopies, 5000 in which the patients were not intubated. In another investigation, an esophageal pH probe failed to reveal reflux in 63 laparoscopy patients [10]. These authors note that tracheal intubation has its own associated morbidity. Stomach decompression by an oral-gastric tube is recommended; it not only improves the surgical field and protects the stomach from instrument injury but lessens the volume and pressure of gastric contents.

Almost any general anesthetic technique may be used. Laparoscopic surgeries do not typically require a deep level of anesthesia. They are short procedures, and the duration from beginning of closure to completion of surgery is brief. A technique that allows for rapid emergence is preferred. Short-acting narcotics, benzodiazepines, and muscle relaxants can aid in serving this purpose. Isoflurane has a lower blood-gas solubility than halothane or enflurane, and it will thus be more rapidly eliminated. The short redistribution half-life of propofol permits rapid emergence. Indeed, DeGrood and coworkers [11] found propofol anesthesia in laparoscopic surgery provided a more rapid emergence than an isoflurane and nitrous oxide anesthetic.

The use of nitrous oxide during laparoscopic procedures remains controversial. The low blood-gas solubility of nitrous oxide allows for its rapid uptake and rapid elimination. Moreover, nitrous oxide is less soluble in blood than the nitrogen and methane normally present in the intestine. Nitrous oxide will, therefore, diffuse more quickly into the intestine than intestinal gases diffuse out. The result is expansion of intestinal gas and distended bowel, which may impede surgical conditions. Equilibrium of intestinal gas with inspired nitrous oxide proceeds at a slower pace than with other closed spaces [12]. Eger and Saidman [12] demonstrated that 4 hours of 70%- inspired nitrous oxide increases intestinal gas volume 200%. The absolute increase in intestinal volume depends directly on the initial intestinal gas volume. The average intestinal gas content is only 100 ml [13]. Larger initial volumes of air in bowel may result from assisted mask ventilation. Taylor and coworkers studied surgical conditions in laparoscopic cholecystectomies with an average duration of 72 minutes. One group of patients inspired 70% nitrous oxide throughout the duration of the anesthetic. In the other group nitrous oxide was omitted. The surgeon was unable to detect a difference in bowel distention, and the authors concluded nitrous oxide administration was not detrimental to surgical conditions [14•].

Muscle relaxants are useful in laparoscopy. Neuromuscular blockade ensures immobility. Visceral injury may occur if the patient moves during laparoscopic instrumentation. Laparoscopic procedures provide less surgical stimulation than their open counterparts. A lighter level of anesthesia may be used with neuromuscular blockers and more rapid emergence achieved. The volume of pneumoperitoneum is important for surgical conditions, but intra-abdominal pressure is primarily responsible for pulmonary and cardiovascular compromise. Relaxation of abdominal musculature increases abdominal compliance so that a greater volume of gas may be insufflated for a given intra-abdominal pressure increase [15].

Fluid replacement requirements are likely less for laparoscopic surgery than for those that require a laparotomy. Evaporative fluid loss is minimized in laparoscopic procedures, and blood loss may be less during laparoscopic procedures using laser instrumentation than during open surgical procedures [16]. A single peripheral intravenous catheter is sufficient in the majority of laparoscopic procedures. Although a urinary catheter is typically placed to ensure that a distended bladder does not interfere with surgical visualization or is not unintentionally entered by a trocar, it also aids in intravascular volume assessment.

Surgical considerations may require one or both arms to be positioned at the patient's side. Brachial plexus stretch and ulnar nerve compression must be avoided during laparoscopy as frequent tilting of the operative table may result in undesirable arm positions. Pelvic procedures require the Trendelenburg position so gravity moves the bowel off pelvic structures. Similarly, for a laparoscopic cholecystectomy, the patient is positioned in the reverse Trendelenburg position to remove the bowel from the operative site.

PHYSIOLOGIC EFFECTS OF PERITONEAL GAS INSUFFLATION

The peritoneal space is a potential space normally containing a small amount of serous fluid. Gaseous insufflation of the peritoneal cavity causes an increase in intra-abdominal pressure, and consequent alterations in cardiac and respiratory physiology. The magnitude of

intra-abdominal pressure elevation is related to volume of gas insufflated and abdominal compliance. Cardiovascular function is affected by this increase in intra-abdominal pressure. Laparoscopy patients were studied using a general anesthetic and ventilated with a constant minute volume [15,17]. Intraperitoneal insufflation proceeded with 1- to 2-L amounts of carbon dioxide, and hemodynamic measurements were obtained after each gaseous injection. A progressive increase in intra-abdominal pressure to approximately 20 mm Hg was accompanied by a progressive increase in central venous pressure (CVP), which exceeded the increase in intrathoracic pressure thereby resulting in an augmented, right-sided filling pressure. In the supine patient, increased filling pressure was associated with increased cardiac output (CO). The CVP increased 3.5 mm Hg, and the CO increased 1.1 L/min/70 kg at 20 mm Hg. As intra-abdominal pressure increased over 20 mm Hg, CVP and CO steadily diminished [15,17,18]. Hodgson and coworkers [19] observed similar effects of laparoscopy on central venous pressure but did not study cardiac output.

The biphasic response to CVP and CO to increases in intraperitoneal pressure has been predicted mathematically and confirmed experimentally by Takata and coworkers [20]. The abdominal venous compartment serves as both a capacitor and resistor, depending on the relationship between abdominal pressure and right-atrial pressure. When increases in intra-abdominal pressure are small to moderate yet still less than right-atrial pressure, capacitance properties of the abdominal veins predominate. The effective abdominal venous compliance decreases, with a resultant transfer of blood out of the abdominal compartment, which increases central blood volume and venous return [15,20]. Higher intra-abdominal pressures can cause inferior vena cava compression at its exit from the abdomen when it exceeds right-atrial pressure. The effective inferior vena cava resistance increases, venous return decreases, and hypotension may occur. In effect, a starling resistor or vascular waterfall is created. In the supine hypotensive syndrome caused by a gravid uterus, the physical compression of the inferior vena cava increases venous resistance, which lowers venous return and cardiac output.

The relationship of hemodynamic parameters and increased intraperitoneal pressures has not been studied in the medically compromised patient, nor has it been studied in the reverse Trendelenburg position required for laparoscopic cholecystectomy. Upper abdominal procedures require a larger pneumoperitoneum than that needed for pelvic surgery [21]. Exaggerated physiologic changes in upper abdominal surgery produced by the reverse Trendelenburg position and larger pneumoperitoneum may produce hemodynamic compromise in the patient with preexisting cardiac and pulmonary disease.

The pneumoperitoneum also alters respiratory system mechanics. The development of an intra-abdominal pressure of 25 mm Hg exerts a force equivalent to 50 kg on the diaphragm [22]. Diaphragmatic elevation occurs, thus limiting lung expansion. Functional residual capacity falls, as does total lung volume. Ventilation-perfusion $\dot{V}/\dot{Q}$ inequality and pulmonary atelectasis result [8]. Respiratory compliance is decreased as evidenced by the higher peak airway pressures needed to maintain a constant tidal volume during abdominal insufflation. Peak inspiratory pressure elevation may be of little physiologic importance in young, healthy patients. One investigator observed only an approximate 5-cm H_2O increase and another an approximate 12-cm H_2O increase [18,23•]. But some patients may require an increase in airway pressure of 15 to 20 cm H_2O to compensate for decreased respiratory system compliance [19].

Oxygenation is minimally affected during laparoscopic procedures in healthy patients; no significant change in arterial oxygen pressure (PaO_2) occurs in American Society of Anesthesiologists (ASA) physical status class 1 patients. This result has been demonstrated during spontaneous and controlled ventilation [23•,24]. A study of 10 spontaneously ventilating patients contained two individuals with histories of heavy smoking. Both patients developed arterial desaturation to a PaO_2 of less than 50 mm Hg while breathing gas containing 37% oxygen. Postoperative pulmonary function tests revealed one of these patients had moderate obstructive lung disease and the other had normal pulmonary function. The investigator suggested avoiding spontaneous ventilation during laparoscopy in patients with suspected pulmonary dysfunction [24].

Carbon dioxide is commonly insufflated during laparoscopy and has a blood solubility approximately 20 times that of nitrogen. Gaseous carbon dioxide (CO_2) exchange occurs with intraperitoneal insufflation. The extent of exchange depends upon the partial pressure gradient, blood-gas solubility, peritoneal blood flow, and the diffusion distance between the gas and blood. When the abdomen is insufflated with CO_2 at 1 atm, the pressure gradient for CO_2 across the peritoneum is approximately 660 mm Hg. Yet, calculated intraperitoneal carbon dioxide absorption during insufflation is only 14 mL/min, an addition of 7% to the normal body carbon dioxide production [25]. The relation of $PaCO_2$ to carbon dioxide insufflation during brief gynecologic procedures has been studied extensively. The calculated 7% increase in carbon dioxide would increase $PaCO_2$ 3 mm Hg from 35 mm Hg to 38 mm Hg. This calculation somewhat underestimates the actual $PaCO_2$ increase measured during laparoscopy. In studies of laparoscopic procedures performed on ASA 1 patients with controlled and constant minute ventilation, $PaCO_2$ increased 4.5 to 10 mm Hg [8,19,23•].

Carbon dioxide absorbed from the pneumoperitoneum is both stored in the body and eliminated by the lungs [26]. $PaCO_2$ measurement, therefore, does not accurately reflect total body carbon dioxide content until an equilibrium is achieved between carbon dioxide pressures within blood and tissue. This equilibrium occurs 20 minutes after a perturbation of carbon dioxide homeostasis. In a 30-minute carbon dioxide insufflation during constant minute volume ventilation, $PaCO_2$ rises steadily for 20 minutes and then attains a plateau [19].

Although spontaneously breathing patients under general anesthesia increase their minute volume during CO_2 insufflation, $PaCO_2$ increases 10 mm Hg [19]. Patients undergoing laparoscopy with sedation and local anesthesia or with epidural anesthesia maintain a constant $PaCO_2$ during the procedure [3,27]. Thus, absorbed carbon dioxide from the peritoneum appears not to be of sufficient magnitude to grossly affect respiratory homeostasis in the healthy patient. Carbon dioxide can be eliminated effectively with moderate hyperventilation.

In healthy patients, capnometry provides a close estimation of arterial carbon dioxide pressure. End-tidal CO_2 ($EtCO_2$) is normally slightly less than $PaCO_2$. Dead space acts to dilute alveolar gas that has come to an equilibrium with pulmonary capillary blood carbon dioxide. A larger difference between $PaCO_2$ and $EtCO_2$ reflects increased dead space ventilation. Arterial carbon dioxide pressure is 1 to 2 mm Hg higher than $EtCO_2$ in the healthy, awake, spontaneously ventilating patient and is 4 to 5 mm Hg higher during controlled ventilation under general anesthesia [8]. Pneumoperitoneum minimally contributes toward dead space ventilation [23•,28].

Most studies of pneumoperitoneum effects on respiratory and cardiac function use short insufflation times in young, healthy patients. Newer, more complex, laparoscopic surgical techniques have been developed and are now performed on older patients who may have preexisting medical conditions. These procedures require a longer period of peritoneal gas insufflation. ASA class 2 and 3 patients with cardiac or pulmonary disease who underwent laparoscopic cholecystectomies experienced a significant increase in dead space. Although capnometry demonstrated no change in end-tidal carbon dioxide, blood-gas analysis revealed an increase in $PaCO_2$ of 14 mm Hg despite a 20% increase in minute ventilation. In two of the 10 patients studied, hypercapnia and acidosis unresponsive to maximal ventilatory increases forced conversion to open procedures [29•]. Hence, the combination of peritoneal carbon dioxide absorption and pneumoperitoneum-induced alteration of pulmonary mechanics during laparoscopy is not tolerated by some patients. An arterial catheter may facilitate management in some patients with pulmonary disease during laparoscopy; it allows for blood-gas analysis and continuous blood-pressure management.

EFFECTS OF LAPAROSCOPY ON PULMONARY FUNCTION

Less profound changes in pulmonary function occur after laparoscopic procedures than after open surgical procedures. The morning after cholecystectomy via a subcostal incision, forced vital capacity (FVC), forced expiratory volume in one second (FEV_1), and peak expiratory flow decrease to approximately 50% of preoperative values. This decrease compares with a 25% decrement of the above parameters in patients after laparoscopic cholecystectomy. The FEV_1/FVC ratio is not altered in either group [1•,30]. This improvement in pulmonary function may lower the incidence of postoperative respiratory complications especially in the patient with chronic obstructive pulmonary disease [31]. A midline incision causes greater pulmonary dysfunction than a transverse incision [31]. Thus, laparoscopy may prevent further diminution of pulmonary function after procedures traditionally performed via midline incisions. Further studies are necessary to determine if laparoscopic surgery results in fewer postoperative pulmonary complications such as atelectasis or pneumonia.

COMPLICATIONS

Table 1 lists complications associated with laparoscopy. Cardiac arrest is a rare complication. The risk of death associated with laparoscopic tubal ligations is approximately 4/100,000 procedures [32]. A more recent retrospective review found two cases of cardiac arrest in 5018 laparoscopic sterilizations; both occurred during anesthesia induction [33]. Patients undergoing laparoscopy are at risk for a number of potentially life-threatening complications. These complications include venous air embolism, hemodynamic compromise secondary to increased intra-abdominal pressure, cardiac dysrhythmia, pneumothorax, and unrecognized hemorrhage.

A potentially catastrophic complication of laparoscopy is venous carbon dioxide embolism. Carbon dioxide is used for peritoneal insufflation because it has a high solubility in blood and thus can be rapidly excreted via the lungs. Should carbon dioxide enter the circulation as a bubble or embolus, rapid absorption of carbon dioxide into the blood occurs, and the bubble embolus shrinks or is eliminated. The CO_2 is then excreted via the lungs. A hemodynamically significant carbon dioxide venous embolism produces a character-

Table 1. Complications of laparoscopy

Complication	Etiology	Treatment
Venous air embolism	Gas insufflation into a vessel or vascular organ	Evacuate pneumoperitoneum
		Hyperventilate
		Left-side-down position
		Vasopressors as needed
Decreased venous return	Excessive pneumoperitoneum	Evacuate pneumoperitoneum
	Reverse Trendelenburg position	Level operating room table
Cardiac arrhythmia	Hypercarbia	Hyperventilate
	Vagal stimulation	Lidocaine (premature ventricular contractions, ventricular tachycardia)
		Atropine (bradycardia)
Pneumothorax	Gas leak from diaphragmatic defect	100% oxygen
	Barotrauma related to high peak airway pressures	Thoracentesis, chest tube
Hemorrhage	Vessel injury, unrecognized	Crystalloid, colloid, blood replacement
		Vasoactive drugs as temporizing measure

istic millwheel cardiac murmur [34]. A precordial or esophageal stethoscope must be monitored vigilantly, as it may allow early detection and aid in the differential diagnosis of cardiovascular collapse. Capnometry should also be monitored during laparoscopy. A CO_2 embolism causes a decrease in $EtCO_2$ as gas bubbles prevent lung perfusion to affected lung regions and result in increased dead space ventilation. Treatment of venous carbon dioxide embolism includes immediate intraperitoneal gas evacuation, 100% oxygen administration, vasopressor support as needed, and hyperventilation to aid elimination of carbon dioxide. Like other forms of pulmonary embolism, cardiovascular collapse results from obstruction of forward blood flow at the level of the right ventricular outlet. Durant and coworkers describe turning the patient to the left lateral position for suspected air embolism. This position displaces the gas embolism from the right ventricular pulmonary outflow tract into the right ventricle and traps other bubbles in the right atrium, thus relieving or preventing the outflow tract obstruction and allowing unimpeded forward blood flow [35].

Other mechanisms of cardiovascular collapse have been reported. Excessive intra-abdominal pressure may cause acute hemodynamic compromise and can be avoided in most patients by maintaining an intra-abdominal pressure of less than 20 mm Hg [19,36]. A case report notes prompt normalization of hemodynamic parameters with release of peritoneal gas [36]. Additionally, hemorrhage as a cause of cardiovascular collapse may be unrecognized by anesthesia and surgical personnel and must be considered in the differential diagnosis of unexplained hypotension.

Significant bradycardia and asystole may occur during laparoscopy. Sudden peritoneal traction caused by peritoneal insufflation or traction on abdominal viscera can elicit reflex vagal stimulation [37–39]. A sudden decrease in venous return caused by a marked increase in intra-abdominal pressure may also lead to bradycardia via the Bainbridge reflex. Bradycardia may be more prevalent when anticholinergic drugs and nonvagolytic muscle relaxants are not administered. Mobitz type I block during laparoscopy, a rare rhythm in the anesthetized patient, has been reported with a propofol-, fentanyl-, and vecuronium-based anesthetic [40]. An anticholinergic premedication with the above drug combination may be useful [40].

Hypercarbia in combination with a light level of anesthesia increases catecholamine levels and can precipitate other cardiac dysrhythmias. Halothane is perhaps best avoided, as it increases susceptibility to dysrhythmias, including supraventricular tachycardia, premature ventricular contractions, and ventricular bigeminy, under high-catecholamine conditions. The incidence of arrhythmias during laparoscopy using halothane may approach 27% [22,41].

Pneumothorax is a known complication of positive pressure ventilation, usually associated with lung pathology or high peak airway pressures. Pneumothorax is also a complication of laparoscopic-induced pneumoperitoneum [42]. Carbon dioxide may enter the pleural space from a diaphragmatic defect and produce a pneumothorax. Mediastinal emphysema also may occur. Subcutaneous emphysema often accompanies a pneumothorax, and, if noted, gas should be expelled from the abdomen and the possibility of a pneumothorax considered. Subcutaneous gas exclusive of pneumothorax during laparoscopy is most likely caused by direct carbon dioxide insufflation into subcutaneous tissue with initial needle puncture or gaseous dissection into a subcutaneous tissue plane after successful establishment of the pneumoperitoneum.

POSTOPERATIVE PAIN AND ANALGESIA

Although a recent study reported no difference in postoperative pain whether cholecystectomies were performed by laparoscopic or open techniques, a major benefit of laparoscopic surgery over open laparotomy is generally believed to be diminished postoperative pain [2,30]. Definitive postoperative pain studies have not been performed.

Pain after laparoscopy is multifactorial. Incisional pain is largely avoided, but pain results from inflammation, ischemia, and tissue trauma at the surgical site. As expected, the type of surgical procedure influences the degree of discomfort that will be experienced. Postoperative pain is greater after laparoscopic sterilization than after diagnostic laparoscopy [43]. Using clips or bands rather than electrocoagulation for tubal ligations increases pain after surgery [44]. Other laparoscopic procedure pain comparisons have not been made.

Intraperitoneal insufflation is most commonly accomplished with carbon dioxide, but nitrous oxide insufflation may decrease the pain of the procedure. Diagnostic laparoscopy using local anesthesia produces less operative pain when nitrous oxide is used than when carbon dioxide is used [45,46]. The anesthetic effects of absorbed nitrous oxide were assumed negligible in these studies. Carbon dioxide may cause peritoneal irritation secondary to hydrogen ion–mediated vasodilation [46]. Postoperative pain comparisons were not reported. Nitrous oxide supports combustion and *therefore is not to be insufflated in laparoscopic procedures that require electrocautery.* Furthermore, nitrous oxide does not have the favorable solubility characteristics of carbon dioxide; overall, there is probably little benefit to recommend its use.

Although the bulk of insufflated gas is expelled, and the peritoneum can absorb residual carbon dioxide, a small pneumoperitoneum persists at the end of surgery.

Subdiaphragmatic free air has been demonstrated three days postoperatively in a large number of patients [47]. Carbon dioxide–induced irritation of the diaphragm and phrenic nerve is the probable cause of shoulder pain after laparoscopy and of upper abdominal pain in pelvic procedures. Shoulder pain occurs in 35% to 65% of patients after abdominal laparoscopy [47,48]. Interstudy variability of shoulder pain incidence might be explained by differences in efforts to maximally remove intraperitoneal carbon dioxide. The anesthesiologist may assist in this process with a sustained valsalva maneuver during gas expulsion. This procedure increases intra-abdominal pressure and creates a pressure gradient for gas release. An open drain left in the umbilical incision for 6 hours halved the frequency of postoperative pain, presumably by venting residual gas [49].

Ambulation tends to exacerbate shoulder pain because intraperitoneal free air rises to the diaphragm. Dobbs and coworkers [47] document a significant decrease in pain during the first postoperative night for inpatients after diagnostic and sterilization laparoscopies. An equally marked increase in pain occurs the following day when patients return home and resume normal activities. In an effort to decrease gas irritation of the diaphragm, a 30°, head-down position for 30 minutes was attempted. The maneuver did not prove helpful [47]. A subset of patients have their pain alleviated with sitting, which suggests another cause of post-laparoscopic pain. Blood and other fluids that remain in the peritoneal cavity may irritate the diaphragm and peritoneum while the patient is supine; in the sitting position, irritating fluid flows away from contact with sensitive peritoneal surfaces [50].

Table 2 lists analgesic drugs used for laparoscopy. Topically applied local anesthetics may aid in postoperative pain management. Applied to fallopian tubes during a laparoscopic tubal ligation, local anesthetics diminish postoperative pain. Kaplan and coworkers [44] studied the effect of 3 mL of 0.5% bupivacaine applied to the fallopian tubes during sterilization procedures. Pain scores decreased significantly at 15 and 60 minutes postprocedure, but after 5 hours control and local treatment groups experienced similar pain. Although some investigators have stressed the importance of applying local anesthetic prior to tubal ligation and to the entire length of the fallopian tube, Baram and coworkers [51] showed that local anesthetic effects depend upon neither of these factors. Five milliliters of 1% etidocaine topically applied to the banded portion of each fallopian tube decreased postoperative pain at 2

Table 2. Analgesic drugs for laparoscopy

Drug	Side effects	Comment
Narcotics	Respiratory depression	Low doses recommended, as laparoscopy is not particularly painful
	Sedation	
	Nausea	High doses may slow anesthetic emergence
	Pruritus	
	Urinary retention	
Nonsteroidal anti-inflammatory agents	Gastric ulceration	Avoid narcotic side effects
	Bronchospasm	Ketorolac administered via IM or IV route
	Impaired renal function	
	Decreased platelet function	Ketorolac provides analgesia equivalent to narcotics
		Ketorolac equal or superior to other nonsteroidal anti-inflammatory agents in efficacy
Intraperitoneally applied local anesthetic	Local anesthetic toxicity (CNS irritability, cardiac irritability) with large doses	Few side effects if administered in appropriate doses
		Aid in contolling early postoperative pain

CNS—central nervous system; IM—intramuscular; IV—intravenous.

and 6 hours, but these salutary effects had dissipated by 24 hours [51]. Topical application of 2 mg/kg of 1.5% etidocaine results in more profound pain relief in the first 2 hours after laparoscopic sterilization than does application of 1.5 mg/kg of 0.75% bupivacaine [52].

Intraperitoneal installation of local anesthetic has also been proposed for postoperative pain relief. Helvacioglu and Weis [53•] studied pain scores after various operative laparoscopic procedures. Twenty milliliters of 0.5% lidocaine instilled intraperitoneally provided 5 hours of significant pain reduction compared with a control group. Systemic absorption of intraperitoneally administered local anesthetics was studied by Spielman and coworkers [54]. The peak in plasma level after administration of 12 mL of 2% lidocaine occurs 30 minutes after intraperitoneal administration; the level was less than that obtained with epidural or brachial plexus blocks. Twenty milliliters of 0.5% bupivacaine results in a peak plasma level at 60 minutes that was lower than that after epidural or brachial plexus blocks [54]. All of the plasma local anesthetic levels were well below those considered toxic.

Perioperative pain is traditionally managed with narcotics, but narcotics may cause respiratory depression, sedation, nausea, and decreased gastrointestinal motility. Nonsteroidal anti-inflammatory agents can supplement or replace opioids in the perioperative period. The development of a parenterally administered cyclo-oxygenase inhibitor, ketorolac, allows for postoperative administration in patients unable to take medications by mouth. Ketorolac demonstrates equivalent or superior analgesic efficacy compared with various other nonsteroidal anti-inflammatory drugs [55••–57]. A recent study compared ketorolac and morphine with respect to efficacy of postoperative pain relief. Intramuscularly administered ketorolac (30–90 mg) provides equal or superior analgesia to 6 to 12 mg of morphine given via the same route [55••]. A single dose of ketorolac decreases total narcotic required in the postoperative period [58]. Ketorolac given at regular intervals provides equal analgesia to "as-required" morphine administration [55••]. In addition, intramuscular ketorolac and morphine have similar temporal onsets of action [59•]. Because nonsteroidal anti-inflammatory agents decrease prostaglandin-mediated pain in dysmenorrhea, pain after gynecologic surgery may be particularly amenable to nonsteroidal therapy [60•]. Ketorolac in the laparoscopy patient has not been studied, but other anti-inflammatory agents have proven useful in postlaparoscopic analgesia. Ibuprofen administration orally (800 mg) prior to laparoscopy for infertility provides longer-lasting postoperative analgesia than 75 µg of fentanyl given intravenously. The two analgesics are equally effective until 90 minutes postoperatively, when ibuprofen, with its longer half-life, provides significantly greater pain relief. The ibuprofen-treated group also experienced significantly less nausea and vomiting [60•]. One might expect similar results with ketorolac.

Ketorolac does share the adverse effects of other cyclo-oxygenase inhibitors. These include gastric ulceration, bronchospasm, impairment of renal function, and decreased platelet function. The last is of particular concern in the surgical patient. Skin bleeding times do increase after ketorolac administration but do not increase the bleeding time above the upper limit of normal [61–63]. Operative blood loss in abdominal procedures is not increased with administration of ketorolac [61].

POSTOPERATIVE NAUSEA

Postoperative emesis occurs commonly after anesthesia and surgery. Watcha and White [64••] recently wrote a review of the subject. Nausea and vomiting prolong recovery room time, delay patient discharge, and increase hospital costs [65]. The incidence of postoperative nausea and vomiting depends on the type of surgery. The highest incidence of postoperative emesis occurs in women undergoing laparoscopic ovum retrieval (54%) followed by other laparoscopic surgery (35%) [66]. Anxiety may also contribute to higher postoperative nausea and vomiting and may be related to higher serum catecholamine levels [67]. Other risk factors associated with a high postoperative emesis rate include obesity, a previous episode of postoperative emesis, a history of motion sickness, and the female gender. For similar surgical procedures, women are twice as likely to suffer postoperative emesis as are men [68]. The reason for this disparity is unknown, but a relation to the hormonal milieu is suggested [67]. The highest nausea-vomiting rate after laparoscopy occurs when the procedure is performed during menses; it is significantly lower if performed during the remainder of the menstrual cycle [69•]. Bellville [70] found women in the third and fourth weeks of their menstrual cycle had emesis rates equal to men undergoing similar procedures. Few studies have controlled for day of menstrual cycle; this lack may contribute to inconsistencies in reported emesis treatment efficacy.

Variation of anesthetic techniques may contribute to postoperative emesis. The role of nitrous oxide in postlaparoscopy emesis is controversial. Some authors have reported an association of nitrous oxide use and emesis [71]. Nitrous oxide increases sympathetic tone, alters middle ear pressure, and causes abdominal distension, and these effects may be responsible for postoperative emesis [64••]. Other authors have failed to relate nitrous oxide to postoperative nausea and vomiting [72–74]. The three potent inhalational agents halothane, enflurane, and isoflurane are equivalent in regard to postoperative nausea [64••].

Narcotic-based anesthetics are associated with a higher incidence of postoperative nausea than are inhalation-based anesthetics. Isoflurane, 1% to 2%, combined with nitrous oxide, is superior to 300 μg fentanyl and nitrous oxide with respect to the incidence of postlaparoscopic emesis [75]. Ketorolac may be a useful alternative or supplement to narcotics during laparoscopic procedures, as it does not contribute to nausea. Propofol is associated with a remarkably low incidence of nausea after gynecologic surgery (1%–3%) and may have antiemetic qualities [76]. Data from Bridenbaugh [77] show a decreased incidence of nausea or vomiting with epidural anesthesia as compared with general anesthesia. Intraoperative gastric emptying has not been shown to influence emesis rate. Muscarinic receptor stimulation by agents used to antagonize neuromuscular blockade may increase postoperative vomiting [78].

Antiemetic administration is not indicated for all surgical procedures, as the risk of postoperative emesis does not warrant the potential side effects of antiemetic drugs (Table 3). In patients with a high risk for postoperative vomiting, such as those undergoing laparoscopic surgery, prophylactic antiemetic therapy is justified. Although central efferent vagal activity leads to vomiting, multiple afferent receptor-mediated stimuli initiate the nausea-vomiting phenomena. Four distinct substances, dopamine, histamine, acetylcholine, and serotonin, stimulate emesis at the vomiting center, and specific receptor blockers are in use as antiemetic agents.

Phenothiazines, including chlorpromazine and prochlorperazine, and butyrophenones, including droperidol and haloperidol, exert antiemetic effects by dopaminergic receptor antagonism. These drugs all may cause sedation and lethargy and lead to extrapyramidal symptoms. Droperidol at a dose of 20 μg/kg is an effective antiemetic in women undergoing outpatient laparoscopy. A dose of 10 μg/kg is less effective and has a slightly higher rate of emesis. Neither dose delays discharge from the recovery room because of sedation [79].

Metoclopramide also acts via dopaminergic inhibition. At doses of 0.1 to 0.2 mg/kg, metoclopramide inconsistently demonstrates antiemetic properties. The short duration of parenterally administered drug and the increased antiemetic efficacy in men compared with women may account for the differences between studies [64••]. Ten milligrams of metoclopramide administered by mouth 30 minutes prior to laparoscopy had no significant effect on postoperative emesis [79]. Metoclopramide may be more effective in larger doses, but it also increases the incidence of sedation and extrapyramidal reactions.

Scopolamine, an anticholinergic drug, is a unique antiemetic in that it can be administered transdermally. The scopolamine patch is designed to deliver an initial priming dose of scopolamine to rapidly achieve an effective serum concentration and then provide a slow, continuous release of drug to maintain constant plasma

Table 3. Antiemetic drugs

Class	Commonly used drugs	Mechanism of action	Side effects
Phenothiazine	Chlorpromazine	Dopamine-receptor blockade	Lethargy, sedation
Butyrophenone	Prochlorperazine	Dopamine-receptor blockade	Extrapyramidal symptoms
Benzamides	Droperidol	Dopamine-receptor blockade	Lethargy, sedation
Antihistamines	Metoclopramide	Histamine-receptor blockade	Extrapyramidal symptoms
Anticholinergic	Diphenhydramine	Cholinergic-receptor blockade	Lethargy, sedation
Serotonin antagonist	Promethazine	Serotonin-receptor blockade	Extrapyramidal symptoms
	Scopolamine		Sedation
	Ondansetron		Sedation
			Dry mouth
			Amblyopia
			Difficulty urinating
			Exacerbation of narrow-angle glaucoma
			Mild sedation

levels. Outpatient nausea and vomiting after laparoscopy is decreased with transdermal scopolamine applied 8 hours prior to surgery [80]. Side effects include sedation, dry mouth, amblyopia, dysphoria, and confusion. Scopolamine is relatively contraindicated in patients with narrow angle glaucoma and urinary tract obstruction. Antihistamines, including diphenhydramine and promethazine, are another class of antiemetics. Sedation is the principal side effect. Their role in laparoscopic procedures has not been studied.

Serotonin antagonists are a promising new class of antiemetic drugs. The prototype, ondansetron, decreases emetic symptoms after laparoscopy [81]. Preoperative prophylactic administration of ondansetron is superior to droperidol and metoclopramide in prevention of postoperative emesis [82]. A major advantage of serotonin antagonists is that they lack significant adverse effects.

Because few studies compare the efficacy of different antiemetics, one antiemetic cannot be recommended over another. Emesis stimulation may be varied, and thus different antiemetics are appropriate under different circumstances. Furthermore, combining antiemetics with different mechanisms of action may provide synergistic relief of symptoms [64••].

CONSIDERATIONS FOR THORACIC ENDOSCOPIC PROCEDURES

The techniques and benefits derived from laparoscopy in performing abdominal and pelvic surgery are used in mediastinal and thoracic surgery. Mediastinoscopy is a diagnostic procedure. Following a suprasternal notch incision and paratracheal blunt dissection, the superior and middle mediastinum are visualized and biopsied if necessary. Scarring from previous mediastinoscopy may obliterate tissue planes and is a relative but not absolute contraindication to repeat mediastinoscopy [83]. In such situations, the anesthesiologist must be prepared for massive hemorrhage. Prior mediastinal radiation therapy may produce similar fibrotic changes. Other relative contraindications to mediastinoscopy include the superior vena cava syndrome, in which vessel and tissue engorgement increase the technical difficulty of the procedure and risk of hemorrhage. A thoracic aortic aneurysm distorts normal vascular anatomy and may result in vessel injury with mediastinoscopy. Tracheal deviation, tracheotomy, and laryngectomy all introduce more difficult surgical conditions [84].

Special preoperative considerations exist in the patient undergoing mediastinoscopy. A mediastinal mass may cause airway compression during general anesthesia and result in an inability to ventilate despite proper endotracheal tube position [85]. Tracheal deviation may make intubation difficult. Patients with superior vena cava compression syndromes benefit from lower extremity intravenous catheters, as fluid and drug administration in an upper extremity vein may not reach the central circulation. Prolonged neuromuscular paralysis may occur in the patient with bronchogenic carcinoma and associated Eaton-Lambert syndrome. Similarly, patients with previously undiagnosed myasthenia gravis undergoing mediastinoscopy for a mediastinal mass may have prolonged duration of neuromuscular blockade [86].

Complications of mediastinoscopy in decreasing order of frequency include hemorrhage, pneumothorax, recurrent laryngeal nerve injury, phrenic nerve injury, esophageal injury, chylothorax, air embolism, and transient hemiparesis. The overall complication rate is 1.5% to 3% [83,87]. In a series of 9543 mediastinoscopies, nine deaths were reported that were directly attributable to the procedure or anesthetic [87].

Hemorrhage may be massive and result from arterial or venous injury. If the superior vena cava is the injured vessel, intravascular volume must be replaced via a vessel that is not a tributary of the superior vena cava, *ie*, a lower-extremity vein. Immediate thoracotomy or median sternotomy to control bleeding may prove lifesaving. Pneumothorax may be responsible for decreased oxygen saturation, increased airway peak pressure, or cardiovascular compromise. Recurrent laryngeal nerve injury may result from biopsy of an adjacent lymph node, unintentional electrocautery, or compression by adjacent hematoma. If such injury is suspected, the vocal cords may be visualized during spontaneous ventilation at the completion of surgery.

The mediastinoscope may compress the innominate artery and compromise blood flow to the right cerebral hemisphere. A right radial arterial catheter or pulse oximetry of a right-hand digit can be used to monitor innominate blood flow. Simultaneous left-arm blood pressure measurement serves to distinguish innominate compression from cardiovascular collapse.

Mediastinoscopy may be performed using local anesthesia and allows for constant central nervous system monitoring, but local anesthesia is rarely employed. General anesthesia offers several advantages. Positive pressure ventilation limits lung collapse in the event of mediastinal pleura laceration. General anesthesia allows for more surgical flexibility, including the ability to rapidly perform a median sternotomy or thoracotomy if needed. Like diagnostic laparoscopy, mediastinoscopy is a short procedure, and the anesthetic technique should be tailored accordingly. Intravenous access should be adequate to provide for the possibility of rapid blood loss. Arterial blood pressure is monitored on an individual basis. A nonkinking endotracheal tube will better resist tracheal compression caused by the mediastinoscope and may be used if tracheomalacia is a concern preoperatively [84]. Most often this precaution is not needed.

Thoracoscopy permits direct inspection of the pleura and lung parenchyma. Although primarily a diagnostic and staging procedure, thoracoscopic surgery may be therapeutic; pleurodesis, ablation of spontaneous pneumothoraces, pericardiectomy, and peripheral lung resection have been performed. To permit adequate visualization, a pneumothorax is created. Under positive pressure ventilation the lung on the operative side will still inflate and obscure the surgeon's view; a double-lumen endotracheal tube allows for single lung ventilation and maintains intrapleural air. Gas insufflated into the pleural cavity enlarges the pneumothorax and thus aids visualization; as long as this procedure does not result in increased pleural pressure, the hemodynamic compromise of a tension pneumothorax does not develop. Gaseous absorption is more rapid in the pleural cavity than in the peritoneal cavity and may lead to increased physiologic alterations [12]. Reported complications include hemorrhage into the pleural space and subcutaneous and mediastinal emphysema.

Regardless of the type of anesthesia chosen, intercostal nerve blocks will provide analgesia during the surgery as well as postoperatively. Nitrous oxide administration may be limited by the need to treat hypoxemia related to one-lung ventilation. Additionally, nitrous oxide must be discontinued if pneumomediastinum is suspected. Monitoring is routine; arterial catheter monitoring is useful if one-lung ventilation is used.

REFERENCES

Papers of particular interest, published within the period of review, have been highlighted as:
• Of special interest
•• Of outstanding interest

1.• Frazee RC, Roberts JW, Okeson GC, *et al.*:Open Versus Laparoscopic Cholecystecotomy. *Ann Surg* 1991, 213:651–653.

Open cholecystectomy decreases a patient's pulmonary function parameter's including forced vital capacity and forced expiratory volume in one second, postoperatively to a greater degree than does laparoscopic cholecystectomy. However, a smaller decrement in pulmonary function tests has not correlated with decreased postoperative pulmonary morbidity.

2. Dubois F, Icard P, Berthelot G, Levard H:Celioscopic Cholecystectomy:Preliminary Report of 36 Cases. *Ann Surg* 1990, 211:60–62.

3. Ciofolo MJ, Clergue F, Seebacher J, *et al.*:Ventilatory Effects of Laparoscopy Under Epidural Anesthesia. *Anesth Analg* 1990, 70:357–361.

4. Bridenbaugh LD, Soderstrom RM:Lumbar Epidural Block Anesthesia for Outpatient Laparoscopy. *J Reprod Med* 1979, 23:85–86.

5. Ong BY, Palahniuk RJ, Cumming M:Gastric Volume and pH in Out-patient. *Can Anaesth Soc J* 1978, 25:36–39.

6. Duffy BL: Regurgitation During Pelvic Laparoscopy. *Br J Anaesth* 1979, 51:1089–1090.

7. Carlsson C, Islander G: Silent Gastropharyngeal Regurgitation During Anesthesia. *Anesth Analg* 1981, 60:655–657.

8. Seed TF, Shakespeare TF, Muldoon MJ: Carbon Dioxide Homeostasis During Anaesthesia for Laparoscopy. *Anaesthesia* 1970, 25:223–231.

9. Scott DB: Regurgitation During Laparoscopy. *Br J Anaesth* 1980, 52:559.

10. Roberts CJ, Goodman NW: Gastro-oesophageal Reflux During Elective Laparoscopy. *Anaesthesia* 1990, 45:1009–1011.

11. DeGrood PMRM, Harbers JBM, VanEgmond J, Crul JF: Anaesthesia for Laparoscopy. *Anaesthesia* 1987, 42:815–823.

12. Eger EI, Saidman LJ: Hazards of Nitrous Oxide Anesthesia in Bowel Obstruction and Pneumothorax. *Anesthesiology* 1965, 26:61–66.

13. Levitt MD: Volume and Composition of Human Intestinal Gas Determined by Means of Intestinal Washout Technique. *N Engl J Med* 1971, 284:1324–1328.

14.• Taylor E, Feinstein R, White PF, Soper N: Anesthesia for Laparoscopic Cholecystectomy. Is Nitrous Oxide Contraindicated? *Anesthesiology* 1992, 76:541–543.

The clinical relevance of nitrous oxide mediated bowel distension is studied. During laparoscopic cholecystectomy, 70% nitrous oxide was used in one population and omitted in the other. Surgeons evaluated operating conditions and bowel distension as equivalent in both groups.

15. Kelman GR, Swapp GH, Smith I, *et al.*: Cardiac Output and Arterial Blood-Gas Tension During Laparoscopy. *Br J Anaesth* 1972, 44:1155–1161.

16. Greville AC, Clements EA: Anaesthesia for Laparoscopic Cholecystectomy Using the Nd:Yag Laser. The Implications for a District General Hospital. *Anaesthesia* 1990, 45:944–949.

17. Smith I, Benzie RJ, Gordon NLM, *et al.*: Cardiovascular Effects of Peritoneal Insufflation of Carbon Dioxide for Laparoscopy. *Br Med J* 1971, 3:410–411.

18. Motew M, Ivankovich AD, Bieniarz J, *et al.*: Cardiovascular Effects and Acid-Base and Blood Gas Changes During Laparoscopy. *Am J Obstet Gynecol* 1973, 115:1002–1012.

19. Hodgson C, McClelland RMA, Newton JR: Some Effects of the Peritoneal Insufflation of Carbon Dioxide at Laparoscopy. *Anaesthesia* 1970, 25:382–390.

20. Takata M, Wise RA, Robotham JL: Effects of Abdominal Pressure on Venous Return: Abdominal Vascular Zone Conditions. *J Appl Physiol* 1990, 69:1961–1972.

21. Stanton JM: Anaesthesia for Laparoscopic Cholecystectomy. *Anaesthesia* 1991, 46:317.

22. Scott DB: Some Effects of Peritoneal Insufflation of Carbon Dioxide at Laparoscopy. *Anaesthesia* 1970, 25:590.

23.• Puri GD, Singh H: Ventilatory Effects of Laparoscopy Under General Anaesthesia. *Br J Anaesth* 1992, 68:211–213.

Physiologic dead space does not increase in this study of healthy women undergoing laparoscopy with general anesthesia.

24. Corall IM, Knights K, Potter D, Strunin L: Arterial Oxygen Tension During Laparoscopy with Nitrous Oxide in the Spontaneously Breathing Patient. *Br J Anaesth* 1974, 46:925–928.

25. de Sousa H, Tyler IL: Can Absorption of the Insufflation Gas During Laparoscopy be Hazardous? *Anesthesiology* 1987, 67:A476.

26. Brown DR, Fishburne JI, Roberson VO, Hulka JF: Ventilatory and Blood Gas Changes During Laparoscopy with Local Anesthesia. *Am J Obstet Gynecol* 1976, 124:741–745.

27. Diamant M, Benumof JL, Saidman LJ, *et al.*: Laparoscopic Sterilization with Local Anesthesia: Complications and Blood-Gas Changes. *Anesth Analg* 1977, 56:335–337.

28. Brampton WJ, Watson RJ: Arterial to End-Tidal Carbon Dioxide Tension Difference During Laparoscopy. *Anesthesia* 1990, 45:251–214.

29.• Wittgen CM, Andrus CH, Fitzgerald SD, *et al.*: Analysis of the Hemodynamic and Ventilatory Effects of Laparoscopic Cholecystectomy. *Arch Surg* 1991, 126:997–1001.

End-tidal carbon dioxide is a good estimate of arterial carbon dioxide pressure during laparoscopic cholecystectomies in healthy patients. End-tidal carbon-dioxide, however, may severely underestimate arterial carbon dioxide pressure during laparoscopic cholecystectomies in patients with cardiopulmonary disease. Arterial blood gas monitoring should be considered in these patients.

30. Rademaker BM, Ringers J, Odoom JA, *et al.* Pulmonary Function and Stress Response After Laparoscopic Cholecystectomy: Comparison with Subcostal Incision and Influence of Thoracic Epidural Analgesia. *Anesth Analg* 1992, 75:381–385.

31. Becquemin J-P, Piquet J, Becquemin M-H, *et al.*: Pulmonary Function After Transverse or Midline Incision in Patients with Obstructive Pulmonary Disease. *Intensive Care Med* 1985, 11:247–251.

32. Peterson HB, DeStefano F, Rubin GL, *et al.*: Deaths Attributable to Tubal Sterilization in the United States, 1977 to 1981. *Am J Obstet Gynecol* 1983, 146:131–136.

33. Cunanan RG Jr, Courey NG, Lippes J: Complications of Laparoscopic Tubal Sterilization. *Obstet Gynecol* 1980, 55:501–506.

34. Clark CC, Weeks DB, Gusdon JP: Venous Carbon Dioxide Embolism During Laparoscopy. *Anesth Analg* 1987, 56:650–652.

35. Durant TM, Long J, Oppenheimer MJ: Pulmonary (Venous) Air Embolism. *Am Heart J* 1947, 33:269–281.

36. Lee CM: Acute Hypotension During Laparoscopy: A Case Report. *Anesth Analg* 1975, 54:142–143.

37. Carmichael DE: Laparoscopy—Cardiac Considerations 1971, 22:69–70.

38. Doyle DJ, Mark PWS: Laparoscopy and Vagal Arrest. *Anaesthesia* 1989, 44:448.

39. Shifren JL, Adlestein L, Finkler NJ: Asystolic Cardiac Arrest: A Rare Complication of Laparoscopy. *Obstet Gynecol* 1992, 79:840–841.

40. Ganansia M-F, Francois TP, Ormezzano X, *et al.*: Atrioventricular Mobitz I Block During Propofol Anesthesia for Laparoscopic Tubal Ligation. *Anesth Analg* 1989, 69:524–525.

41. Harris MNE, Plantevin OM, Crowther A: Cardiac Arrhythmias During Anaesthesia for Laparoscopy. *Br J Anaesth* 1984, 56:1213–1216.

42. Kent RB: Subcutaneous Emphysema and Hypercarbia Following Laparoscopic Cholecystectomy. *Arch Surg* 1991, 126:1154–1156.

43. Davis A, Millar JM: Postoperative Pain: A Comparison of Laparoscopic Sterilization and Diagnostic Laparoscopy. *Anaesthesia* 1988, 43:796–797.

44. Kaplan P, Freund R, Squires J, Herz M: Control of Immediate Postoperative Pain with Topical Bupivacaine Hydrochloride for Laparoscopic Falope Ring Tubal Ligation. *Obstet Gynecol* 1990, 76:798–802.

45. Sharp JR, Pierson WP, Brady CE: Comparison of CO_2 and N_2O-Induced Discomfort During Peritoneoscopy Under Local Anesthesia. *Gastroenterology* 1982, 82:453–456.

46. Minoli G, Terruzzi V, Spinzi GC, *et al.*: The Influence of Carbon Dioxide and Nitrous Oxide on Pain During Laparoscopy: A Double-Blind, Controlled Trial. *Gastrointest Endosc* 1982, 28:173–175.

47. Dobbs FF, Kumar V, Alexander JI, Hull MGR: Pain After Laparoscopy Related to Posture and Ring Versus Clip Sterilization. *Br J Obstet Gynaecol* 1987, 94:262–266.

48. Kenefick JP, Leader A, Maltby JR, Taylor PJ: Laparoscopy: Blood-Gas Values and Minor Sequelae Associated with Three Techniques Based on Isoflurane. *Br J Anaesth* 1987, 59:189–194.

49. Alexander JI, Hull MGR: Abdominal Pain After Laparoscopy The Valve of a Gas Drain. *Br J Obstet Gynaecol* 1987, 94:267–269.

50. Boheimer NO, Thomas JS, Bowen-Simpkins P: Pain After Laparoscopy. *Anaesthesia* 1990, 45:253–254.

51. Baram D, Smith C, Stinson S: Intraoperative Topical Etidocaine for Reducing Postoperative Pain After Laparoscopic Tubal Ligation. *J Reprod Med* 1990, 35:407–410.

52. McKenzie R, Phitayakorn P, Uy NTL, *et al.*: Topical Etidocaine During Laparoscopic Tubal Occlusion for Postoperative Pain Relief. *Obstet Gynecol* 1986, 67:447–449.

53.• Helvacioglu A, Weis R: Operative Laparoscopy and Postoperative Pain Relief. *Fert Steril* 1992, 57:548–552.

Intraperitoneal lidocaine and incisional bupivacaine effectively reduce postoperative pain following operative laparoscopy.

54. Spielman FJ, Hulka JF, Ostheimer GW, Mueller RA: Pharmacokinetics and Pharmacodynamics of Local Analgesia for Laparoscopic Tubal Ligations. *Am J Obstet Gynecol* 1983, 146:821–824.

55.•• Buckley MM, Brogden RN: Ketorolac: A Review of its Pharmacodynamic and Pharmacokinetic Properties, and Therapeutic Potential. *Drugs* 1990, 39:86–109.

The anesthetic properties of ketorolac are compared with other nonsteroidal anti-inflammatory agents and narcotics. Therapeutic trials are reviewed; side effects are discussed.

56. Bloomfield SS, Mitchell J, Cissell GB, *et al.*: Ketorolac Versus Aspirin for Postpartum Uterine Pain. *Pharmacotherapy* 1986, 6:247–252.

57. Sunshine A, Richman H, Cordone R, *et al.*: Analgesic Efficacy and Onset of Oral Ketorolac in Postoperative Pain. *Clin Pharmacol Ther* 1988, 43:159.

58. Parker RK, Holtmann B, White PF: Effect of Ketorolac on the Postoperative Opioid Requirement and Recovery Profile [abstract]. *Anesthesiology* 1991, 75:A758.

59.• Rice ASC, Lloyd J, Miller CG, *et al.*: A Double-Blind Study of the Speed of Onset of Analgesia Following Intramuscular Administration of Ketorolac Tromethamine in Comparison to Intramuscular Morphine and Placebo. *Anaesthesia* 1991, 46:541–544.

Intramuscular ketolac (30 mg) and 10 mg intravenous morphine have comparative analgetic onset time.

60.• Rosenblum M, Weller RS, Conard PL, *et al.*: Ibuprofen Provides Longer Lasting Analgesia than Fentanyl After Laparoscopic Surgery. *Anesth Analg* 1991, 73:255–259.

Ibuprofen (800 mg) provides equivalent and longer duration pain relief than 75 µg of fentanyl following laparoscopic surgery. Additionally, ibuprofen treated patients had a lower incidence of nausea.

61. Power I, Noble DW, Douglas E, Spence AA: Comparison of I.M. Ketorolac Trometamol and Morphine Sulphate for Pain Relief After Cholecystectomy. *Br J Anaest* 1990, 65:448–455.

62. Spowart K, Greer IA, McLaren M, *et al.*: Haemostatic Effects of Ketorolac with and without Concomitant Heparin in Normal Volunteers. *Thromb Haemost* 1988, 60:382–386.

63. Conrad KA, Fagan TC, Mackie MJ, Mayshar PV: Effect of Ketorolac Tromethamine on Hemostasis in Volunteers. *Clin Pharmacol Ther* 1988, 43:542–546.

64.•• Watcha MF, White PF: Postoperative Nausea and Vomiting. *Anesthesiology* 1992, 77:162–184.

An excellent review of postoperative nausea and vomiting. Anesthetic and nonanesthetic factors contributing to emesis are discussed as is antiemetic therapy.

65. Metter SE, Kitz DS, Young ML, *et al.*: Nausea and Vomiting After Outpatient Laparoscopy:Incidence, Impact on Recovery Room Stay and Cost. *Anesth Analg* 1987, 66:S116.

66. Pataky AO, Kitz DS, Andrews RW, Lecky JH: Nausea and Vomiting Following Ambulatory Surgery: Are All Procedures Created Equal? *Anesth Analg* 1988, 67:S163.

67. Palazzo MGA, Strunin L: Anaesthesia and Emesis. I: Etiology. *Can Anaesth Soc J* 1984, 31:178–187.

68. Boulton TB, Chir B: Oral Chlorpromazine Hydrochloride. *Anaesthesia* 1955, 10:233–246.

69.• Beattie WS, Lindblad T, Buckley DN, Forrest JB: The Incidence of Postoperative Nausea and Vomiting in Women Undergoing Laparoscopy Is Influenced by the Day of Menstrual Cycle. *Can J Anaesth* 1991, 38:298–302.

The incidence of postoperative nausea and vomiting after laparoscopic tubal ligation is highest during the first week of the menstrual cycle and is lowest during the third week at the menstrual cycle.

70. Bellville JW: Postanesthetic Nausea and Vomiting. *Anesthesiology* 1961, 22:773–780.

71. Lonie DS, Harper NJN: Nitrous Oxide Anaesthesia and Vomiting. *Anaesthesia* 1986, 41:703–707.

72. Hovorka J, Korttila K, Erkola O: Nitrous Oxide Does Not Increase Nausea and Vomiting Following Gynaecological Laparoscopy. *Can J Anaesth* 1989, 36:145–148.

73. Scheinin B, Lindgren L, Scheinin TM: Perioperative Nitrous Oxide Delays Bowel Function After Colonic Surgery. *Br J Anaesth* 1990, 64:154–158.

74. Sengupta P, Plantevin OM: Nitrous Oxide and Day-Case Laparoscopy: Effects of Nausea, Vomiting and Return to Normal Activity. *Br J Anaesth* 1988, 60:570–573.

75. Rising S, Dodgson MS, Steen PA: Isoflurane v Fentanyl for Outpatient Laparoscopy. *Acta Anaesth Scand* 1985, 29:251–255.

76. Gunawardene RD, White DC: Propofol and Emesis. *Anaesthesia* 1988, 43:65–67.

77. Bridenbaugh LD: Regional Anaesthesia for Outpatient Surgery—A Summary of 12 Years Experience. *Can Anaesth Soc J* 1983, 30:548–552.

78. King MJ, Milazkiewicz R, Carli F, Deacock AR: Influence of Neostigmine on Postoperative Vomiting. *Br J Anaesth* 1988, 61:403–406.

79. Pandit SK, Kothary SP, Pandit UA, et al.: Dose- Response Study of Droperidol and Metoclopramide as Antiemetics for Outpatient Anesthesia. *Anesth Analg* 1989, 68:798–802.

80. Bailey PL, Streisand JB, Pace NL, et al.: Transdermal Scopolamine Reduces Nausea and Vomiting After Outpatient Laparoscopy. *Anesthesiology* 1990, 72:977–980.

81. Wetchler BV, Sung YF, Duncalf D, Joslyn AF: Ondansetron Decreases Emetic Symptoms Following Outpatient Laparoscopy. *Anesthesiology* 1990, 73:A35.

82. Alon E, Himmelseher S: Ondansetron in the Treatment of Postoperative Vomiting: A Randomized, Double-Blind Comparison with Droperidol and Metoclopramide. *Anesth Analg* 1992,. 75:561–565.

83. Puhakka HJ: Complications of Mediastinoscopy. *J Laryngol Otol* 1989, 103:312–315.

84. Benumof JL: Anesthesia for Thoracic Surgery. Philadelphia:WB Saunders; 1987:335–339.

85. Prakash UBS, Abel MD, Hubmayr RD: Mediastinal Mass and Tracheal Obstruction During General Anesthesia. *Mayo Clin Proc* 1988, 63:1004–1011.

86. Rock P: Mediastinoscopy and Thoracoscopy. In Current Practice in Anesthesiology, 2nd ed. Edited by Rogers MC. St. Louis: BC Decker; 1992:290–294.

87. Ashbaugh DG: Mediastinoscopy. *Arch Surg* 1970, 100:568–573.

Chapter 4

A Better Understanding of Monopolar Electrosurgery and Laparoscopy

C. Randle Voyles
Robert D. Tucker

The challenge of laparoscopy is to perform complex operations within the peritoneal cavity from external sites. Tissue transection and hemostasis can be accomplished either mechanically or thermally. An ongoing evaluation of electrical, laser, and recently, ultrasonic transfer of energy appears to have settled on radio-frequency (RF) electrical energy as the "gold standard" for energy source [1•,2•,3]. The arguments for bipolar versus monopolar electrosurgery vary according to the surgical task. Laser dissection has fallen into disfavor because of efficacy, cost, and time.

When electrosurgery is combined with laparoscopy (versus laparotomy), a better understanding of the biophysics involved is essential to improve the efficacy and safety of the procedure. First, minimal access to the surgical site mandates maximum utility of the energy source. Second, the peritoneal cavity is viewed incompletely during laparoscopy. Third, the introduction of surgical electrodes through or near other closely aligned metal devices may induce currents that are less significant with open operations.

The term *electrocautery* is unimodal and strictly refers to heating a wire to cauterize, brand, or burn tissue but not to cut it. *Electrosurgery*, a more definitive term, encompasses different tissue effects caused by passing varying waveforms of RF current through tissue. Tissue effects can be modified further by variables of the generator, surgical technique, and active-electrode design.

The incidence of unrecognized electrosurgical injury during laparoscopic electrosurgery is low, but the occasional complication leaves the surgeon groping for an explanation [4–6]. Understanding and preventing the occasional, unexpected burn—out of the view of the laparoscope—is impossible without a better appreciation of the science associated with RF energy. Our purpose is to provide an overview of the biophysics of electrosurgery necessary to improve efficacy and to outline the potential mechanisms of "stray current" outside the view of the laparoscope.

BASIC SCIENCE OF ELECTROSURGERY

A complete review of the biophysics of electrosurgery is beyond the scope of this chapter; more complete references are available [7••,8,9]. In general terms, the effect of RF electrical energy occurs because electrons or, more accurately, electrical charges are driven through a section of tissue, the tissue resists the current flow, and heat is generated. All the tissue effects of electrosurgery (and laser energy) occur as a result of conversion of electrical energy (or laser energy) to heat. Electrons or electrical charges are transmitted most readily by tissue with a high electrolyte content, such as blood and muscle; such tissues have a low resistance to the transmission of electrical charges.

The force pushing electrons through tissue (measured in volts) is analogous to the head of pressure forcing water through a pipe. The current reflects a quantity of electrical charge that is pushed through a tissue and is measured as charge per unit time, or amperes (amps). Current can be increased by increasing voltage (height of water tower) or decreasing resistance (enlarging the diameter of the water pipe).

In the electrosurgical generator unit (ESU), the voltage "pushing" the electrical charge is not constant but alternates between positive and negative (Fig. 1). The tissue effect occurs as a result of the rapid continuous change in the charge per unit time and not the net change, which is zero at the completion of a complete cycle. In Figure 1, the voltage shift varies between a positive 2000 V and a negative 2000 V (a "peak-to-peak" 4000 voltage or a "peak" voltage of 2000 V). For practical purposes, tissue resistance, voltage, and current can be considered as if there were a continuous flow rather than alternating currents.

The electrical power for your home is provided by an alternating current at 60 cycles per second, but typical ESUs in the operating room provide an alternating current with a frequency of 300,000 to 2 million cycles per second. (One complete alternation, or cycle per second, is referred to as a Hertz (Hz). 1000 cps = 1 KiloHertz = 1 KHz; 1,000,000 cps = 1 megaHertz = 1 MHz.) The high frequency from the generator (radio frequency) is essential to prevent neuromuscular stimulation.

The ESU generates the RF energy that is delivered to

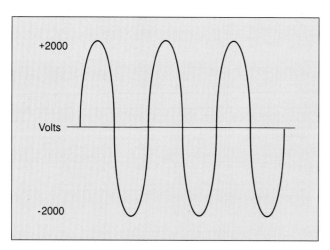

Figure 1. Alternating current with voltage changes.

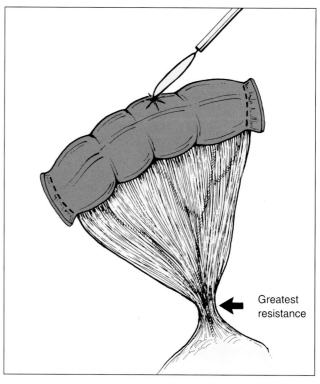

Figure 2. Potential for "pedicle injury" increases when current is concentrated in distal high resistance tissue.

the tissue by a surgical electrode. From the surgical site, the RF energy traverses tissue en route to the dispersive, or return, electrode (more commonly referred to as a ground pad). Because of the alternating current, there is really no "flow" but a rapid alternation of electrical charge at all points in the circuit. The desired tissue effect occurs because most of the heat is dissipated at the electrode-tissue interface, the point in the circuit with the greatest resistance. Burns at the ground-pad site (the most common electrosurgical injury 10 years ago) have been virtually eliminated by specifically designed ground pads that are actively monitored by the ESU for adequacy of skin contact to prevent burns.

A watt is a unit of power delivered by the ESU but specifically reflecting the power that is dissipated by resistance at the electrode-tissue interface as well as all other points within the circuit. The wattage is the product of continuously changing voltage and current:

$$P = IV \qquad (1)$$

Where P = power (watts), I = current (amperes), V voltage. Although the generator may be set at 40 watts "coag," the voltage and current change continuously as a function of varying tissue or circuit resistance. As tissue is desiccated, resistance increases and current decreases. To maintain a given power, voltage increases. Engineers analyze electrosurgical current flow in terms of "average" (root mean square, or RMS) values. This method allows waveform differences to be simply averaged and direct comparisons made between cut and coag powers. Manufacturers usually perform these averages and label the generators accordingly. The maximum voltage varies according to manufacturer and product line (Table 1).

The ohm is a unit of resistance and is equal to one volt per amp (Ohm's law). The total resistance (R) of a homogenous circuit (*ie*, a wire) increases with length of the circuit and decreases with area and conductivity of the conductor.

$$R = \frac{V}{I} = \frac{length}{(conductivity)\,(area)} \qquad (2)$$

Equation 2 explains the potential for a pedicle injury (Fig. 2). The point of maximum resistance in the circuit is typically the point of tissue-electrode contact. A scenario can be created, however, in which an elevated pedicle of tissue has a sufficiently narrowed base that power can be concentrated at a point remote to the electrode, thus creating a burn. Tissue conductivity can be varied significantly by surgical manipulation or the presence of blood or saline.

The rate of change in tissue temperature correlates with the concentration of current or power per unit of tissue. As the RF current spreads from the electrode through the tissue, the concentration of current (and temperature change) decreases dramatically. Theoretically, tissue heating at the tissue-electrode interface occurs as follows [7••]:

$$\Delta T = (I^2/r^4)\,R\,t \qquad (3)$$

(I = current, r = radius of tissue electrode contact, R=tissue resistance, t=time). Thus, the most important determinant of tissue heating is the radius of the electrode contact; current is secondary in importance. (Doubling the current increases heating by a factor of four; doubling the radius leads to a change of 16.) Accordingly, the skilled surgeon controls the radius of contact (through electrode size and contact area) to obtain the desired tissue effect with the least wattage. Large contact areas within the electrical circuit (*ie*, the dispersive ground pad or perhaps, the all-metal trocar-cannula) may exhibit minimal temperature change.

The above analysis does not entirely correspond to reality. Radio-frequency currents do not flow uniformly through tissue; they follow the path of least resistance,

Generator	Peak to peak voltage, W	Frequency, kHz
Valleylab SSE2L	4070	450
Valleylab Force 2	7000	500
Valleylab Force 4B	8000	750
Valleylab Force 40	9000	500
Aspen Excalibur	10500	417

Table 1. Maximum peak to peak voltage and frequency of commonly used generators

which is typically blood vessels. The current densities and tissue resistance vary from millisecond to millisecond. The situation is further complicated by the fact that the generator power output varies by millisecond as the tissue resistance changes. The prediction of the extent of tissue damage is at best difficult. We do know, however, that if cellular temperatures of 70°C or greater are reached, collagen is denatured. Above 100°C, liquids are converted to vapor. Above 200°C, tissues are carbonized. It may be surprising how little power can cause unintended, serious burns. Overt tissue necrosis and full-thickness bowel burns have been created experimentally by only 12 W of capacitively coupled power coming off the trocar-cannula after 5 seconds [10•].

ELECTROSURGICAL WAVEFORMS

Examples of the varying waveforms created by the ESU are depicted in Figure 3. The operating modes of ESUs vary by the following: voltage, current, frequency, and waveform.

The "cut" waveform has a continuous cycle with a peak voltage of about 500 V at 50-W power. Although the precise mechanism of cutting is not fully understood, the uninterrupted movement of ions within cells is believed to generate intense intracellular heat, which causes the cellular contents to boil (liquid converted to gas), thereby vaporizing the cell. "Sparking" from the electrode to the tissue seems essential for the cutting effect. A bubble or layer of steam from erupting cells provides a high concentration of conductive ions

between the electrode and the tissue that facilitates the process of energy exchange. It is critical to understand that cut waveforms typically have a lower voltage than the coag or "blend" waveforms (given the same wattage, as in Fig. 3). Conversely, the cut waveform has a higher current than the coag waveform.

Cut waveforms work best when a fine edge or tip of an electrode is in close proximity to, but not touching, the tissue. With apposition of the electrode to the tissue, there is no steam layer—and no cutting—as the energy is directly transferred into the tissue with drying or desiccation rather than cutting. Thus, the most effective use of cutting is with a light stroking action and a fine-edged electrode: a rapid temperature rise occurs as the electrode comes within range of the target tissue. The surgeon's feedback for controlling precise cutting is visual not tactile sensation.

The cut mode cuts best when the electrode has a fine edge or point to provide a concentration of current or power. Power density is simply the power per cross sectional area (*A*) of tissue.

$$\text{Power density} = \frac{power}{A} \qquad (4)$$

Appropriate tension and counter-tension of tissue increases power density by decreasing the amount of tissue that receives the electrical or mechanical energy; tension makes the knife or electrode appear "sharper." The depth of necrosis (and, indeed, the safety of using monopolar electrosurgery) is dependent on the rapid dispersal of power at points remote from the tissue-electrode interface.

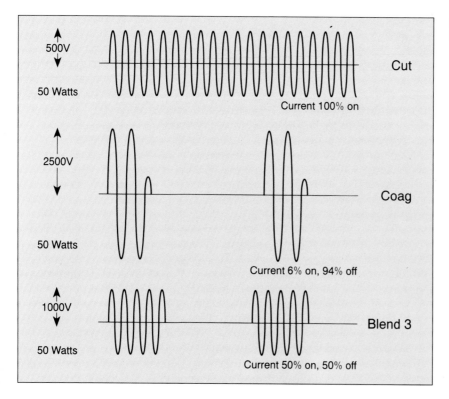

Figure 3. Diagram of cut, coag, and blend currents.

Why does the cut mode give poor hemostasis? With appropriate use of the cutting mode, superficial cells vaporize, erupt, and dissipate heat into the atmosphere rather than the surrounding tissue. The lower voltage of this modality also generates less force to push the charge into deeper tissues. Since little heat is transferred to deeper tissue, there is very little coagulation of tissue and very little hemostasis.

The labels of cut and coag incompletely describe the full application of RF energy. The cut mode will coagulate quite well when a broad-based electrode-tissue contact is maintained in static position. The coagulate mode will also cut given an adequate concentration of power.

Why does the coag mode lead to tissue desiccation? The previous diagram (Fig. 3) shows the high-voltage, low-current waveform of the coag mode. Note the initial burst of electrical activity with a voltage that is greater than the peak-to-peak voltage change with cutting current. The current is "on" for only 6% of the time; however, the balance of time, the generator is not generating a current. (This coag waveform is often called a "dampened waveform.") The base frequency of both cut and coag is typically 500 kHz, varying with different generators and models. The initial short burst of high-voltage energy leads to cellular insult (but not vaporization as with the continuous waveform of cutting). During the "off" interval, a drying effect, or cellular desiccation, occurs. In the subsequent electrical burst, the "dry" cells have an increased resistance to electron flow, which leads to more local heat dissipation and further cellular desiccation. The progressive insult to deeper layers of tissue from the higher voltage leads to tissue coagulation and hemostasis. As the desiccation increases, tissue resistance continues to increase until the current may actually cease. We see this principle demonstrated when charred tissue coats the electrode and renders the coag mode ineffective. (With a "charred" electrode, why does coag work better than cut? If you don't know the answer, reread this section.)

Coaptive coagulation is a useful electrosurgical technique. A vessel is grasped by a hemostat (or atraumatic dissector) and compressed. In open surgery, the hemostat is touched by the activated electrode; in laparoscopy, the atraumatic dissector electrode is activated. As a result of compression of the tissue, the tissue is rendered less vascular, and tissue resistance is increased. Electrical energy, locally applied to the tissue, promotes a collagen weld of the vessel. Larger arteries can be controlled with coaptive coagulation than by simple application of electrical energy to a bleeding vessel. When coaptive coagulation is used, less lateral tissue damage is present (and less chance for inadvertent damage) if cut current is used rather than coag. By using the cut mode, the surgeon selects a low-voltage waveform that coagulates with a more local tissue effect than the coag mode would because of the lower voltage.

Fulguration (Webster's definition: to give off flashes like lightning) is accomplished by setting the generator in the coag mode and holding the electrode off the tissue. Sparks ("mini lightning") are given off from the electrode and strike through the path of least resistance. As with lightning, the burst of energy burns, dries, or desiccates the target tissue. The key point for the surgeon is that the tissue desiccation is very superficial because the current actually delivered to the tissue is low and the energy is rapidly dissipated (by the tissue as well as by heat and light that you see in the flashes). Tissue contact causes a deeper desiccation. The use of the argon beam may help to distribute the energy over a broader area; the blowing effect of the argon also clears fluid from the target tissue.

With proper fulguration, the surgeon can desiccate and avoid mechanical disruption of friable tissue. Fulguration is enhanced by a higher wattage from the ESU. However, as fulguration occurs with open circuit and with the high voltage of the coag mode, stray current of capacitive coupling and insulation failure will also be increased (fully discussed below in "Type 2 Problem: Capacitive coupling").

The blend modes offer varying combinations of the cut and coag waveforms (Fig. 4). As the relative amount of the coag current is increased in different blend settings, tissue desiccation is enhanced and tissue cutting is lessened.

POTENTIAL PROBLEMS OF MONOPOLAR ELECTROSURGERY

Our early editorial [1•] describing the advantages of electrosurgery over laser was followed by criticism from surgeons preferring lasers [11]. Attacks were based on safety concerns referencing early gynecologic laparoscopy. Unfortunately, both electrosurgical and laser injuries have been recognized [4–6] in the past two years. Features common to these injuries include

1) Mechanism of injury is frequently unknown
2) Site of injury is not observed during procedure
3) Recognition of injury is delayed
4) Poor outcome is likely; a mortality rate with unrecognized bowel injury may exceed 25%
5) Litigation is common

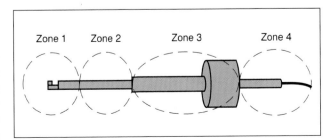

Figure 4. Zones of insulation failure.

6) The biophysical principles of the energy source are not fully appreciated

7) Surgeons are reluctant to discuss the poorly understood complications

Because of the difficulties in retrospectively studying the characteristics and mechanisms of bowel injury during laparoscopy, the potential mechanisms of energy transfer should be categorized to prevent injuries. The rest of this chapter attempts to provide such categorization. The authors contend that most of the bowel injuries can be avoided with education and relatively simple engineering advances.

To be simplistic, the two sites where injury can occur are either within the view of the laparoscope or outside the view of the laparoscope. Injuries within the view of the laparoscope are related to surgical technique and can be reduced by a better understanding of the energy source. Electrosurgical injuries outside the view of the laparoscope may occur because of three different types of "stray" energy: insulation failure, capacitive coupling, and direct coupling. Though specific documentation of each mechanism is impossible (for obvious reasons), unexplained morbidity and deaths have occurred. Emphasis must be placed on biophysics and prevention of injury rather than epidemiology. As will become apparent, the potential problems have an appropriate preventive measure with minimal, if any, increase in cost.

TYPE 1 PROBLEM: INSULATION FAILURE

The operating surgeon is able to deliver RF energy to the target tissue because of the insulation surrounding the active electrode. There is no standard for insulation of laparoscopic instruments. Several variables are important in evaluating insulation: thickness, dielectric strength (the characteristic of insulating capability), hardness (how readily it is damaged) and porosity (whether it retains moisture). Insulation defects can be acquired from cannula valve or other mechanical trauma, repeated heating through use or sterilization, manufacturing flaws, or capacitively coupled meltdown. An unrecognized defect in the insulation—too small to be seen—can deliver 100% of the RF energy to a site outside the view of the scope.

The hazard of insulation failure is dependent on the location of the point of failure (Fig. 4). Defects in the handle of the electrode (zone 4) are generally a result of poor engineering with exposed metal (particularly trumpet valves) that can burn the surgeon. Zone 1 insulation failure occurs as a result of trauma during insertion through cannula valves and repeated intraoperative use. Insulation breakdown in zone 1 appears to be more common with the newer instruments, which have more complete distal insulation (as opposed to the earlier instruments with exposed metal shoulders). Zone-1 defects may cause injury or may "ground out" (on the liver during laparoscopic cholecystectomy) with a loss of efficacy at the target tissue.

Zone 2 represents the shaft of the electrode that is neither within view of the laparoscope nor inside the cannula. Even the most careful surgeon receives no clue that insulation failure and thermal injury have occurred in zone 2. The incidence of zone-2 injury will increase as the general surgeon pursues operations outside the right upper quadrant.

The signs of insulation failure within zone 3 depend on whether a metal or plastic cannula is used. If a metal cannula is used, there is often a current flow between the metal of the electrode and the metal of the cannula;

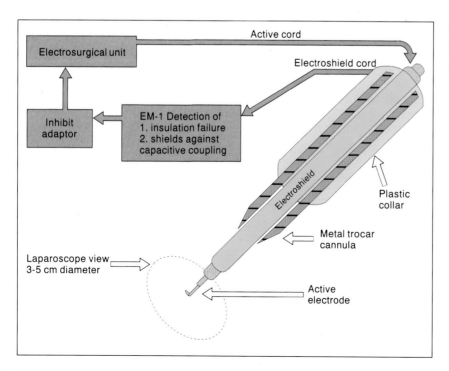

Figure 5. Diagram of the dynamically monitored electrode to guarantee insulation and prevent capacitive coupling to the cannula or biologic tissue.

the resulting arcing of the current creates a lower-frequency current (referred to as a demodulated frequency) as low as a few cycles per second. With this lower frequency, there may be neuromuscular stimulation [12] and jerking of the abdominal wall or diaphragm as well as possible interference with the video monitor. These clues suggest insulation failure to the informed surgeon. Unfortunately, insulation failure and subsequent bowel burn can occur without any clues prior to the development of an ileus, infectious complications, or peritonitis. Because no clues indicate insulation failure if the electrode is within a plastic cannula, the need for metal cannulas is apparent. The stray current, once transferred to the metal cannula, should be dissipated harmlessly by the broad contact area at the abdominal wall; more prolonged energy transfer via the cannula may lead to tissue desiccation at the level of the skin and abdominal wall. Plastic anchoring devices over a metal shaft must be avoided; they will insulate the abdominal wall at the expense of the viscera.

What are the solutions to problems of insulation failure? Superficial logic suggests that disposable instruments might be advantageous. The insulation of some disposables is thinner than that of most new, reusable instruments, however. Additionally, many surgeons consider the cost of disposable instruments prohibitive [13,14].

All forms of conventional insulation (plastic, teflon, etc.) are based on a passive system, with layers of nonconductors around the electrode. Defects within a passive system may not be detected before injury can occur. A new concept of insulation is based on dynamic monitoring of insulation integrity [10] (Electroscope, Boulder, CO) (Fig. 5). The actively monitored electrode is constructed with a central metal conductor (the electrode), a nonconductive layer, and an outer conductor that is assessed for any electrical current. Continuous monitoring of insulation should eliminate bowel burns from insulation failure with the same efficacy that

dynamically monitored return electrodes or ground pads eliminated burns to the thigh.

TYPE 2 PROBLEM: CAPACITIVE COUPLING

Capacitive coupling is a mechanism whereby electrical current in the electrode (intended) induces a current in nearby conductors (unintended) despite otherwise intact insulation. Some degree of capacitive coupling occurs with all standard monopolar electrosurgical instruments because the electrode is passed either through or near other conductors within the abdomen [10,15,16]. Whether or not the stray energy of capacitive coupling causes any clinical injury depends on the total amount of current that is transferred and the concentration of the current (*ie*, the power density) as it makes its way back to the patient return electrode (ground pad).

Figure 6 shows a simple diagram demonstrating a capacitor with two parallel plates. A capacitor is defined as two conductors separated by a dielectric (an insulator), which is air in the diagram. The charge from the ESU is transmitted to the left side of a plate that is separated by a short distance from the right plate. Even if an insulating material is placed between the plates, the charge on the left plate affects the right plate and "induces" an equal and opposite charge on the right side conductive plate. This net transfer of energy is because of the capacitance effect. A simple insulator between the two conductors does not eliminate the effect. As an analogy, consider how a paper between two oppositely charged magnets has little effect on the attractive force between the two magnets.

Typically, 5-mm electrodes are introduced into the abdomen through either 5-mm cannulas or 5-mm reducers within 10-mm cannulas. The cannulas are all metal, all plastic, or metal with a plastic abdominal wall anchor. The conductive active electrode within its insulation and the conductive tubular cannula represent a capacitor. The capacitance of this system is given by the formula:

$$C = \frac{2\pi e_o k \, L}{\ln (b/a)} \qquad (5)$$

where L = the length of the metal cannula-electrode interface; e_o is an engineering constant, k = the dielectric constant of the insulation, b = radius of trocar cannula; and a radius of the active electrode. Thus, the induced current into the surrounding cannula is increased in any system in which the length of the surrounding cannula is increased and the distance between the electrode and the surrounding cannula is decreased.

It may be useful to think of the electrode as a "transmitter" of radio-frequency electrical energy (much like a radio antenna). The energy can be transmitted through the intact insulation (such as teflon, carbon dioxide, or air) to any outer surrounding "receiver." The reception

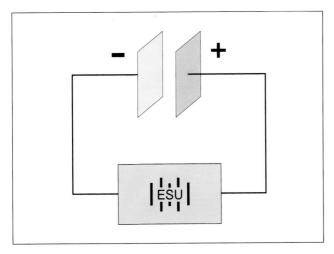

Figure 6. Capacitive coupling between two parallel plates.

will be greater if the transmitter and receiver are closer together or if the enface surface areas of the transmitter or receiver are increased, Thus, the efficiency of transfer is related to the geometric interface of the two conductors. The 10-mm electrode will transfer more current to a surrounding 10-mm cannula than would a 5-mm electrode. There is also more coupled current if a 5-mm electrode is passed through a 5-mm cannula instead of a 10 mm cannula.

Capacitive coupling is increased by higher wattage but also by generators with higher voltage and frequencies (Table 1). The low-voltage cut mode exhibits less coupling than the coag mode. The low-voltage generator (such as the Valleylab SSE2L) exhibits very little coupling compared with the higher voltage generators (Force 2 or 4B). Higher-voltage generators, however, also have a greater efficacy for cutting and desiccation. Surgeons must recognize that open-circuit activation (electrode not touching tissue) increases voltage and capacitive coupling dramatically. Accordingly, try to limit noncontact activation of the ESU and use wattage as low as possible.

Clinically, capacitive coupling can lead to laparoscopic complications. In an experimental model, only 12 watts of power from capacitive coupling for 5 seconds can cause full-thickness intestinal injury to the dog [10•]. Documentation in patients is difficult, however, because bowel injury from capacitive coupling occurs outside the view of the laparoscope.

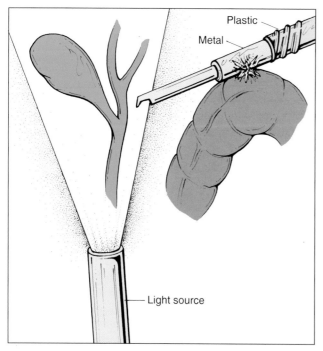

Figure 7. Capacitive coupled current can create a burn when a hybrid plastic/metal cannula is used.

Cannula selection and design is important to reduce capacitively coupled injuries [10•,15]. If a trocar cannula is employed that has a metal sheath and a plastic tissue anchor, the abdominal wall may be in contact only with the nonconducting plastic anchor. Although this apparatus does hold the cannula in place, it also electrically isolates the metal cannula from the abdominal wall (Fig. 7). Therefore, induced current from the cannula could be discharged to an internal organ such as the bowel within close proximity of the isolated metal trocar cannula. A preferable method for fixing the cannula at the abdominal wall would be a conductive metal anchor or a rubber wafer–adhesive barrier at the skin level.

Another potentially dangerous scenario with capacitive coupling can occur with a small electrode that is passed through a metal suction-irrigator. As might be anticipated from Equation 5, the length and proximity of the two conductors promote effective capacitive coupling (almost 70% of the intended power is available as stray current). If the device is introduced into the peritoneal cavity through a plastic nonconductive cannula, all of the stray current may be concentrated at a narrow point on the transverse colon (Fig. 8). An all-metal cannula at the abdominal wall will "bleed off" the stray current through the abdominal wall, but the use of metal also decreases the resistance of the capacitively coupled pathway and increases the net coupling. High-amperage, capacitively coupled currents from the electrode to the metal suction-irrigation sleeve can cause considerable heating to the instrument through corona heating. Thus, the authors recommend that the metal-sleeved suction-irrigation electrodes not be used; if they are used, they should be introduced only through a metal trocar-cannula, never a plastic one.

Capacitive coupling is demonstrated quite dramatically when the surgeon receives a burn to the hand from "buzzing" a hemostat during open operations [17•]. Surgeons generally attribute the injury to a hole in their gloves, but few recognize that the hole may have been created by capacitively coupled current. The same energy that can burn a hole in the surgeon's glove can also cause a melt-down of the insulation of some instruments, particularly if the insulation is thin [17•]. Fluid, blood, or a bit of tissue on the electrode surface provide the secondary conductor to create an effective capacitor and can melt a hole completely through the insulation. The extremely thin insulation of some instruments can markedly decrease the separation of the electrode from the surrounding conductor and increase coupling logarithmically (Eq. 5). In brief, thinly insulated instruments provide more coupling than thickly insulated ones.

The potential for injury from capacitive-coupled currents can be reduced with an understanding of the biophysics involved and good electrosurgical technique. Avoid using hybrid cannulas, suction-irrigation electrodes (with exposed metal suction-irrigator), and thinly insulated instruments. The surgeon should use low-wattage and low-voltage power when possible (use cut versus coag, minimize open-circuit activation). Higher voltage is helpful and open circuit activation is inevitable, however, during electrosurgical dissection. Accordingly, capacitive coupling will inevitably occur when conventional electrosurgical instruments are used. Capacitive coupling can be eliminated only by use of recently designed electrosurgical instruments that "collect" the stray current, remove it from the surgical site, and monitor the total amount of current before returning it to the ground pad [10•] (Electroscope, Boulder, CO). This system confines capacitive coupling to the collecting sheath and monitoring circuit, thereby eliminating transmission to either the cannula or biologic tissues.

TYPE 3 PROBLEM: DIRECT COUPLING
Direct coupling refers to the condition in which the activated electrode touches other metal instruments (in particular, the laparoscope) within the abdomen, creating a situation whereby the energy can be unknowingly trans-

ferred (coupled) to tissue outside the view of the laparoscope (Fig. 9). The active electrode is typically within 2 cm of the end of the laparoscope and occasional contact (or close proximity to allow arcing without physical contact) with the laparoscope is a reality [18]. An electrode that has been placed more parallel than perpendicular to the laparoscope may be much closer to the laparoscope than is apparent on the video monitor. When the laparoscope becomes activated inadvertently, a metal cannula through which the laparoscope is passed helps disperse the energy at the abdominal wall and markedly reduces the chance for injury. Plastic, nonconductive cannulas should be avoided around the laparoscope [7••,10•,15,19]; they concentrate the energy away from the abdominal wall and increase the risk of burn to the bowel.

ENHANCED ELECTROSURGERY, 1993
The primary deficiency of laparoscopic electrosurgery is not technologic but relates to surgical education regarding the underlying biophysics. The fully developed art of electrosurgery is reflected by the surgeon's ability to manipulate fine electrodes and tissue to achieve results,

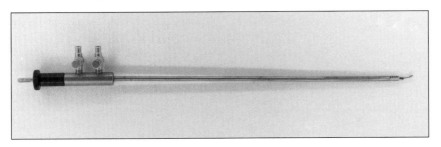

Figure 8. A surgical electrode introduced through a metal suction irrigator creates an effective capacitor. The chance for injury is increased with a plastic cannula.

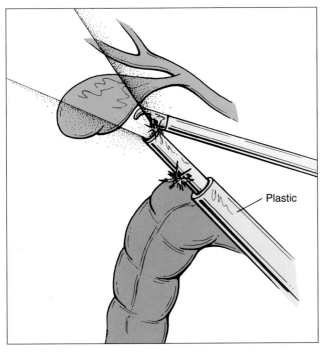

Figure 9. Unrecognized contact between the electrode and the laparoscope may transmit 100% of power to the laparoscope. A plastic cannula increases the risk of bowel burns if this occurs.

Plastic

with an appropriate wattage. The informed surgeon understands the relative merit and disadvantages of both high- and low-voltage waveforms; if only cutting is needed, a low-voltage, pure cut waveform is appropriate. High voltage and high wattage may be useful for deeper desiccation, however, especially for noncontact, superficial arc-fulguration. Current should be applied with bursts rather than with continuous ESU activation. In summary, safety issues in electrosurgery are impossible to understand without a better understanding of the biophysics involved. Injuries related to stray currents (insulation failure, capacitive coupling, and direct coupling) can be reduced or eliminated with all-metal cannulas and recent developments with dynamically monitored electrodes. The following specific instruments should be avoided: standard metal-sleeved suction-irrigators containing electrodes, hybrid cannulas, and thinly insulated electrodes. Finally, the laparoscope should always be introduced through a metal cannula. The recent interest in the art and science of electrosurgery is timely; for the informed surgeon, the term "enhanced electrosurgery" seems appropriate.

REFERENCES

Papers of particular interest, published within the period of review, have been highlighted as:
• Of special interest
•• Of outstanding interest

1.• Voyles CR, Meena AL, Petro AB, *et al.*: Electrocautery is Superior to Laser for Laparoscopic Cholecystectomy. *Am J Surg* 1990, 160:457.
This editorial documented the relative benefits of electrosurgery and temporally correlated with change from laser to electrosurgery in the United States.

2.• Bordelon BM, Hobday KA, Hunter JG: Laser vs Electrosurgery in Laparoscopic Cholecystectomy. *Arch Surg* 1993, 128:233–236.
This well-designed study outlined, in a prospective randomized trial, the merit of electrosurgery compared with laser dissection.

3. Wetter LA, Payne JH, Kirshenbaum G, *et al.*: The Ultrasonic Dissector Facilitates Laparoscopic Cholecystectomy. *Arch Surg* 1992, 127:1195–1199.

4. Deziel DJ, Millikan KW, Economou SG, *et al.*: Complications of Laparoscopic Cholecystectomy: A National Survey of 4,292 Hospitals and an Analysis of 77,604 Cases. *Am J Surg* 1993, 165:9–14.

5. Park YH, Oskanian Z: Obstructive Jaundice after Laparoscopic Cholecystectomy with Electrocautery. *Am J Surg* 1992, 58:321–323.

6. Larson GM, Vitale GC, Casey J, *et al.*: Multipractice Analysis of Laparoscopic Cholecystectomy in 1,983 Patients. *Am J Surg* 1992, 163:221–226.

7.•• Voyles CR, Tucker RD: *Essentials of Monopolar Electrosurgery for Laparoscopy.* Jackson, MS: Electrosurgical Concepts; 1992.
This video and syllabus represent a single resource outlining the essential biophysics and potential complications related to monopolar electrosurgery. The video is an invaluable aid in presenting concepts that are somewhat difficult to comprehend in the written form.

8. Pearce JA: *Electrosurgery.* London: Chapman & Hall; 1986.

9. Serway RA: *Physics for Scientists and Engineers.* Philadelphia: Saunders; 1990: 714.

10.• Voyles CR, Tucker RD: Education and Engineering Solutions for Potential Problems with Laparoscopic Monopolar Electrosurgery. *Am J Surg* 1992, 164:57–62.
This article and reference 15 within measure and document the effects of capacitive-coupled currents in laparoscopic scenarios. The potential for injury during laparoscopy is presented along with preventive measures.

11. Wiley C: Are General Surgeons Ignoring Lessons of Gynecology? *Clin Laser Monthly* 1991, 9:1–4.

12. Tucker RD, Schmitt OH, Sievert CR, Silvis SE: Demodulated Low Frequency Currents From Electrosurgical Procedures. *Surg Gynecol Obstet* 1984, 159:39–43.

13. Voyles CR, Petro AB, Meena AL, *et al.*: A Practical Approach to Laparoscopic Cholecystectomy. *Am J Surg* 1991, 161:365–371.

14. Voyles CR: The Laparoscopic Dividend. *JAMA* 1992, 267:1469.

15. Tucker RD, Voyles CR, Silvis SE: Capacitive Coupled Stray Currents During Laparoscopic and Endoscopic Electrosurgical Procedures. *Biomed Instrum Technol* 1992, 26:303–311.

16. Barlow DE: Endoscopic Applications of Electrosurgery: A Review of Basic Principles. *Gastrointest Endosc* 1982, 28:73–76.

17.• Tucker RD, Fergusson S: Do Surgical Gloves Protect Staff During Electrosurgical Procedures? *Surgery* 1991, 110:892–895.
The concept of capacitive-coupled current with enough power density to burn a surgical glove is presented.

18. Soderstrom RM: [Letter]. *JAMA* 1974, 227:1261.

19. Federal Registry 45: 12701, Feb 26, 1980.

Chapter 5

Laparoscopic Cholecystectomy

Nathaniel J. Soper

E. Mühe of Böblingen, Germany, performed the first laparoscopic cholecystectomy in 1985 [1]. However, most authors have assigned the credit to P. Mouret of Lyon, France, who in 1987 facilitated the procedure by rotating the entire right lobe of the liver in a cephalad direction with traction applied to the gallbladder itself. This maneuver allowed the gallbladder and porta hepatis to be viewed from a telescope, placed at the umbilicus, that was directed cranially toward the under-surface of the liver. Surgeons in Paris and Bordeaux subsequently learned the procedure and initiated the first clinical series of laparoscopic cholecystectomies [2,3]. This procedure was first performed in the United States in mid-1988 and has since been reported by Reddick and Olsen [4] and Spaw and coworkers [5], as well as many others [6,7••,8–13]. Because of the competitive, free-market medical system, patients' preference for less invasive procedures, and marketing efforts by individuals and hospitals, laparoscopic cholecystectomy was adopted at a rate unprecedented in American surgery and rapidly became the new "gold standard" therapy for symptomatic cholelithiasis [6].

Laparoscopic cholecystectomy has many potential advantages over traditional "open" cholecystectomy [14•] (Table 1). Postoperative pain and intestinal ileus are diminished. The small size of the fascial incisions allows rapid return to heavy physical activities. The multiple small incisions are cosmetically more appealing than the large incision used during traditional cholecystectomy. The patient can usually be discharged from the hospital within 24 hours of operation and can return to full activity within a few days [15,16••]. These factors lead to a decreased overall cost of the procedure [17,18]. However, laparoscopic cholecystectomy also has several disadvantages. Patients must be acceptable candidates for general anesthesia. Three-dimensional depth perception is limited by the monocular image of the video telescope, and the operative field being viewed is determined by an individual other than the surgeon; some patients may be excluded from undergoing this therapy by virtue of their anatomy or intra-abdominal adhesions. The common bile duct is more difficult to visualize and instrument during laparoscopy than during traditional open surgery. It is technically difficult to remove the gallbladder from the fundus to the infundibulum, and control of brisk hemorrhage is diminished using laparoscopy compared with laparotomy. In the ensuing discussion, I review the current status of laparoscopic cholecystectomy, focusing on preoperative, intraoperative, and postoperative considerations.

PREOPERATIVE CONSIDERATIONS

INDICATIONS

The ability to perform laparoscopic cholecystectomy should not expand the indications for removing the gallbladder. In general, patients should have documented cholelithiasis and symptoms attributable to a diseased gallbladder. Occasionally, individuals with gallstones and no symptoms (porcelain gallbladder, immunosuppression, lack of access to medical care) or those with no stones but typical biliary symptoms (low gallbladder ejection fraction on cholecystokinin-stimulated biliary scintigraphy) may be considered for this therapy. Recent studies suggest that symptoms develop in less than 20% of individuals with asymptomatic gallstones over a prolonged period and that the risk of "prophylactic" operation outweighs the potential benefit of surgery [19,20]. In an individual with typical biliary colic, the only diagnostic test necessary is a high-quality ultrasound. This study demonstrates the stone size and number, the thickness of the gallbladder wall, and the diameter of the common bile duct. It may also give clues to nonbiliary disorders, such as hepatic lesions or fatty infiltration, masses in the pancreas, or renal tumors. If atypical symptoms are present, a more extensive work-up, including upper gastrointestinal contrast radiographs or endoscopy, computed tomography, or cardiac evaluation, may be appropriate.

CONTRAINDICATIONS

Contraindications to the elective performance of laparoscopic cholecystectomy have changed tremendously as experience with this technique has grown. Absolute contraindications include the following (Table 2): inability to tolerate general anesthesia, uncorrectable coagulopathy, diffuse peritonitis, a frozen abdomen, cholecystoenteric fistula, and gallbladder cancer. Numerous relative contraindications, which are primarily dictated by the

Table 1. Comparison of laparoscopic cholecystectomy to open cholecystectomy

Advantages	Disadvantages
Smaller incisions	**Technical limitations**
Less pain	More difficult to control hemorrhage and explore common bile duct
Shorter hospitalization	Monocular vision controlled by assistant
More rapid return to full activity	Less tactile discrimination
Decreased total cost	Expensive, technologically advanced instruments
	Anatomic limitations
	Inflammation/adhesions restrict application
	Antegrade removal of gallbladder difficult
	Incidence of bile duct injury may be increased

surgeon's philosophy and experience, also exist. Many of the relative contraindications shown in Table 2 had previously been considered absolute. Certainly, for the novice laparoscopic surgeon, it would be wise to avoid such patients for the first few cases. Despite scattered reports of laparoscopic cholecystectomies having been performed during pregnancy [21], the effects of the prolonged carbon dioxide pneumoperitoneum on the fetus are unknown, and the position of the gravid uterus itself may also present a problem.

OPERATING ROOM PREPARATION

Chapter 2 details the equipment necessary for safe performance of laparoscopic cholecystectomy. Set-up of the operating room and its personnel also requires consideration. Performance of laparoscopic biliary surgery requires more personnel than open operations. The surgeon stands to the left of the patient for cross-table access to the right upper quadrant (Fig. 1). The French

prefer to operate with the patient in the lithotomy position, with the surgeon standing or sitting between the patient's legs [2,3]. The first assistant stands to the patient's right to manipulate the gallbladder and provide exposure. A laparoscopic video camera operator, who stands below the surgeon, assumes the important responsibility of being the surgeon's eyes. The camera operator must maintain the proper orientation of the camera and scope, particularly if an angled laparoscope is used; keep the surgeon's instruments in the center of the video monitor; follow (or guide) all instruments as they enter or exit the operative field; and assist with instruments or trocar valves as needed. No sharp instruments should be moved unless under direct vision. The camera operator must also take care of any obstruction to vision, such as wiping off condensation or blood that may cloud the lens. Condensation on the lens itself can be minimized by heating the laparoscope before its insertion into the warm, moist abdominal cavity.

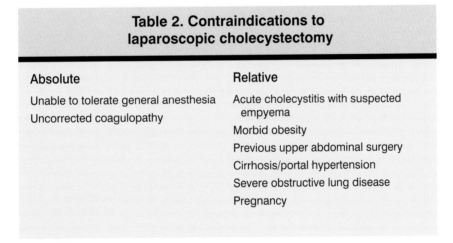

Table 2. Contraindications to laparoscopic cholecystectomy

Absolute	Relative
Unable to tolerate general anesthesia	Acute cholecystitis with suspected empyema
Uncorrected coagulopathy	Morbid obesity
	Previous upper abdominal surgery
	Cirrhosis/portal hypertension
	Severe obstructive lung disease
	Pregnancy

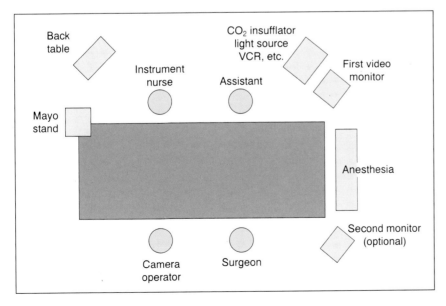

Figure 1. The organization of the operating room for laparoscopic biliary surgery. The patient's head is to the right, the surgeon stands at the patient's left, and the first assistant is to the patient's right. The electronic laparoscopic equipment is placed on protective carts, and the monitors are positioned to allow clear visualization by the entire surgical team. (From Soper [14]; with permission.)

PREOPERATIVE CARE AND ANESTHESIA

As for any abdominal operation, patients are fasted from midnight before the operation. Patients without other major medical problems are admitted to the hospital the morning of operation and are given preoperative sedatives and histamine-2 blockers. All patients are administered a single dose of broad-spectrum intravenous antibiotics. Upon arrival in the operating room, sequential compression stockings are placed on both legs to avoid pooling of blood in the lower extremities caused by the reverse Trendelenburg position. We have not routinely used minidose heparin, but this can be used safely in patients at risk for venous thromboembolism. After induction of anesthesia, a bladder catheter and orogastric tube are placed to decompress these hollow organs. The abdomen is prepared in standard fashion, except that particular care is taken to clean the umbilicus of all detritus.

Although diagnostic laparoscopy can be performed with either local or regional anesthesia, laparoscopic cholecystectomy is generally performed using inhalation anesthesia and controlled ventilation. Important considerations for the optimal anesthetic management are as follows: adequate depth of anesthesia, complete muscle relaxation, administration of amnesics, and administration of an antiemetic, such as droperidol, before conclusion of the operation. Appropriate patient monitoring during therapeutic laparoscopy using general anesthesia includes electrocardiography, blood pressure, precordial stethoscope, airway pressure, and capnography (specifically to assess end-tidal oxygen). Invasive monitoring (arterial line, Swan-Ganz catheter) may be indicated in selected high-risk individuals [22,23]. (See Chapter 3 for a detailed discussion of anesthesia for therapeutic laparoscopy).

There are scattered reports of performing laparoscopic cholecystectomy using thoracic epidural (bupivacaine) anesthesia supplemented with intravenous sedation and local anesthetics. Referred shoulder pain may be troublesome with this technique, but it can be diminished by insufflating the peritoneal cavity slowly or maintaining a lower abdominal pressure (<10 mm Hg). Regional anesthesia may be appropriate for high-risk patients or those who want to avoid a general anesthetic. However, we use general anesthesia in all cases because of the potential need for rapid conversion to an open laparotomy.

CREATION OF PNEUMOPERITONEUM AND TROCAR INSERTION

A pneumoperitoneum, which is established by instilling gas, is usually used to allow visualization of the abdominal cavity. Recently, devices that elevate the abdominal wall by external retraction to create the working space have been described [24–26]. This technology would potentially eliminate the adverse local and systemic effects of the pneumoperitoneum and allow the use of instrumentation free of the design limitations imposed by maintenance of an airtight system. This novel instrumentation may ultimately replace peritoneal insufflation for abdominal wall lift during laparoscopy. Prospective randomized trials will be necessary to assess whether perioperative pain or morbidity is increased when these traction devices are used.

For diagnostic laparoscopy, both carbon dioxide and nitrous oxide are applicable. Nitrous oxide is not usually used to create the pneumoperitoneum for laparoscopic cholecystectomy; despite being nonflammable, it supports combustion. Carbon dioxide has the advantage of being noncombustible and is eliminated rapidly from the body; most carbon dioxide disappears within 4 hours postoperatively. However, it is readily absorbed into the blood stream and may lead to hypercarbia in high-risk patients or in those with chronic obstructive pulmonary disease [27•]. Also, carbon dioxide is converted to carbonic acid on the moist peritoneal surfaces and may therefore cause mild postoperative discomfort. Because of these adverse effects, ongoing studies are establishing whether other gases (such as helium or argon) may be preferable for use during laparoscopic surgery [28]. Nevertheless, absorption of carbon dioxide from the blood is ordinarily rapid; the body can safely absorb it (without formation of gas emboli) when infused into a systemic vein at a rate less than 1 L per minute [29].

The pneumoperitoneum can be established by either a closed or an open technique. In the closed technique, carbon dioxide is insufflated into the peritoneal cavity through a needle; the initial laparoscopic trocar and sheath are then placed blindly into the abdominal cavity. Using the open technique, a small incision is made, and a laparoscopic sheath without the sharp trocar is inserted under direct vision into the peritoneal cavity. The pneumoperitoneum is established only after ensuring safe peritoneal entry. There are advantages and disadvantages to both techniques, and surgeons performing laparoscopy should learn both and use them on a selective basis.

When using the closed technique, carbon dioxide is insufflated through a Veress needle or one of its disposable counterparts. Before insertion, the pneumoperitoneum needle should be checked to ensure that the spring-loaded stylet is functioning properly and that the lumen is patent to the injection of water. The patient is then placed in a 10° to 15° Trendelenburg position, and a small incision is made into the subcutaneous tissue of the infraumbilical skinfold. The surgeon stands to the left of the patient and grasps the lower abdomen, elevating and stabilizing the abdominal wall. The Veress needle is then inserted at a right angle to the abdominal wall, usually at a 45 ° angle off the vertical axis toward the pelvis. The surgeon will hear one or two "clicks" of the obturator as the needle passes into the peritoneal cavity. Various tests to assure the safety of the needle insertion are then performed. A syringe containing 5 mL normal saline solution is attached to the Luer lock connector to aspirate and demonstrate the absence of blood, urine, or stool. If the aspiration is negative, it is repeated after injecting a few milliliters of saline. If blood-stained fluid or frank blood is recovered, the needle should be removed and its position changed. If no fluid is aspirated, an assessment is made of the ease with which saline flows by gravity into the relatively negative pressure of the peritoneal cavity. Manually elevating the lower abdominal wall will decrease intra-abdominal pressure and enhance free flow; the fluid will flow much slower if the needle is in the preperitoneal space.

In patients who have had previous abdominal surgery, an alternative site for initial puncture may be required. With an upper midline scar, the insertion should be in the right or left lower quadrant, two thirds the distance from the umbilicus to the iliac crest. A lower midline scar favors an initial puncture in the right or left upper abdomen at the lateral edge of the rectus muscle. If this approach is used, the position of the liver and spleen must be ascertained before needle insertion. The tubing from the insufflator is then connected to the Veress needle, and insufflation of carbon dioxide is initiated at a flow rate of 1 L per minute. The abdomen should be percussed to confirm symmetrical tympany associated with the intraperitoneal gas. The abdomen is then inflated with the insufflator's upper pressure limit set at 15 mm Hg pressure, which usually requires 3.5 to 6 L of carbon dioxide, depending on the size of the abdominal cavity and the weight of the abdominal wall. Obese or muscular patients tend to have heavier abdominal walls and higher abdominal pressures, and sometimes the pressure limit needs to be raised to allow for an adequate pneumoperitoneum.

During the early phase of insufflation, the patient must be monitored closely for signs of gas embolism (hypotension, "millwheel" heart murmur), vagal reaction (hypotension or bradycardia), ventricular arrhythmias, and hypercarbia with acidosis. Most of these complications require immediate treatment by allowing the carbon dioxide to escape and then gradually reestablishing the pneumoperitoneum after the patient's condition has stabilized. Gas embolism results in an "air-lock" right ventricular outflow obstruction. When suspected, this entity should be treated by placing the patient in Trendelenburg position with the left side down and inserting a central venous catheter to aspirate the carbon dioxide. When the intra-abdominal pressure exceeds 20 mm Hg, central venous pressure and blood pressure fall in association with the diminished cardiac output. Adequate muscle relaxation helps minimize the rise in intra-abdominal pressure. After the pneumoperitoneum has been established, the Veress needle is removed.

The initial large (10- to 11-mm) trocar and sheath are placed in the infraumbilical incision previously created. This is inserted with a gentle "drilling" motion for controlled entry into the peritoneal cavity. The sheath is inserted at the same angle as that of the Veress needle while stabilizing the lower abdominal wall manually. With practice, it is generally apparent when the resistance of the fascia and peritoneum is overcome and the sheath enters the abdominal cavity. With a nondisposable trocar, the hissing noise of escaping carbon dioxide indicates that the trocar tip is correctly positioned in the pneumoperitoneal space. With a disposable sheath, the safety shield can be heard springing into place over the trocar tip. The trocar is then removed, and the telescope is inserted.

Creation of the pneumoperitoneum by the open technique is performed similarly to open diagnostic peritoneal lavage [30]. A 1.5-cm skin incision (either vertical or horizontal) is made in the infraumbilical skinfold (Fig. 2A). Dissection of the subcutaneous tissue should be performed deep to the skin of the umbilicus to reach the fascia quickly, even in obese patients, as this is the thinnest part of the abdominal wall. Kocher clamps are then applied to both sides of the midline of the linea alba, and a small vertical incision is made into the peritoneal cavity. A finger is placed into the wound to assure that the free peritoneal cavity has been entered and to sweep away any adhesions present. If Hasson trocars (Weck & Co., Research Triangle Park, NC) are available, two heavy absorbable sutures are placed on both sides of the fascial incision and are tied to the "wings" of the olive-tipped trocar after it is inserted into the peritoneal cavity under direct vision (Fig. 2B). Alternatively, standard laparoscopic sheaths can be used after placing two concentric purse-string stitches of heavy monofilament suture around the fascial incision (Fig. 2C and D). The laparoscopic sleeve without its sharp trocar is then inserted into the peritoneal cavity, and the purse-string sutures are tightened down by using a section of red rubber catheter similar to a vascular tourniquet. At the conclusion of the case after removing the sheath, the outer purse-string suture is removed and the inner one tied down. Open insertion of the initial port takes a few minutes longer than its closed counterpart. However, extraction of the gallbladder at the conclusion of the operation is easier. We perform open insertion of the sheath on a selective basis, in patients with previous periumbilical incisions, patients in whom insertion of the Veress needle is not performed satisfactorily, and in those with large (>2.5 cm) gallstones or acute cholecystitis.

TECHNIQUE OF LAPAROSCOPIC CHOLECYSTECTOMY

A 10.5-mm laparoscope is inserted into the abdomen. The retroperitoneum immediately posterior to the umbilicus and the pelvis is first viewed to assure that there is no injury as a result of insertion of the trocar or sheath. The pelvic viscera are examined for other pathologic abnormalities before evaluating the upper abdomen. The anterior surface of the intestines, omentum, and stomach are examined for abnormalities. The patient is then placed in a reverse Trendelenburg position of 30° to 40° while the table is rotated to the patient's left by 15° to 20°. This maneuver generally allows the colon and duodenum to fall away from the liver edge. The falciform ligament and both lobes of the liver are closely examined for abnormalities. The inferior margin of the liver is then visualized to determine the location of the gallbladder; usually, the gallbladder can be seen protruding beyond the liver edge, but sometimes the gallbladder is not visible without carefully elevating the right liver lobe.

The two small accessory subcostal ports are then placed under direct vision. The first trocar is placed in the anterior to middle axillary line between the 12th rib and the iliac crest. This sheath should be placed inferior (caudad) to the gallbladder fundus and liver edge. A second 5-mm port is then inserted under direct vision

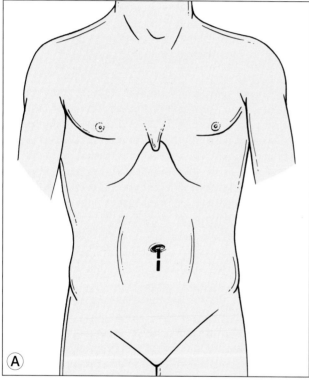

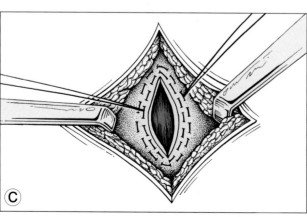

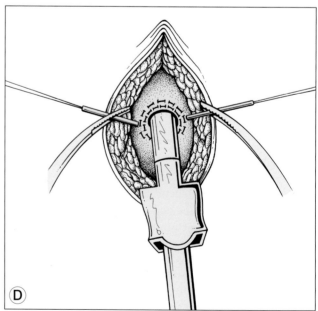

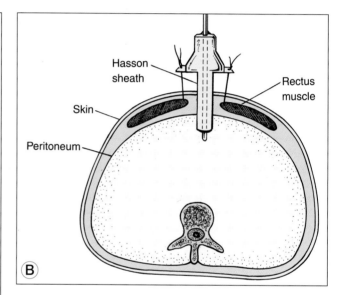

Figure 2. Techniques for open insertion of the initial laparoscopic sheath. **A,** Site of skin incision. **B,** Placement of Hasson sheath through the abdominal wall and secured in place with sutures between the fascia and the wings of the sheath. **C** and **D,** An alternative technique using a standard laparoscopic sheath and two concentric purse-string sutures placed in the abdominal fascia. (*From* Soper [14]; with permission.)

approximately midway between the axillary sheath and the xiphoid process. It should be possible to avoid major abdominal wall blood vessels during trocar insertion by a combination of transillumination and direct examination of the parietal peritoneum. Grasping forceps are then placed through these two sheaths, and the gallbladder is secured. The assistant (standing on the right side of the table) manipulates the lateral grasping forceps, which are used to elevate the liver edge to expose the fundus of the gallbladder. The surgeon (standing to the left of the patient) uses a dissecting forceps to raise a serosal "fold" of the most dependent portion of the fundus. The assistant's heavy grasping forceps are then locked onto this fold by using either a spring or ratchet device. Using these axillary grasping forceps, the fundus of the gallbladder is then pushed in a lateral and cephalad direction, so that the entire right lobe of the liver rolls cranially. The successful performance of this maneuver is critical to expose the porta hepatis and gallbladder. In patients with high- or low-lying livers, the position of these trocars is quite different than in the "standard" patient. In patients with a fixed, cirrhotic liver or a heavy, friable liver due to fatty infiltration, this maneuver is complicated.

In patients with few adhesions to the gallbladder, pushing the fundus cephalad exposes the entire gallbladder, cystic duct, and porta hepatis. Most patients, however, have adhesions between the gallbladder and the omentum, hepatic flexure, or duodenum. These adhesions are generally avascular and may be lysed bluntly by grasping them with a dissecting forceps at their site of

attachment to the gallbladder wall and gently "stripping" them down toward the infundibulum. After exposing the infundibulum, blunt grasping forceps are placed through the midclavicular trocar for traction on the neck of the gallbladder. The operative field is thereby established, and the final working port is then inserted.

The last 10- to 11-mm trocar is placed through a transverse incision in the midline of the epigastrium. In general, this is placed 5 cm below the xiphoid process, but the position depends on the location of the gallbladder, as well as on the size of the medial segment of the left liver lobe. When uncertain about the appropriate position for this trocar, a Veress needle may first be placed at the proposed site to ascertain whether its location and angle of insertion are optimal. The trocar is then inserted with a "drilling" motion; the surgeon angles its tip just to the right of the falciform ligament while aiming toward the gallbladder.

The basic positions for placement of the various ports are shown in Figure 3. The accessory sheaths should be separated as far as possible so that the external portions of the instruments do not cross or interfere with one another. The orientation of the laparoscope is generally parallel to that of the cystic duct when the fundus is elevated, whereas the instruments placed through the axillary and epigastric sheaths enter the abdomen at right angles to this plane. Finally, the midclavicular sheath is anterior to the gallbladder, thereby making the instruments passing through it perpendicular to the cystic duct. Thus, all of the accessory sheaths are placed at right angles to the axis of the cystic duct

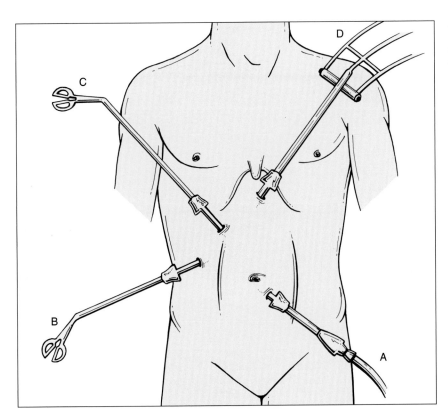

Figure 3. Positions for insertion of the initial (**A**) and accessory sheaths (**B–D**) for biliary surgery. (*From* Soper [14]; with permission.)

while the surgeon's vision is directed along its axis. The French prefer to elevate the liver lobe with a rod placed in a medial right subcostal position and operate through a left paramedian port [2,3].

Having established the positions of all sheaths, the first assistant places the fundus and infundibulum of the gallbladder under tension away from the common bile duct in a superior and lateral direction. Then, either a one-handed or two-handed dissection technique may be used, depending on whether the surgeon or the assistant manipulates the gallbladder infundibulum. With the fundus and neck of the gallbladder under tension, fine-tipped dissecting forceps are used to dissect away the overlying fibroareolar structures from the infundibulum of the gallbladder and Hartmann's pouch. This is done with a blunt stripping action, always starting on the gallbladder and pulling the tissue toward the porta hepatis.

During this initial dissection around the neck of the gallbladder, the peritoneum is lysed with the blunt dissector similar to the technique by which the peritoneum is incised and pushed bluntly with a Kittner dissector during a traditional open cholecystectomy. With the laparoscopic dissection performed under two-dimensional optics, it is critical to clear and identify the structures contained within two triangles: Calot's triangle and its reverse side. Calot's triangle is the ventral aspect of the area bounded by the cystic duct, hepatic duct, and liver edge. The reverse side is the dorsal aspect of this space. Calot's triangle is placed on tension and maximally exposed by retracting the infundibulum of the gallbladder inferiorly and laterally while pushing the

fundus superiorly and medially (Fig. 4A). A lymph node usually overlies the cystic artery, and occasionally a brief application of electrical current must be used to obtain hemostasis as the lymph node is swept away. The assistant then places the infundibulum of the gallbladder on stretch in a superior and medial direction while pushing the fundus superiorly and laterally, thereby exposing the reverse of Calot's triangle, an area defined by the cystic duct, the inferior lateral border of the gallbladder, and right lobe of the liver (Fig. 4B). Further blunt dissection is used to identify precisely the junction between the infundibulum and the origin of the cystic duct. Identification of this junction is the critical maneuver in the operation; certainly, no structure should be sharply divided until the cystic duct is clearly identified. The strands of peritoneal, lymphatic, neural, and vascular tissue are stripped away from the cystic duct to gain as much length as possible. Curved dissecting forceps are helpful in creating a "window" around the posterior aspect of the cystic duct to skeletonize the duct itself (Fig. 4). Alternatively, the tip of a hook-shaped cautery probe can be used to encircle and expose the duct. The cystic artery may be separated from the surrounding tissue by similar blunt dissection either at this time or later, depending on its anatomic location. In the usual position, the cystic duct is dissected and divided first, as it is the structure presenting most anteriorly in the field. If the cystic artery crosses anterior to the duct, the artery may require dissection and division before the cystic duct can be approached. An additional maneuver, which is often helpful during dissection of the duct, is to use the

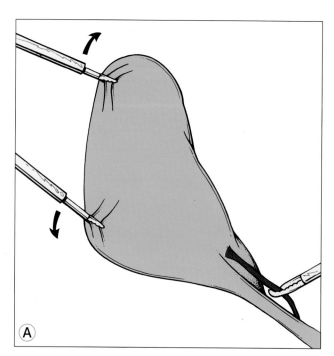

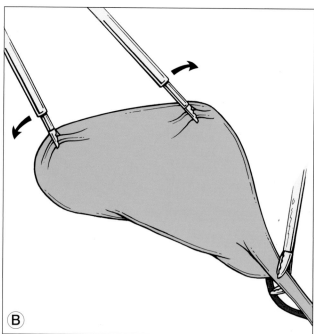

Figure 4. A, Calot's triangle is exposed by manipulating the gallbladder with traction applied by the assistant's grasping forceps. The surgeon's curved instrument is encircling the cystic artery; the cystic duct is anterior. *Arrows* indicate vector of forceps movement. **B,** The reverse (dorsal aspect) of Calot's triangle is displayed. *Arrows* indicate vector of forceps movement. (*From* Soper [14]; with permission.)

blunt concave blade of the spatula-tipped cautery as a Kittner dissector. Gentle irrigation through its central lumen while pushing away the periductal structures aids precise visualization.

After initial dissection of the cystic duct, a cholangiogram may be performed. Cholangiograms may be performed selectively or routinely, using static or fluoroscopic imaging, as detailed in Chapter 6. We perform cholangiography through the cystic duct, although other techniques may be applicable. In brief, the dissecting forceps are used to squeeze gently the cystic duct in the direction of the gallbladder, thereby "milking" cystic duct stones back into the gallbladder. A clip applier placed through the epigastric sheath is used to apply a single clip at the junction of the cystic duct with the gallbladder. A scissors inserted through the axillary or midclavicular trocar is used to incise the anterolateral wall of the cystic duct, and a 4 or 5 F catheter is inserted into the duct and fixed in place. The cholangiograms should be inspected to ascertain the following: 1) the size of the common bile duct; 2) the location of the junction between the cystic and common bile ducts; 3) the presence of intraluminal filling defects; 4) free flow of contrast media into the duodenum; 5) the anatomy of the proximal biliary tree; and 6) aberrant biliary radicles entering the gallbladder directly.

After removing the cholangiocatheter, the cystic duct is doubly clipped near its junction with the common bile duct and divided. The posterior jaw of the clip applier must be visualized before applying each clip to avoid injury to surrounding structures. Great care should be taken so that the common bile duct is not tented up into the clip. If the cystic duct is particularly large or friable, it may be preferable to replace one of the clips with a suture, either hand-tied or preformed.

Attention is then directed to the cystic artery. The assistant places the infundibulum of the gallbladder on tension, and the surgeon dissects the cystic artery bluntly from the surrounding tissue. The surgeon must ascertain that the structure is the cystic artery and not the right hepatic artery looping up onto the neck of the gallbladder, as may be seen. After an appropriate length of cystic artery has been separated from the surrounding tissue, it is doubly clipped both proximally and distally and divided sharply. Electrocautery should not be used for this division, as the current may be transmitted to the proximal clips, thus leading to subsequent necrosis and hemorrhage. A common error is to dissect and divide the anterior branch of the cystic artery, mistaking it for the main cystic artery. This may result in hemorrhage from the posterior branch during dissection of the gallbladder fossa.

The ligated stumps of the duct and cystic artery are then examined to assure that neither bile nor blood has leaked, that the clips are securely placed, and that the clips compress the entire lumen of the structures without impinging on adjacent tissue. To avoid injury to structures in the porta hepatis, no dissection is undertaken medial to the stumps. A suction-irrigation catheter is used to remove any debris or blood that has accumulated during the dissection of the duct and artery. The heavy grasping forceps traversing the midclavicular trocar are repositioned on the proximal end of the gallbladder at Hartmann's pouch. The infundibulum is retracted superiorly and laterally, as well as distracted anteriorly away from its hepatic bed. The surgeon uses the dissecting forceps to thin out the tissue that tethers the neck of the gallbladder and to assure that no other sizable tubular structures are traversing the space. Dissection of the hepatic fossa is then initiated by using a thermal source to divide and coagulate small vessels and lymphatics. Occasionally, a larger blood vessel or aberrant small bile duct will require placement of a clip for control.

Once the appropriate plane has been identified, the separation of the gallbladder from its bed is performed with either electrocautery or laser-based instruments (Fig. 5). With the tissue connecting the gallbladder to its fossa placed under tension, the surgeon uses an electrocautery spatula or hook in a gentle sweeping motion with low power wattage (25 to 30 W) to coagulate and divide this tissue. Using the cautery probe, the surgeon can also perform blunt dissection, pushing the tissue to facilitate exposure of the proper plane. Occasionally, hemorrhage from the liver bed or gallbladder obscures precise identification of the anatomy. Frequent irrigation through the port of the electrocautery instrument

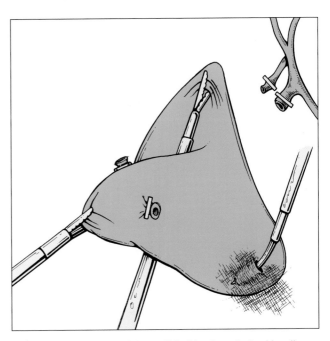

Figure 5. Separation of the gallbladder from its bed by dissecting with a blunt-tipped thermal energy probe. The neck of the gallbladder is placed on traction in a superior direction and then twisted to the left and right to place tension on the junction between the gallbladder and hepatic fossa. (*From* Soper [14]; with permission.)

during this dissection clarifies visualization of the plane.

Dissection of the gallbladder fossa continues from the infundibulum to the fundus, intermittently moving the midclavicular grasping forceps to a position closer to the plane of dissection to allow maximal countertraction. The dissection proceeds until the gallbladder is attached by only a thin bridge of tissue. At this point, before losing visualization of the operative field afforded by cephalad traction applied to the gallbladder, the hepatic fossa and porta hepatis are once again inspected for hemostasis and bile leakage. Small bleeding points are coagulated with the electrocautery. The right upper quadrant is then liberally irrigated and aspirated dry. The final attachments of the gallbladder are lysed, and the liver edge is once again examined for hemostasis.

After thus performing cholecystectomy, the gallbladder must be removed from the abdominal cavity. The gallbladder is usually removed through the umbilicus, as there are no muscle layers and only one fascial plane to traverse. Also, if the fascial opening needs to be enlarged because of large or numerous stones, extending the umbilical incision causes less postoperative pain than enlarging the subxiphoid entry site. The laparoscope is removed from the umbilical port and placed into the epigastric sheath. The pelvis and lower abdomen are inspected for evidence of unappreciated injury to the bowel, bladder, or retroperitoneal blood vessels. The umbilical trocar insertion site is examined for hemorrhage. Large "claw" grasping forceps are introduced through the umbilical sheath and guided to the right upper quadrant. The assistant presents the gallbladder neck into the jaws of the grasper so that it is lined up parallel to the axis of the forceps. The assistant

then releases the gallbladder, and its infundibulum is pulled up into the umbilical sheath. The forceps, sheath, and gallbladder neck are then retracted as a unit through the umbilical incision. The neck of the gallbladder is thus exposed on the anterior abdominal wall, with the distended fundus remaining within the abdominal cavity (Fig. 6).

If the gallbladder is not distended with bile or stones, it can be simply withdrawn with gentle traction. In most cases, a suction catheter is introduced into the gallbladder to aspirate bile and small stones. A stone forceps can be placed into the gallbladder to extract or crush calculi if necessary. Occasionally, the fascial incision must be extended to deliver larger stones. The laparoscopic sheaths are opened to deflate the abdomen. Placing the patient in a slight Trendelenburg position may facilitate escape of carbon dioxide trapped under the diaphragm. The sheaths are then removed.

Each incision is infiltrated with 0.5% bupivacaine and irrigated with saline solution. The fascia of the umbilical incision is closed with one or two large absorbable sutures. The skin of the subxiphoid and umbilical incisions is closed with subcuticular absorbable sutures, and Steri-strips (3M Health Care, St. Paul, MN) are applied to each incision.

ANATOMIC HAZARDS

The surgeon performing laparoscopic cholecystectomy must be aware of anatomic hazards that may lead to complications. The common bile duct may be "tented-up" because of the vigorous superolateral traction placed on the gallbladder, thereby making it susceptible to injury during placement of clips. Likewise, dissection in the region of the lateral wall of the common bile duct

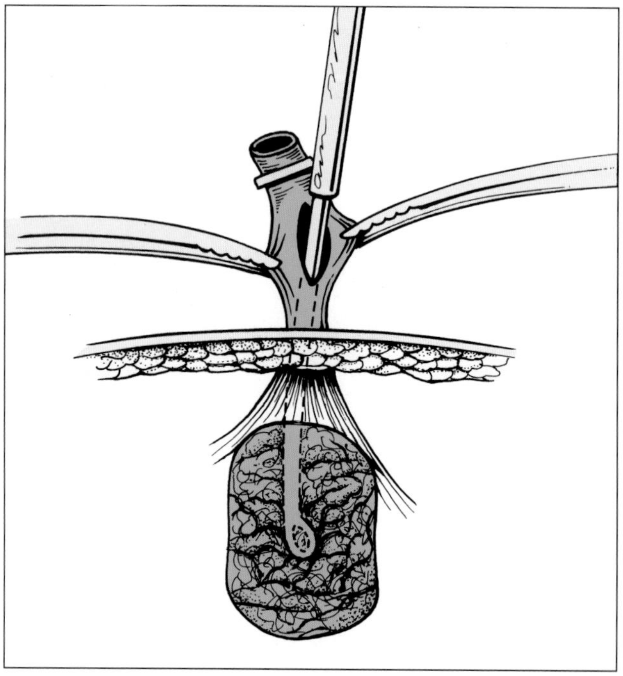

Figure 6. Gallstones contained within the fundus may be crushed or removed after delivering the neck of the gallbladder through the umbilical incision. (*From* Soper [14]; with permission.)

may cause bleeding from its nutrient vessels. Application of electrocautery in this area must be avoided, as subsequent devascularization and stricture may occur. Second, absent or extremely short cystic ducts may lead to two potential problems. The surgeon must recognize this anomaly and not mistake the common bile duct for the cystic duct. Also, it may be extremely difficult to occlude the cystic duct with a clip of insufficient length. The surgeon may need to convert to an open cholecystectomy in these circumstances, or possibly close a small portion of gallbladder infundibulum with a laparoscopic suture.

Aberrant bile ducts may also be present. If not recognized and ligated, direct communications between the biliary system and the gallbladder bed may lead to postoperative bile collections [11]. Aberrant origin of the right hepatic duct is not uncommon and must be ruled out in every case. Anomalous hepatic and cystic arteries may also be present. The most common anomaly in our experience has been a right hepatic artery that loops up onto the infundibulum of the gallbladder. In this situation, the cystic artery must be dissected up onto the gallbladder wall, clipped and divided to allow the hepatic artery to retract away from the operative field. Finally, patients with a large left hepatic lobe may pose special problems. The epigastric trocar must be placed in an appropriate location so that instruments enter the operative field from an angle that does not lacerate the left liver lobe, as occurred in one of our cases. If needed, an extra 5-mm port can be placed for insertion of a blunt probe to retract the left hepatic lobe during the operation.

CONVERSION TO OPEN OPERATION

Surgeons performing laparoscopic cholecystectomy should not hesitate to convert to a traditional open cholecystectomy if the anatomy is unclear or if complications arise (Table 3). It is better to "open one too many than to open one too few." Some complications requiring laparotomy are obvious, such as massive hemorrhage, bowel perforation, or major injury to the bile duct. An additional indication for open laparotomy is anatomy that, because of inflammation, adhesions, or

anomalies, cannot be delineated. Fistulas between the biliary system and bowel are not common [3], but generally require laparotomy for optimal management. Finally, the demonstration of potentially resectable carcinoma dictates open exploration.

ACUTE CHOLECYSTITIS

Acute cholecystitis may complicate the performance of laparoscopic cholecystectomy. Intervention during the early phase reveals an inflamed, thick-walled, tensely distended organ. To gain purchase for the grasping forceps, it may be necessary to decompress the gallbladder by aspirating it with a large-gauge needle. As long as the inflammation is limited to the gallbladder, laparoscopic cholecystectomy is usually technically feasible. However, if inflammation extends to the porta hepatis, great care must be taken in proceeding with the operation. The normally thin, minimally adherent tissue that invests the cystic duct and artery is markedly thickened and edematous and may not readily separate from these structures with the usual blunt dissection techniques. The duct wall may also be edematous, thus making its external diameter similar to the gallbladder neck and common bile duct. If the anatomy is unclear, a cholangiogram must be performed before clipping or dividing tissue. When acute inflammation has been present for several days or weeks before operation, the pericholecystic tissue planes may be obliterated by thick, "woody" tissue that is impossible to dissect bluntly. The surgeon may therefore need to convert to open cholecystectomy if laparoscopic surgery is initiated during this subacute phase.

The ability to perform laparoscopic cholecystectomy should not influence the management of patients with acute cholecystitis [32]. Antibiotics and bowel rest are initiated on admission to the hospital, and operation undertaken within 24 to 48 hours. There is no harm in inserting the laparoscope and assessing the right upper quadrant. The subcostal working ports are placed, and the initial dissection performed. If the anatomy is obliterated, a laparotomy is performed; if laparoscopic dissection is possible, the operation is completed. The decision to convert to an open operation is a matter of

Table 3. Reasons to convert to open cholecystectomy

Known or suspected injury to major blood vessel, viscus, or bile duct

Unclear anatomy

Unexpected pathology not amenable to laparoscopic management

Common bile duct stone that cannot be removed laparoscopically with
  little chance of subsequent endoscopic extraction (Billroth II
  anastomosis, duodenal diverticulum, previously failed ERCP)

judgment, based on the existing anatomy and the surgeon's experience. Several authors have reported performing laparoscopic cholecystectomy in the face of acute inflammation [33–35]. Despite a greater incidence of conversion to open surgery, the procedure may be completed safely in most patients.

INTRAOPERATIVE GALLBLADDER PERFORATION

Perforation of the gallbladder with bile or stone leakage can be a distressing problem, but should not necessarily require conversion to an open cholecystectomy. Perforation may occur secondary to traction applied by the grasping forceps or because of thermal injury during removal of the gallbladder from its bed. Almost one third of our patients had some intraoperative spillage of bile or stones. Patients with a bile leak did not experience an increased incidence of infection, or prolongation of hospitalization, or postoperative disability [36]. The only difference between those with and without bile leakage was that the operating time for patients with a gallbladder perforation was approximately 10 minutes longer, presumably because of the time spent cleaning up the operative field. When perforation does occur, the bile should be aspirated completely and irrigation used liberally. The stones should be retrieved and removed, if at all possible. Escaped stones composed primarily of cholesterol pose little threat of infection. However, pigment stones frequently harbor viable bacteria and may lead to infectious complications if allowed to remain in the peritoneal cavity [37].

POSTOPERATIVE CARE

Patients may be observed in the hospital or discharged later the same day following laparoscopic cholecystectomy. We routinely keep patients overnight to monitor for immediate complications. It seems reasonable to perform this operation on an outpatient basis for responsible individuals who live near the hospital with another person and for those without evidence of acute cholecystitis, urinary retention, or persistent nausea. Orders are written for antiemetics and analgesics as needed. The patient is allowed clear liquids in the immediate postoperative period and advanced to a regular diet as tolerated. Nausea and shoulder pain due to diaphragmatic irritation may occur in the early postoperative period. No activity restrictions are placed on the patient, as functional status depends entirely on the degree of abdominal tenderness, which usually subsides by the 2nd or 3rd postoperative day. The patient may return to work as soon as the abdominal discomfort is tolerable, but is encouraged to do so within 1 week. We routinely evaluate the patients in the office 1 month after the operation, or sooner should they have cause for concern.

RESULTS OF LAPAROSCOPIC CHOLECYSTECTOMY

AUTHOR'S PERSONAL SERIES

Between November 1989 and January 1993, more than 2000 laparoscopic cholecystectomies were performed at Washington University's affiliated hospitals, and I was personally involved with more than 650 of them. Our early results have been previously reported [6]. There has been no mortality within 30 days of surgery; major morbidity has occurred in 1.6% of patients, and minor morbidity in 2.1% of patients (Table 4). The postoperative course in most patients has been uneventful, with 90% of patients being discharged from the hospital within 24 hours of surgery and only 11% requiring parenteral narcotics after leaving the recovery room. Similarly, the duration of disability is minimal; the average

Table 4. Compiled results of laparoscopic cholecystectomy

Study	Patients, n	Converted,* %	Mortality, %	Major complications, %	Bile duct injury, %
The Southern Surgeons Club [7]	1518	4.7	0.07	1.5	0.5
Cuschieri et al. [10]	1236	3.6	0	1.6	0.3
Soper et al. [6]	618	2.9	0	1.6	0.2
Spaw et al. [5]	500	1.8	0	1	0
Wolfe et al. [12]	381	3	0.9	3.4	0
Bailey et al. [8]	375	5	0.3	0.6	0.3
Graves et al. [13]	304	6.9	0	0.7	0.3
Peters et al. [11]	283	2.8	0	2.1	0.4
Schirmer et al. [9]	152	8.5	0	4	0.7

*Converted to open laparotomy.

postoperative interval to return to full activity is 8 days. These results compare favorably with those of traditional open cholecystectomy, after which hospitalization for 3 to 5 days and return to work 1 month after surgery are standard [15].

OTHER REPORTED SERIES

Our data reflect those of most series of laparoscopic cholecystectomies reported to date (Table 4). Mortality is rare after this procedure, usually being attributed to unrelated events. However, death due to bile duct or intestinal injury has been reported [12]. The rate of conversion from laparoscopy to an open operation ranges from 1.8% to 8.5% and is generally greater early in the surgeon's experience with the procedure. Major complications, such as bile duct injury, are relatively rare in these series of cases performed by surgeons who have been performing laparoscopic cholecystectomy since its description. Complications of laparoscopic cholecystectomy are detailed in Chapter 8.

RESULTS OF NATIONAL INSTITUTES OF HEALTH CONSENSUS DEVELOPMENT CONFERENCE

Because of the prevalence of gallstones in the US population, the cost borne by the health system for this disease, and the rapid employment of laparoscopic cholecystectomy, the National Institute of Diabetes and Digestive and Kidney Diseases held a Consensus Development Conference entitled "Gallstones and Laparoscopic Cholecystectomy" September 14–16, 1992 [38]. The purpose of the conference was to evaluate and compare the data available on laparoscopic cholecystectomy versus traditional surgical and nonsurgical treatments of gallstones. The consensus panel, composed of surgeons, endoscopists, hepatologists, gastroenterologists, radiologists, epidemiologists, and representatives of the general public, considered the scientific evidence presented by several experts in relevant fields. The panel's conclusions included the following:

1) Most asymptomatic patients with cholelithiasis should not be treated; however, once symptoms develop, treatment should be initiated promptly.

2) Laparoscopic cholecystectomy has become the treatment of choice for many patients, because it offers decreased pain and disability and potential substantial costs savings; however, the outcome of laparoscopic cholecystectomy is greatly influenced by the surgeon's training, experience, skill, and judgment.

3) Open cholecystectomy is a safe and effective operation for symptomatic gallstone disease and remains the standard against which new treatments should be judged; conversion from laparoscopic to open cholecystectomy should not be considered a complication of laparoscopic cholecystectomy.

4) Nonresective therapies for gallstones have limited clinical applicability and require further development.

5) Management of common bile duct stones depends on the local availability of technical expertise, and the valid treatment options include preoperative, intraoperative, or postoperative identification and removal of stones.

6) Future research should focus on refining the techniques of laparoscopic cholecystectomy and laparoscopic common bile duct exploration to maximize safety and cost effectiveness.

7) Strict guidelines for training in laparoscopic surgery and determination of competence and monitoring of quality should be developed and implemented promptly.

8) Safe, noninvasive, cost-effective strategies to prevent gallstones should be actively sought.

CONCLUSIONS

Laparoscopic management of gallstones has rapidly become the new gold standard therapy in the United States and throughout the world. Most cases of symptomatic gallstones can be treated laparoscopically. Occasionally, anatomic or physiologic considerations will preclude the laparoscopic approach, and conversion to an open operation reflects sound surgical judgment and should not be considered a complication.

REFERENCES

Papers of particular interest, published within the period of review, have been highlighted as:
• Of special interest
•• Of outstanding interest

1. Mühe E: Die Erste Cholecystektomie Durch Das Laparoskop. *Langenbecks Arch Chir* 1986, 369:804–.

2. DuBois F, Icard P, Berthelot G, Levard H: Coelioscopic Cholecystectomy: Preliminary Report of 36 Cases. *Ann Surg* 1990, 211:60–62.

3. Perissat J, Collet D, Belliard R: Gallstones: Laparoscopic Treatment: Cholecystectomy, Cholecystostomy, and Lithotripsy. *Surg Endosc* 1990, 4:1–5.

4. Reddick EJ, Olsen DO: Laparoscopic Laser Cholecystectomy: A Comparison with Mini-Lap Cholecystectomy. *Surg Endosc* 1989, 3:131–133.

5. Spaw AT, Reddick EJ, Olsen DO: Laparoscopic Laser Cholecystectomy: Analysis of 500 Procedures. *Surg Laparosc Endosc* 1991, 1:2–7.

6. Soper NJ, Stockmann PT, Dunnegan DL, Ashley SW: Laparoscopic Cholecystectomy: The New "Gold Standard"? *Arch Surg* 1992, 127:917–921.

7.•• The Southern Surgeons Club: A Prospective Analysis of 1518 Laparoscopic Cholecystectomies. *N Engl J Med* 1991, 324:1073–1078.

Dr. William Meyers organizes a group of surgeons in the US Southeast to publish the first large multi-institutional series of laparoscopic cholecystectomies in a widely read medical journal.

8. Bailey RW, Zucker KA, Flowers JL, *et al.*: Laparoscopic Cholecystectomy: Experience with 375 Consecutive Patients. *Ann Surg* 1991, 214:531–540.

9. Schirmer BD, Edge SB, Dix J, *et al.*: Laparoscopic Cholecystectomy: Treatment of Choice for Symptomatic Cholelithiasis. *Ann Surg* 1991, 213:665–676.

10. Cuschieri A, DuBois F, Mouiel J, *et al.*: The European Experience with Laparoscopic Cholecystectomy. *Am J Surg* 1991, 161:385–387.

11. Peters JH, Gibbons GD, Innes JT, *et al.*: Complications of Laparoscopic Cholecystectomy. *Surgery* 1991, 110:769–778.

12. Wolfe BM, Gardiner BN, Leary BF, Frey CF: Endoscopic Cholecystectomy: An Analysis of Complications. *Arch Surg* 1991, 126:1192–1196.

13. Graves HA, Ballinger JF, Anderson WJ: Appraisal of Laparoscopic Cholecystectomy. *Ann Surg* 1991, 213:655–662.

14.• Soper NJ: Laparoscopic Cholecystectomy. *Curr Probl Surg* 1991, 28:585–655.

The author gives an extensive overview of laparoscopic cholecystectomy, including indications and contraindications, instrumentation, detailed technique, and early results.

15. Soper NJ, Barteau JA, Clayman RV, *et al.*: Laparoscopic vs. Standard Open Cholecystectomy: Comparison of Early Results. *Surg Gynecol Obstet* 1992, 174:114–118.

16.•• Barkun JS, Barkun AN, Sampalis JS, *et al.*: Randomized Controlled Trial of Laparoscopic vs. Mini-Cholecystectomy. *Lancet* 1992, 340:1116–1119.

The Montreal group publishes the first (and perhaps the only) prospective randomized trial of laparoscopic versus open cholecystectomy, demonstrating a clear improvement in early outcome following laparoscopic cholecystectomy.

17. Anderson ER, Hunter JG: Laparoscopic Cholecystectomy Is Less Expensive than Open Cholecystectomy. *Surg Laparosc Endosc* 1991, 1:82–84.

18. Fisher KS, Reddick EJ, Olsen DO: Laparoscopic Cholecystectomy: Cost Analysis. *Surg Laparosc Endosc* 1991, 1:77–81.

19. Gracie WA, Ransohoff DF: The Natural History of Silent Gallstones: The Innocent Gallstone Is not a Myth. *N Engl J Med* 1982, 307:798–800.

20. Ransohoff DF, Gracie WA, Wolfenson LB, Neuhauser D: Prophylactic Cholecystectomy or Expectant Management for Silent Gallstones: A Decision Analysis to Assess Survival. *Ann Intern Med* 1983, 99:199–204.

21. Soper NJ, Hunter J, Petrie RH: Laparoscopic Cholecystectomy in Pregnancy. *Surg Endosc* 1992, 6:115–117.

22. Spoelting RK, Miller RD: Monitoring. In *Basics of Anesthesia*. New York: Churchill Livingstone; 1989:211–227.

23. Gravenstein JS, Paulus PA, Hayes TJ: Carbon Dioxide and Monitoring. In *Capnography in Clinical Practice*. Boston: Butterworth; 1989: 3–10.

24. Kitano S, Tomikawa M, Iso Y, *et al.*: A Safe and Simple Method to Maintain a Clear Field of Vision During Laparoscopic Cholecystectomy. *Surg Endosc* 1991, 6:197–198.

25. Hashimoto D, Nayeem SA, Kajiwara S, Hoshino T: Laparoscopic Cholecystectomy: An Approach Without Pneumoperitoneum. *Surg Endosc* 1993, 7:54–56.

26. Banting S, Shimi S, Velpen GV, Cuschieri A: Abdominal Wall Lift: Low Pressure Pneumoperitoneum Laparoscopic Surgery. *Surg Endosc* 1993, 7:57–59.

27.• Fitzgerald SD, Andrus CH, Baudendistel LJ, *et al.*: Hypercarbia During Carbon Dioxide Pneumoperitoneum. *Am J Surg* 1992, 163:186–190.

The authors demonstrate that hypercarbia with acidosis may develop during laparoscopic cholecystectomy performed with a carbon dioxide pneumoperitoneum. This was most likely to occur with high-risk patients and highlighted the need for alternatives to the standard carbon dioxide pneumoperitoneum.

28. Leighton TA, Bongard FS, Liu SY, *et al.*: Comparative Cardiopulmonary Effects of Helium and Carbon Dioxide Pneumoperitoneum. *Surg Forum* 1991, 42:485–487.

29. Graff TD, Arbgast NR, Phillips OC, *et al.*: Gas Embolism. A Comparative Study of Air and Carbon Dioxide as Embolic Agents in the Systemic Venous System. *Am J Obstet Gynecol* 1959, 78:259–265.

30. Fitzgibbons RJ Jr, Schmid S, Santoscoy R, *et al.*: Open Laparoscopy for Laparoscopic Cholecystectomy. *Surg Laparosc Endosc* 1991, 1:216–222.

31. Remine WH: Biliary-Enteric Fistulas: Natural History and Management. *Adv Surg* 1973, 7:69–75.

32. Hermann RE: Surgery for Acute and Chronic Cholecystitis. *Surg Clin North Am* 1990, 70(6):1263–1275.

33. Cooperman AM: Laparoscopic Cholecystectomy for Severe Acute, Embedded, and Gangrenous Cholecystitis. *J Laparosc Endosc Surg* 1990, 1:37–40.

34. Reddick EJ, Olsen D, Spaw A, *et al.*: Safe Performance of Difficult Laparoscopic Cholecystectomies. *Am J Surg* 1991, 161:377–381.

35. Unger SW, Edelman DS, Scott JS, Unger HM: Laparoscopic Treatment of Acute Cholecystitis. *Surg Laparosc Endosc* 1991, 1:14–16.

36. Soper NJ, Dunnegan DL: Does Intraoperative Gallbladder Perforation Influence the Early Outcome of Laparoscopic Cholecystectomy? *Surg Laparosc Endosc* 1991, 1:156–161.

37. Stuart L, Smith AL, Pellegrini CA, *et al.*: Pigment Gallstones Form as a Component of Bacterial Microcolonies and Pigment Solids. *Ann Surg* 1987, 206:242–249.

38. National Institutes of Health Consensus Development Conference Statement on Gallstones and Laparoscopic Cholecystectomy. *Am J Surg* 1993, 165:390–398.

Chapter 6

Laparoscopic Cholangiography

John G. Hunter

Laparoscopic surgery has offered us the opportunity to reexamine our approaches to many standard surgically treated disease processes. This examination has been extremely fertile. We have relearned many lessons from surgical history and successfully challenged much unsubstantiated surgical dogma. In this "postmodern" era of minimally invasive surgery, reexamining the role of cholangiography performed in conjunction with laparoscopic cholecystectomy is appropriate.

One hundred years ago, Ludwig Courvosier [1] of Basel, Switzerland reported the performance of choledochotomy to remove a bile duct stone. For the next 40 years, surgeons relied on their eyes and fingers to determine who needed choledochotomy and common bile duct exploration. The clinical findings of jaundice, cholangitis, bile duct dilatation, and a palpable stone indicated the need for choledochotomy. In 1932, Mirizzi [2] added one more absolute indication to the list, a positive intraoperative cholangiogram. Nearly 30 years passed before surgeons understood the value of operative cholangiography. The evidence of its value was reported in several papers dating from the late 1950s to the 1980s that showed a dramatic decrease in unnecessary bile duct exploration after operative cholangiography [3–5]. Although no one discounted the value of operative cholangiography, in the late 1980s the pendulum began to swing back, as much data were collected that demonstrated that noninvasive tests and clinical observations could reduce the number of unnecessary cholangiograms performed [6–8]. Thus, as laparoscopic cholecystectomy entered the arena, surgical sentiment was swinging toward accepting a policy of selective cholangiography. Because of perceived difficulty in performing laparoscopic cholangiography, this shift was good news. However, as data on the overuse of preoperative endoscopic retrograde cholangiopancreatography and unrecognized bile duct transections became available, the tide began swinging back toward routine operative cholangiography. The arguments for both approaches are presented later in this chapter. Even the strongest advocates of selective cholangiography agree that surgeons performing laparoscopic cholecystectomy should also be able to perform cholangiography.

TECHNIQUE OF LAPAROSCOPIC CHOLANGIOGRAPHY

ESTABLISHING ACCESS TO THE BILIARY SYSTEM

When laser laparoscopic cholecystectomy was developed, some surgeons performed cholecystocholangiography to delineate biliary anatomy [9]. This technique was used because it was considered easier than cystic duct cholangiography. The shortcomings of cholecystocholangiography are several: In 15% to 20% of all cases, the cystic duct or gallbladder infundibulum is occluded with a stone or edema. Judging the amount of contrast required to inject to adequately but not excessively opacify the common bile duct is difficult. Contrast in the gallbladder may obscure visualization of the common bile duct. Last, if cholecystocholangiography is performed before dissection of the cystic duct, the cystic and common bile ducts can still be confused during subsequent dissection. One circumstance in which cholecystocholangiography may be helpful is when preliminary dissection reveals a duct that could be either cystic or common. If the surgeon puts a clip next to the dissected duct and performs a cholecystocholangiogram through the infundibulum of the gallbladder, the true nature of the duct will be revealed.

Cystic duct cholangiography long ago gained popularity during open cholecystectomy for the reasons mentioned above. Before laparoscopic cholecystectomy had become widespread, the techniques of cystic duct cholangiography were described [10]. Initially, access to the cystic duct was gained through the lateral-most trocar, after the grasper on the fundus of the gallbladder was removed. Soon surgeons realized that maintaining cephalic retraction on the fundus would aid in the performance of cholangiography, so the trocar in the midclavicular line was used. The initial placement of this trocar was generally too low and too medial, which caused the surgeon to try to insert the catheter at right

angles to the cystic duct. With time, the ideal trocar position for performance of cholangiography became apparent: immediately beneath the right costal margin at the anterior axillary line [11]. This placement allows alignment of the cystic duct with the trocar shaft and easier cannulation of the cystic duct. With the trocar high and wide, cystic duct access is gained using a microscissor by making a nick at the junction of the cystic duct and gallbladder infundibulum (after a clip has been placed across the gallbladder infundibulum). This nick should involve no more than one third of the circumference of the cystic duct, and it should be placed on the inferior aspect of the cystic duct. If the nick is placed anteriorly or posteriorly, attempts at catheter placement will result only in rolling the cystic duct. Similarly, a greater than 50% transection of the cystic duct risks its accidental division and may make catheter placement extremely difficult. The catheter is then loaded into a specialized cholangiography clamp (Fig. 1). This clamp has a central channel for passage of the catheter and two wings to clamp down on the cystic duct. The only drawback to this system is that the clamp needs to be supported at all times. If the clamp is released, the weight of the trocar and clamp handle will exert sufficient torque on the cystic duct to pull the catheter out much of the time.

Because this clamp was in short supply, a method of percutaneous cholangiography was developed [12]. With this system, a long thin-walled needle, generally 14 or 16 gauge, is placed directly through the abdominal wall, close to the subcostal port. The needle guide is brought close to the cystic ductotomy, and a 4F or 5F catheter is passed through the guide into the cystic duct. A grasper through the mid-subcostal port is used to maintain traction on the gallbladder infundibulum, while a clipper is placed through the epigastric port and closed snugly down around the catheter to prevent its displacement. A good system of ensuring adequate but not excessive clip pressure is for the surgeon to inject saline through the catheter with the left hand while tightening down a clip held in the right hand. As soon as the flow in the catheter stops, release of pressure with the right hand usually allows sufficient clip relaxation that flow in the system resumes, yet the catheter will not be dislodged easily. The advantages of this system are that the surgeon, because of using a long extension tube, can be far from the radiation source behind a lead screen and that the percutaneous access site can be chosen after the cystic duct anatomy has been defined, thereby ensuring optimal placement for coaxial alignment of the catheter and cystic duct. The disadvantage of percutaneous cholangiography is that another, albeit small, hole is made in the abdominal wall, and two-handed coordination is frequently necessary to guide the catheter into the cystic duct.

CATHETERS

During open cholecystectomy, access to the cystic duct is obtained with short, soft catheters, usually placed using a Debakey forceps. Because of the greater distance between the surgeon and the cystic duct during laparoscopic cholecystectomy, a stiffer catheter was necessary. One of the original cholangiography catheters, a Taut catheter (Taut, Genera, IL), was used because it had a fine-pointed conical tip that allowed easy cannulation. The disadvantage of this catheter was that the cone-shaped tip was effectively a barb that created difficulty in catheter extraction. Although some surgeons still use the original Taut catheter, the most popular cholangiographic catheter is a ureteral catheter. The whistle-tipped ureteral catheter has the advantage of a tapered tip and markings, so the surgeon knows how far into the duct the catheter tip is located. The disadvantage of the whistle-tipped catheter is that most have many side holes, which means that the catheter has to be at least 3 cm into the cystic duct to make sure all the side holes are covered. More recently, end-hole-only ureteral catheters have gained popularity, because the problem with side holes is eliminated and guide wires may be passed through them easily. A major disadvantage of ureteral catheters is that they tend to be somewhat thick walled. The 5F catheter that allows the passage of a 0.089-cm (0.035 inches) guide wire does not have a tapered tip. Thinner-walled catheters with equivalent rigidity have been manufactured for angiographic and endoscopic retrograde cholangiopancreatography use. The 5F catheter of this type is tapered, yet will accommodate a 0.089-cm guide wire. In my estimation, this type is the ideal cholangiographic catheter.

Yet another type of cholangiocatheter has been designed that requires neither a specialized clamp nor a clip to hold it in place. These are balloon catheters; the cholangiocatheter is placed in the cystic duct, and a balloon is inflated to hold the catheter in position. Although these catheters may provide some technical advantages, they are much less versatile. Specifically, they cannot be used with a short cystic duct, as the balloon will slip into the common bile duct and obstruct the flow of contrast into the proximal biliary system. Also, the balloon may be mistaken for a stone. The other shortcoming of this system is its expense.

Occasionally, no catheter can be threaded into the common bile duct. This situation occurs usually because of a poor cannulation angle, but it may reflect the presence of spiral valves in the cystic duct or a cystic duct stone. In response to this problem, the surgeon should first "milk back" the cystic duct from the common duct junction to the cystic ductotomy to make sure that there are no cystic duct stones. Then, if a long cystic duct is present, a ductotomy may be made closer to the common bile duct. Alternatively, a hydrophilic guide wire may be passed through the catheter into the common bile duct, and the cholangiocatheter may then be passed over the guide wire. The hydrophilic coating, polyethylene oxide, makes this type of guide wire particularly slippery when wet (slime wire) and allows more successful passage through the narrow, tortuous cystic duct. Once the guide wire has been removed, the catheter is full of air. Attempts to aspirate the air back are usually unsuccessful, and the patient must be placed in steep Trendelenburg position and the common bile duct flushed with 50 mL of normal saline, thereby forcing the air out of the system into the duodenum. The patient is returned to the supine position, and a fluoroscopic cholangiogram is obtained.

IMAGING

One of the primary contributions of laparoscopic cholecystectomy to the field of biliary surgery was the ability to recognize the virtues of fluoroscopic cholangiography. Before laparoscopic cholecystectomy, most surgeons relied on static images of the bile duct to look for

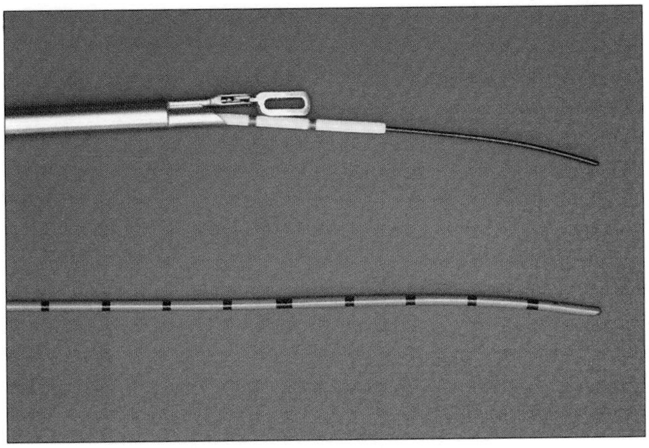

Figure 1. Inexpensive access to the cystic duct may be gained with ureteral catheters and a specialized clamp. Hydrophilic guide wires slip through the tight spinal valves, and are extremely useful in difficult cannulations.

common bile duct stones. This examination generally takes 15 to 20 minutes, from the time the cholangiocatheter enters the cystic duct to the time the roentgenographic images are back on the light board. After that wait, 20% of the films are found to be inadequate because they were overexposed, underexposed, or misaligned, or the contrast did not fill the entire biliary system and duodenum. Under these circumstances another 20 minutes is needed to reshoot the roentgenogram. When the static cholangiogram shows a filling defect that the surgeon thought represented a stone, the surgeon was wrong 20% of the time. Therefore, 20% of common bile duct explorations were performed unnecessarily [6]. With laparoscopic cholecystectomy, the difficulties in obtaining an adequate static cholangiogram are compounded by the amount of instrumentation that could obscure the extrahepatic biliary system, the air-water interface at the hepatic plate, and the frequent inability to visualize the intrahepatic ducts with the patient in the reverse Trendelenburg position. To summarize, the shortcomings of static cholangiography are length of procedure, frequently inadequate cholangiograms, and a high rate of false-positive cholangiograms, erroneously predicting the presence of choledocholithiasis.

Cholangiography was performed exclusively by surgeons after its description by Mirizzi, until it also became the domain of radiologists (transhepatic cholangiography) and gastroenterologists (retrograde cholangiography) in the 1970s. When these individuals perform cholangiography, they rely on fluoroscopy to guide the examination and determine which images best represent biliary anatomy and pathology. These images are made into standard roentgenographic "spot films." Such an ideal system has been difficult to duplicate in the operating room because it requires the ability to perform fluoroscopy and the intermittent placement of an emulsion film in the line of the roentgen ray beam. Expensive radiolucent operating tables, synchronized with the C-arm, would be necessary to allow this kind of performance.

Image-intensifier cholangiography has served as a poor alternative to static films for some time. The disadvantage of this type of cholangiography is in image processing and resolution. The only good way to record the image for review is with videotape, which is cumbersome to store in the permanent medical record. Static films made from these videotapes are clearly inferior in resolution to plain emulsion roentgenograms.

Adequate film quality has been achieved by the use of computer-driven, digitally enhanced fluoroscopy. With this technology, a standard fluoroscopic C-arm is connected to a computer that digitizes the information obtained. The image can be stored on computer disk for review and further processing. In addition, if the computer software is developed correctly, the quality of the cholangiogram can be enhanced to approximate the resolution attainable with emulsion film (Fig. 2). As well, digital processing allows the magnification of certain portions of the field to obtain fine detail. For the medical record and for examination by radiologists, the image can be recorded on videotape or exported to a matrix or laser printer to produce an image quality rivaling static films.

The advantages of fluoroscopic cholangiography are many. The first is that the time necessary to perform cholangiography can be cut in half. The time necessary to position the C-arm is the same as that for taking a plain roentgenogram from an overhead tube. As soon as the field is located, the contrast is injected, and the

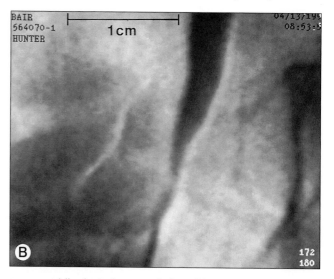

Figure 2. A, Digital operative cholangiogram demonstrating normal anatomy. **B,** Enlargement of the finally tapered distal common bile duct gives resolution of features 1 mm and larger.

plain roentgenogram from an overhead tube. As soon as the field is located, the contrast is injected, and the cholangiogram is reviewed as it is performed. This procedure ensures a complete cholangiogram in 100% of cases; reduces the waiting period for cholangiographic results, during which common bile duct injuries may occur; and as discussed below reduces the incidence of false-positive cholangiograms. A major limitation of fluoroscopic cholangiography is that the surgeon must be near the operating table. If the cholangioclamp system is used, the surgeon generally needs to be dressed in a lead apron or positioned behind a lead screen immediately adjacent to the operating field. If the percutaneous system is used, long extension tubing may allow the surgeon to move a little farther from the radiation source but not enough to be unshielded. If the surgeon moves six feet from the table side, the exposure risk is minimal [13]. Particularly vulnerable are the surgeon's head and eyes, which are difficult to shield with lead. Leaded glasses should be worn for eye protection if the surgeon stands at tableside.

TECHNIQUE OF FLUOROSCOPIC CHOLANGIOGRAPHY

For the majority of cholangiograms, a guide wire is unnecessary. If two surgeons are performing laparoscopic cholecystectomy, the cholangiogram is generally performed by the assistant surgeon on the patient's right. As mentioned earlier, success requires that the transcutaneous access site be high and lateral (Fig. 3). Through this high, lateral port the cystic duct is incised with a pair of microscissors. The surgeon on the patient's left (primary surgeon) holds tension on the gallbladder neck and aligns the cystic duct, as viewed on the video monitor, parallel to the microscissors. Usually the cystic duct must be pushed back toward the liver slightly to produce an angle between the cystic duct and scissors, in the axial plane, of approximately 30°. A cystic ductotomy is clearly impossible to make if scissors and duct are completely parallel. A nick large enough to allow insertion of a 5F catheter is made, the microscissors are removed, and the saline-flushed cholangiography catheter is brought into the abdomen with 1 cm of catheter exposed beyond the tip of the clamp. With the cystic duct held in the same orientation as for creation of the ductotomy, the surgeon should be able to advance the catheter into the cystic duct unless impeded by cystic duct stones or valves of Heister. Once all side holes are in the duct, the catheter is secured and irrigated. The technique of guide-wire cholangiography was described above.

If percutaneous access is used, the skin puncture site should be very close to the trocar used for making the cystic ductotomy. This technique is easier for a single surgeon, as it can be performed from the left side of the table, using the left hand to guide the catheter through the skin and the right hand to advance the catheter into the cystic duct using a grasper. The grasper is then exchanged for a clipper, and saline is injected as the clip is squeezed together (see above).

The two most frequent difficulties in fluoroscopic cholangiography are differentiating stones from air bubbles and obtaining filling of the entire biliary system. Several techniques may be used to differentiate bubbles from stones. One technique is to place the patient in Trendelenburg position and flush the bubbles into the duodenum. Alternatively, if the patient is in a reverse Trendelenburg position, the air bubbles will float into the liver, where they frequently break into smaller bubbles in the segmental hepatic ducts. Clearly, stones will not move as such. Gravity is useful in distinguishing stones from air bubbles, as stones usually sink and air bubbles rise. If the common duct is capacious and the catheter is in the common bile duct, aspirating the air bubble back into the cholangiography catheter is occasionally possible. Using these techniques, only once have we had the surgeon and the radiologist, after

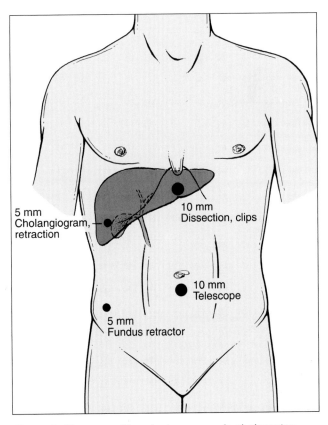

Figure 3. Trocar positions for laparoscopic cholecystectomy. Note the high, lateral position of the subcostal port.

reviewing the cholangiogram, disagree on whether the filling defect was a stone or an air bubble.

With the patient in reverse Trendelenburg position, the contrast flows preferentially into the distal bile duct and duodenum. Filling of the intrahepatic ducts can always be obtained using one of three maneuvers. A rapid bolus infusion of contrast frequently flows retrograde into the liver. If this maneuver fails, the patient is placed in the supine or Trendelenburg position to obtain filling of the liver. As a last resort, morphine can be administered to put the sphincter of Oddi into spasm. Nonfilling of the duodenum may be obviated by the use of intravenous glucagon. Generally, 1 mg of glucagon produces complete sphincter relaxation within one circulation time (less than one minute), and this effect lasts for 10 to 15 minutes. If the duodenum still does not fill after glucagon administration, a small stone or ampullary stricture (benign or malignant) is suspected. Last, the cholangiogram occasionally reveals the pancreatic duct starting to fill. Real-time monitoring of cholangiography can help limit overfilling of the pancreatic duct and possibly reduce the incidence of postoperative pancreatitis.

RESULTS OF LAPAROSCOPIC CHOLANGIOGRAPHY

The most frequent reason for cholangiographic failure is failure to access the cystic duct. Two reasons stand out. The first, and most frequent, is inexperience. If a policy of extremely selective cholangiography is used, or if a surgeon infrequently performs laparoscopic cholecystectomy, the rate of success may be less than 50%. During our initial experience with laparoscopic cholangiography, cystic duct cannulation was successfully performed in 88 out of 99 attempts [14•]. Failure occurred most frequently in the first 20 cases and was attributed to a small cystic duct, tenacious valves of Heister, accidental cystic duct transection, or excessive cystic duct incision. With experience and the occasional use of guide wires, cholangiography can be successful in close to 100% of cases. In our first 100 laparoscopic cholecystectomies, laparoscopic cholangiography altered our operative plan in 10% of our patients [14•]. The finding of common bile duct stones led to bile duct exploration in three patients. In three patients we detected the common or segmental right hepatic ducts inserting into the cystic duct or low common hepatic duct. This finding increased our vigilance in positively identifying the cystic artery before clipping. A third finding of interest was excessive proximity of the dissection to the common bile duct. In one case, the presumed cystic duct proved to be the common bile duct; in another case, a clip on the cystic artery was compressing the wall of the common hepatic duct. In a third case, the direct insertion of the gallbladder into the common bile duct was

correctly identified and appropriately managed. With increased experience, we have found the variations of right hepatic duct anatomy more a curiosity than a concern. The knowledge of the distance between the cystic ductotomy and the common bile duct provided by cholangiography has been very helpful in accurately placing clips so as not to narrow a tented common bile duct. Currently, the most important and useful feature of routine cholangiography is identification of common bile duct stones, suspected and incidental, so that they can be removed concurrently and not require separate procedures and hospitalizations.

False-positive results occur in 1% to 3% of cases, but if a policy of transcystic bile duct exploration is used, a false-positive cholangiogram does not obligate the surgeon to perform choledochotomy and T-tube placement. Choledochoscopy or basket exploration through the cystic duct will reveal the error and allow a primary cystic duct closure. In our initial series of 100 laparoscopic cholecystectomies, one false-positive study resulted from an air bubble and a second resulted from papillary stenosis [15]. The latter diagnosis was revealed on choledochoscopy. A false-negative study has occurred only once in 350 cases (0.3%) to the best of our knowledge. In this patient, the initial cholangiogram showed two stones, only one of which was recovered at the time of bile duct exploration. The second stone was believed to have been flushed into the duodenum, as the completion cholangiogram did not show the stone. The patient passed the stone that evening. The error resulted from an excessively concentrated dye column. Full-strength contrast can be used with fluoroscopic cholangiography, but only if the contrast is injected slowly so that mixing with bile allows detection of small stones.

COMPLICATIONS

The most frequent complication of cholangiography has been perforation of the cystic duct. This complication occurs when an excessively stiff catheter is used or an excessively friable cystic duct is encountered. The perforation should be identified by visualization of the catheter tip in Calot's triangle or by extravasation of contrast on the cholangiogram. Under these circumstances, the surgeon may need to dissect the cystic duct down the common bile duct junction to obtain adequate closure below the level of perforation. In manipulating the common bile duct, we have had three perforations in 350 cases (0.8%). Two of these injuries were guide-wire perforations through friable cholangitic common bile ducts. In both patients, postoperative drainage of the gallbladder bed did not reveal bile leaks. The use of an extremely floppy-tipped guide wire has prevented further occurrence of this complication. In the third patient, a 5F whistle-tipped ureteral catheter penetrated the left wall of the common bile duct rather than turning the corner into the distal common bile duct. This perforation was repaired with a single interrupted suture and protected with a drain. There was no further leakage.

ROUTINE VERSUS SELECTIVE CHOLANGIOGRAPHY

The argument as to whether cholangiography during *open* cholecystectomy should be performed selectively or routinely was never settled, and it is no closer to being settled for laparoscopic cholecystectomy. Although an excellent case for routine operative cholangiography was advanced at the National Institutes of Health Consensus Panel [16•], equally eloquent arguments for selective use of cholangiography were advanced at the Southern Surgical Society Meeting in 1991 [17•]. No aspect of laparoscopic cholecystectomy has raised a more boisterous debate. Unfortunately, in most forums the debate has been like a comparison of apples and oranges. Most surgeons who advocate selective cholangiography discuss the shortcomings of routine static cholangiography. Advocates of routine cholangiography uniformly argue for fluoroscopic cholangiography. Some proponents of selective cholangiography have joined the routine cholangiography camp once given access to modern fluoroscopic equipment.

The most persuasive arguments for selective cholangiography are those that have documented the high expense of routine cholangiography (operating room time, radiologist fee, equipment fee) and the infrequent revelation of useful information. Some reports have stated that common bile duct stones and biliary misadventures are overlooked in less than 1% of cases in which cholangiograms are performed selectively [6–8]. The error of such an argument is that in lieu of cholangiography, the surgeon has no way of knowing whether late-appearing phenomena, such as a retained stone or a biliary stricture, have been overlooked. From our previous review, the incidence of important information that has been missed with selective cholangiography is closer to 5% [14•]. A third argument for selective cholangiography is the rate of false-positive studies (20%), obligating unnecessary duct exploration or endoscopic retrograde cholangiopancreatography. As previously discussed, fluoroscopic cholangiography largely eliminates these problems.

The arguments for routine cholangiography are that it prevents bile duct transection by illuminating confusing anatomy, that it detects unsuspected stones, that it reduces the number of unnecessary preoperative endoscopic retrograde cholangiopancreatographies, and that it allows training of residents and surgeons in the performance of cholangiography so that they will be adept at accessing the common bile duct for stone extraction.

Review of the literature reveals that cholangiography was rarely performed or interpreted correctly in cases where a bile duct transection occurred [18,19]. Possible conclusions from this data are that surgeons do not perform cholangiography in the difficult cases, inept surgeons do not perform cholangiography, or cholangiography does reduce severe biliary injury. Data from Cedars Sinai Medical Center suggest that cholangiography does not reduce small lateral injuries to the bile duct (because duct misidentification occurs before the cholangiogram), but that it reduces the severity of the injury and allows for identification of confusing anatomy before the duct is transected or excised (Phillips, Personal communication).

Routine fluoroscopic cholangiography allows the identification of all common bile duct stones larger than 1 mm. Although some surgeons argue that all clinically significant stones cause ductal dilatation or elevation of pancreatic or liver enzymes, the truth is that one half of common bile duct stones do not create ductal dilatation or enzyme elevation. The majority of these stones will probably be passed without clinically significant sequelae, but some of these overlooked stones will cause cholangitis, biliary obstruction, or pancreatitis, and there is no way to predict which stones will pass uneventfully. Thus the prudent course seems to be to attempt to identify all common bile duct stones at the time of cholecystectomy and leave only small stones, 2 mm or less, in normal common bile ducts. For surgeons who are comfortable and confident in their abilities to perform operative cholangiography, the frequency of unnecessary preoperative endoscopic retrograde cholangiopancreatography drops dramatically. No matter how high the clinical suspicion of choledocholithiasis, half of all retrograde cholangiograms do not show bile duct stones [20]. Before surgeons had developed confidence in their ability to perform operative cholangiography and bile duct stone extraction, the rate of unnecessary endoscopic retrograde cholangiopancreatography was as high as 85% [21]. Routine cholangiography not only detects unsuspected bile duct stones but allows the surgeon the opportunity to develop transcystic bile duct exploration techniques in easy cases and increase his skills to the point where he can handle large, impacted stones at the time of laparoscopic cholecystectomy.

In training institutions, routine cholangiography ensures that residents become as facile with cholangiography as with cystic duct dissection and gallbladder resection. A surgeon who is incapable of performing a laparoscopic cholangiogram is capable of performing only half of the job of the biliary surgeon. A biliary surgeon should be able to deal as effectively with common bile duct stones as he or she can with gallbladder stones.

ALTERNATIVES TO CHOLANGIOGRAPHY

Fluoroscopic cholangiography is safe, easily applied, and capable of revealing most biliary pathology. Intraoperative ultrasonography has been advocated for use in open cholecystectomy to evaluate the common bile duct [22]. The argument is that ultrasonography is more sensitive than cholangiography for detecting bile duct stones and can be performed without risking bile duct injury, misidentification of anatomy, contrast reaction, or radiation exposure. Radiation exposure is most important to avoid in pregnant patients. Initial reports on the use of ultrasonography in determining laparoscopic biliary anatomy show a promising future [23]. The current generation of surgeons is unlikely to be as comfortable with ultrasonography as with cholangiography, but the prospect of defining biliary anatomy before performing potentially damaging dissection is enticing.

Choledochoscopy could conceivably supplant cholangiography, but this possibility is less likely. Conceptually, after making a cystic ductotomy the surgeon could slip a choledochoscope no bigger than a cholangiocatheter into the common bile duct. The distal duct could be examined rapidly and the catheter turned up into the liver with an articulating mechanism to examine the intrahepatic radicals. Choledochoscopy has been shown to be more accurate than cholangiography in avoiding retained stones. Thus, with the development of appropriate technology and skills, the endoscope could replace fluoroscopy in a fashion similar to that in which upper endoscopy has largely replaced the upper gastrointestinal barium examination.

FUTURE OF CHOLANGIOGRAPHY

The future of cholangiography in association with laparoscopic cholecystectomy will be based largely on medical economics. Most surgical procedures are or will soon be subjected to outcomes analysis, in which the cost of the procedure and its morbidity is balanced against improvement in patient outcome. The cost of a single hepatic bifurcation bile duct transection, including medical and legal expenses, is clearly at least twice as high as the cost of purchasing a digital fluoroscopic unit. If fluoroscopic cholangiography is capable of preventing one of these injuries per machine sold, it is well worth the price of technology. As surgeons have become more proficient with laparoscopic cholecystectomy, the bile-duct injury rate has fallen. This improvement may partly result from increasing use of fluoroscopic cholangiography.

REFERENCES

Papers of particular interest, published within the period of review, have been highlighted as:
• Of special interest
•• Of outstanding interest

1. Courvosier LG: *Kasvistisch-statistische Beitrage zur Pathologie und Chirurgie de Gallenwege.* Leipzig: Few Vogel; 1890:57–58.

2. Mirizzi PL: *La Cholangiograffia Durante las Operacions de las via Biliare. Bol Trab Soc Cirug* (B. Aires) 1932, 16:1133–1161.

3. Hutchinson WB, Blake T: Operative Cholangiography. *Surgery* 1957, 41:605–612.

4. Hight D, Lindley JR, Hurtubuse F: Evaluation of Operative Cholangiography as a Guide to Common Duct Exploration. *Ann Surg* 1959, 150:1086–1091.

5. Doyle PJ, Ward-McQuaid JN, McEwen Smith A: The Value of Routine Preoperative Cholangiography—A Report of 4000 Cholecystectomies. *Br J Surg* 1982, 69:617–619.

6. Grogono JL, Woods WGA: Selective Use of Operative Cholangiography. *World J Surg* 1986, 10:1009–1013.

7. Gregg RO: The Case for Selective Cholangiography. *Am J Surg* 1988, 155:540–544.

8. Hauer-Jensen M, Karesen R, Nygaard K, *et al.*: Prospective Randomized Study of Routine Intraoperative Cholangiography During Open Cholecystectomy: Long-Term Follow-Up and Multivariate Analysis of Predictors of Choledocholithiasis. *Surgery* 1993, 113 (3):318–323.

9. Graber JN, Schultz LS, Pietrafitta JJ, Hickok DF: Complications of Laparoscopic Cholecystectomy. *Lasers Surg Med* 1992, 12:91–97.

10. Berci G, Sackier JM, Paz-Partlow M: Routine or Selected Intraoperative Cholangiography During Laparoscopic Cholecystectomy. *Am J Surg* 1991, 161:355–360.

11. Hunter JG, Soper NJ: Laparoscopic Management of Bile Duct Stones. *Surg Clin North Am* 1992, 72(5):1077–1097.

12. Petelin JB: Laparoscopic Approach to Common Duct Pathology. *Surg Laparosc Endosc* 1991, 1:33–41.

13. Early D: Radiation Hazard. In *Operative Biliary Radiology.*. Edited by Berci G, Hamlin JA. Baltimore: Williams & Wilkins, 1981; 27–36.

14. • Bruhn EW, Miller FJ, Hunter JG: Routine Fluoroscopic Cholangiography During Laparoscopic Cholecystectomy: An Argument. *Surg Endosc* 1991, 5:111–115.

Presents the information learned from 88 consecutive routine cholangiograms.

15. Goodman GR, Hunter JG: Results of Laparoscopic Cholecystectomy in a University Hospital. *Am J Surg* 1991, 162:576–579.

16. • Phillips EH: Routine Vs. Selective Cholangiography. *Am J Surg*, 1993, 165:505–507.

Presents a cogent argument for routine cholangiography.

17. • Lilemoe KD, Yeo CJ, Talamini MA, *et al.*: Selective Cholangiography: Current Role in Laparoscopic Cholecystectomy. *Ann Surg* 1992, 215(6):669–676.

The counterpoint, an argument for selective cholangiography.

18. Moosa AR, Easter DW, Van Sonnenberg E, *et al.*: Laparoscopic Injuries to the Bile Duct: A Cause for Concern. *Ann Surg* 1992, 215(3):203–208.

19. Davidoff AM, Pappas TN, Murray EA, *et al.*: Mechanisms of Major Biliary Injury During Laparoscopic Cholecystectomy. *Ann Surg* 1992, 215(3):196–202.

20. Gaisford WD: Endoscopic Retrograde Cholangiopancreatography in the Diagnosis of Jaundice. *Am J Surg* 1976, 132:699–702.

21. Southern Surgeons Club: A Prospective Analysis of 1518 Laparoscopic Cholecystectomies. *N Engl J Med* 1991, 324(16):1073–1078.

22. Jakimowicz JJ, Rutton H, Jurgens PJ, Carol EJ: Comparison of Operative Ultrasonography and Radiography in Screening of the Common Bile Duct for Calculi. *West J Surg* 1987, 11:628–634.

23. Stiegmann GV, McIntyre R: Laparoscopic Intracorporeal Ultrasound: A Rapid and Accurate Alternative to Cholangiography? *Surg Endosc* 1993, 7:124.

Chapter 7

Laparoscopic Choledocholithotomy

Joseph B. Petelin

Choledocholithiasis is present in approximately 10% of patients hospitalized for cholecystectomy. Definitive treatment of these patients includes not only cholecystectomy, but clearance of the entire ductal system. Clearance may be accomplished laparoscopically by techniques described in this chapter. Such intervention proves to be both cost effective and efficient in returning patients to their former lifestyles with the least financial or social disruption (Fig. 1).

Choledocholithotomy may involve the application of numerous technical maneuvers. They include glucagon administration, dilatation of the distal common bile duct, balloon catheter manipulation, basket manipulation with or without fluoroscopic guidance, and choledochoscopic manipulations [1••,2•,3•,4–7•,8•,9,10]. All these techniques are used on the assumption that intraoperative cholangiography has been performed, whether or not preoperative ductal evaluation (chemical, radiographic, or endoscopic) has been used to evaluate or treat the common duct pathology prior to that time.

This chapter explores the techniques and technology currently available for laparoscopic treatment of common duct pathology. However, even as this material is being published, new developments are occurring that may render some of these leading-edge concepts and technologies obsolete. Understanding that the field of telescopic surgery is undergoing heretofore inconceivable expansion and development, the reader is encouraged to entertain these ideas with the following in mind: what is state of the art today will most likely not be state of the art tomorrow.

PATIENT MANAGEMENT

Clinical situations may be divided into two main groups: those in which choledocholithiasis is suspected preoperatively and those in which it is discovered intraoperatively.

In the former case the clinician must decide whether to attempt ductal treatment—endoscopic retrograde cholangiography and extraction with or without sphincterotomy (ERC±S) before operating—or to proceed directly with laparoscopic cholecystectomy and laparoscopic common duct exploration (LCDE) [1••]. ERC±S has been shown to be successful in clearing the common duct in over 90% of cases [11••,12–14]. LCDE is equally successful in clearing the duct [2•,3•,15]. The choice of clearance method is based on the local availability of expert endoscopists capable of a high degree of success with ERC±S, the availability of laparoscopic and choledochoscopic equipment, the surgeon's own expertise in laparoscopic surgery, and the general condition of the patient [11••,16].

In the latter case the decision is much easier to make. The surgeon proceeds with LCDE, converts the case of "open" common duct exploration and choledocholithotomy, or leaves the stones in place for subsequent ERC±S [1••,7•]. Although any of these alternatives is acceptable, it would seem wise in most situations to attempt LCDE unless the patient's condition warrants termination of the anesthetic as soon as possible. If LCDE is unsuccessful or not attempted, the decision regarding conversion to "open" common duct exploration versus postoperative ERC±S will depend on the local availability of expert endoscopists. These considerations are graphically demonstrated in Figure 2.

EQUIPMENT

In addition to the basic set of equipment used to perform laparoscopic cholecystectomy, several other instruments are required to facilitate LCDE.

A standard 2-inch-long 14-gauge intravenous catheter is used to gain access to the peritoneal cavity for intraoperative cholangiography (Fig. 3). This device can be said to present a "fifth port," for introduction of the cholangiography catheter, and subsequently of balloon catheters and baskets [17].

Fogarty embolectomy catheters are often useful for LCDE. A standard vascular type of catheter is preferred because the "biliary" Fogarty catheter is not long enough. Most commonly a 4 French size proves ade-

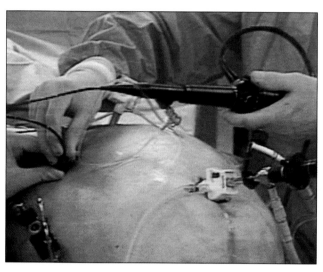

Figure 1. Laparoscopic common bile duct exploration.

Figure 2. Protocol for management of common bile duct stones.

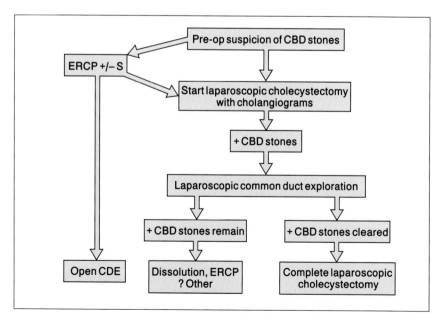

quate, but occasionally a 3 or 5 French model may be required.

Stone retrieval baskets are usually essential. They are available in straight and helical configurations, with either flat or round wires. The straight flat-wire basket, with its natural ability to expand the duct, presents large interstices for stones to enter (Fig. 4). The helical round-wire basket is used by surgeons who prefer a torquing maneuver to capture stones while trolling through the duct. Although I prefer a four-wire straight basket, all surgeons develop their own preferences. Models with variations of the distal tip offer a wide variety of baskets from which to choose.

A flexible choledochoscope is necessary to perform LCDE in over 60% of cases. The most versatile scopes feature a maximum outside diameter of 3 mm, tip deflection in at least one direction, a working channel of less than 1 mm, excellent optics, and camera-ready capability. The scope requires a light source with automatic intensity control (Fig. 5).

Although not essential, a second camera directly connected to the scope significantly improves the performance of LCDE. This second camera allows the surgeon to use both hands during manipulation because it is not necessary to hold the scope to the eye during the exploration. Projection of the choledochoscopic image onto the video monitor allows other members of the operative team to assist more effectively. Obviously, projection requires either an additional monitor or video-mixing equipment.

A video mixer is a useful adjunct in this setting. Using a picture-in-picture effect, the laparoscopic and choledochoscopic images may be viewed on the same monitor simultaneously (Fig. 6). This device reduces clutter in the surgery department by eliminating the need for an additional trolley and monitor. It also improves the efficiency of the operating surgeon who must look at only one monitor instead of two [15,18•].

Lithotripters may be used to disintegrate large stones in the ductal system. Electrohydraulic and laser models

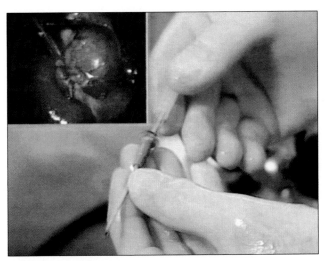

Figure 3. 14 gauge IV sheath used for percutaneous cholangiographic access.

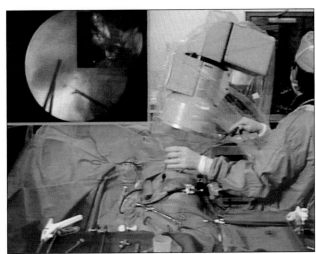

Figure 4. Four-wire straight flat basket.

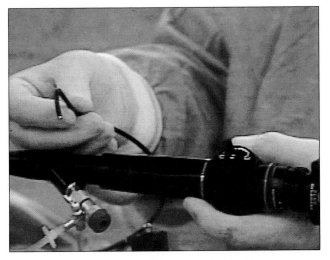

Figure 5. Flexible choledochoscope—the Olympus URF P2.

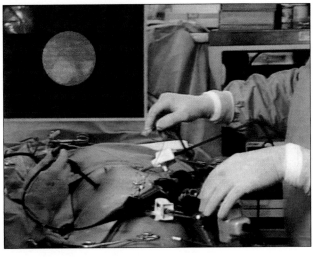

Figure 6. Picture in picture effect used to overlay two images on the same video monitor.

are available, but the latter are prohibitively expensive. The energy from either of these sources is delivered to the stone via wires or optical fibers introduced through the working channel of the choledochoscope. I find both types to be of limited value in most cases because of the multiplication of the debris produced within the duct. Nevertheless, in the infrequent case of distal impaction of a stone, they can be very useful [8•,11••].

Dilators are often used to enlarge the cystic duct to a 12 French diameter to allow easy introduction and manipulation of the choledochoscope. Graduated over-the-wire mechanical dilators have the advantage of being inexpensive and readily available in most urology departments. Pneumatic dilators are slightly more expensive but allow excellent control of the dilatation process (Fig. 7).

In cases requiring choledochotomy, a laparoscopic scalpel or scissors is necessary to open the duct [1••,19•]. Standard T-tubes suffice for subsequent drainage of the duct and are most easily introduced through a 10-mm portal using an 8-mm introduction sleeve [20,21]. Laparoscopic needle holders facilitate closure of the choledochotomy.

OPERATIVE TECHNIQUE

OVERVIEW

Many maneuvers compose the repertoire of the laparoscopic biliary tract surgeon who is clearing the common duct of stones. These maneuvers are discussed in the order in which I employ them, which is the order of increasing invasiveness.

This discussion assumes that laparoscopic access for cholecystectomy has already been established employing a four-port technique [22]. (Note: Many surgeons, including myself, usually use a three-port configuration for uncomplicated laparoscopic cholecystectomy, *ie*, one camera port and two working ports, eliminating the most lateral ports, which is used to retract the fundus of the gallbladder. When choledochoscopic LCDE is considered, the most lateral port is needed.) The "American" portal configuration is demonstrated in Figure 8.

The patient is usually placed in the supine position. For better visualization of the right upper quadrant of the abdomen, the operating table is placed in a reverse Trendelenburg position and rotated to a semi–left-lateral decubitus position. This orientation helps displace the hepatic flexure of the colon and the duodenal sweep away from the porta hepatis.

The performance of laparoscopic common duct exploration may be divided into the following segments:
Dissection of the porta hepatis
Initial maneuvers to clear the duct
Preparation and placement of the equipment
Dilatation of the cystic duct or choledochotomy
Insertion and manipulation of the scope
Insertion of the basket and entrapment of the stone
  or stones
Lithotripsy if necessary
Sphincterotomy if indicated
Placement of the T-tube and closure of the choledo-
  chotomy
Completion of cholangiograms
Completion of the cholecystectomy
In each segment, employment of specific maneuvers and precautions increases the likelihood of a successful exploration without mishap.

DISSECTION OF THE PORTA HEPATIS

Although some dissection in the triangle of Calot will have occurred prior to the initiation of cholangiograms, further delineation of the anatomy in this area is usually required before the common bile duct can be explored.

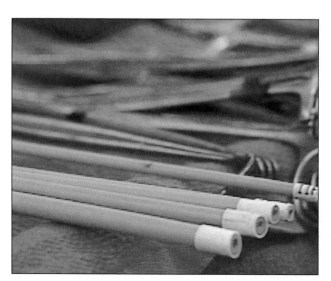

Figure 7. Graduated mechanical over-the-wire dilators.

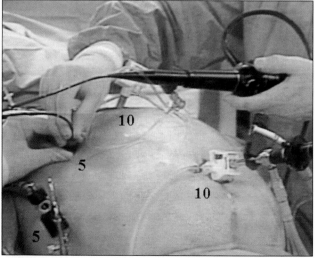

Figure 8. American 4-port configuration for laparoscopic cholecystectomy.

The lateral aspect of the infundibulum of the gallbladder and the cystic duct is approached first (Fig. 9) [23]. The peritoneum in this area is incised and reflected, displaying the junction of the cystic and common ducts, and in some instances allowing the surgeon to "unwrap" a posteriorly located junction. Occasionally the lateral peritoneal attachments of the duodenum must also be served (the Kocher maneuver) to achieve this effect. This maneuver facilitates introduction of instruments into the common duct via the cystic duct. The importance of these maneuvers cannot be overestimated.

The triangle of Calot is then approached again. During dissection of the triangle of Calot, the common duct may be temporarily located by depressing the duodenal sweep inferiorly with atraumatic forceps introduced through the midclavicular port. This maneuver stretches the common duct into a taut band that is easily identified. If the cystic artery has not been divided yet and if it obscures visualization of the common hepatic duct, it may be divided at this time. Extension of the incision in the peritoneum lying medial to the neck of the gallbladder is also helpful in some cases. It often allows the extrahepatic ductal system to be delivered into a more anterior location as the gallbladder is displaced toward the right hemidiaphragm. Dissection must be done carefully here to avoid hemorrhage from small vessels on or around the common duct.

INITIAL MANEUVERS TO CLEAR THE DUCT

If cholangiograms demonstrate no flow of contrast material into the duodenum but no stones are seen in the ductal system, and if spasm of the sphincter of Oddi is the suspected cause of the obstruction, glucagon 1 to 2 mg intravenously, may be given to relax the sphincter. Glucagon also facilitates flushing of small debris (<3mm) into the duodenum. Flushing often yields a normal cholangiogram [7•].

The next step involves the use of a standard 4 French Fogarty balloon catheter (Fig. 10). It is inserted into the abdomen through the 14-gauge sleeve used to perform the percutaneous cholangiograms. The sleeve is located 3 cm medial to the midclavicular port [1••,17]. Forceps introduced through the medial epigastric port guide the catheter into the common duct through the cystic duct. The catheter is advanced into the duodenum if possible. The balloon is inflated and the catheter is withdrawn until resistance is met at the sphincter; the duodenum is observed to move with the catheter at this point. The balloon is dilated, the catheter is withdrawn 1 cm and the balloon is reinflated. This should position it in the most distal portion of the duct, just proximal to the sphincter. The catheter is then withdrawn through the cystic duct using the forceps from the medial epigastric port. Although it would seem unlikely for the stones or debris to be preferentially directed out of the cystic duct rather than into the common hepatic duct, the surgeon is frequently rewarded with delivery of this material out of the cystic duct orifice. It can then be removed with forceps introduced through the medial epigastric port. The surgeons must use great care and gentle manipulations with the catheter to avoid perforating the ductal system during these maneuvers, especially when a stone is impacted in the distal duct.

Stone retrieval baskets may also be inserted through the 14-gauge sleeve used for cholangiography. The basket is advanced into the common duct through the cystic duct using forceps introduced through the medial epigastric port. If no fluoroscope is used during this maneuver, the surgeon must estimate the location of the basket tip in the common duct. Estimation can be relatively accurate when the length of the duct has already been measured with the balloon-tipped catheter. When the basket is located in the distal common duct, it is opened and the entire basket unit is moved back and

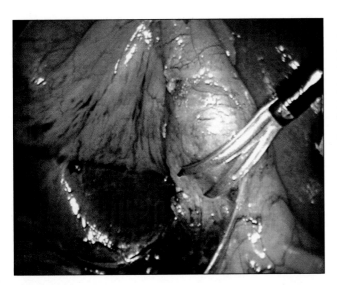

Figure 9. Dissection lateral to the infundibulum of the gallbladder first.

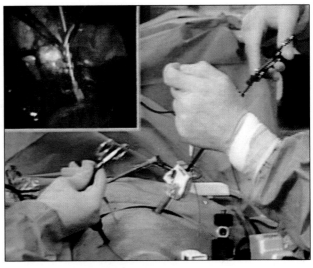

Figure 10. Fogarty balloon catheter manipulation.

forth in small increments while slowly being withdrawn as the wires of the basket are being closed. Capture of a stone is identified when the basket fails to close completely. The device is removed though the cystic duct, and the stones are delivered from the abdomen as described above. Great care must be exercised with this method so that accidental "capture" of the papilla of Vater does not occur.

A more accurate method of determining the exact location of the stone and the basket employs a fluoroscope [2•]. In the contrast-filled common duct, the manipulations required for stone capture with the basket may be monitored in real time. This technique, however, requires positioning of the fluoroscope to avoid interference with movements of the forceps in the medial epigastric port (Fig. 11). In some individuals, especially obese ones, adequate fluoroscope position cannot be achieved. The surgeon must then decide whether to pursue basket extraction without it or use a choledochoscope to monitor the procedure.

PREPARATION AND PLACEMENT OF EQUIPMENT FOR CHOLEDOCHOSCOPY

The conservative measures described above are usually employed while the choledochoscope and its related equipment are being prepared. In many hospitals preparation usually requires 20 to 30 minutes if the scope has not already been sterilized. (The choledochoscope may be either gas sterilized on the day prior to surgery or soaked in gluteraldehyde for 20 minutes at the time of the procedure.) The ancillary disposable equipment, such as irrigation tubing for the choledochoscope and saline solutions, should be readily available in the surgery department. It is wise to have all these materials, including balloon-tipped catheters and baskets located on a cart or trolley, in the department, so that in case of an abnormal cholangiogram they may be accessed without delay.

A separate Mayo stand, placed either at the foot of the table or above the patient's head is useful for storing the choledochoscope and related equipment in the sterile field. The various cables and tubes should be routed to minimize clutter in the operative field. Additionally, nursing staff or biomedical engineering personnel should be available to connect the choledochoscope to its light source, the choledochoscopic camera to its processing unit, and the video cable to the appropriate location on the video mixer or monitor.

These considerations are often overlooked in most surgery departments, resulting in a chaotic environment when LCDE becomes necessary. Prior time spent in planning for equipment preparation and placement during LCDE scenarios is well worth the effort, and should be given the same importance as preparation of the surgeon's skills to carry out the maneuvers once the equipment is available.

DILATATION OF THE CYSTIC DUCT OR CHOLEDOCHOTOMY

Although some authors prefer common access via a choledochotomy [24–26], laparoscopic common duct exploration may be carried out through cystic duct access in over 90% of cases [1••,2•,3•,8•]. When choledochoscopic maneuvers are needed, the cystic duct will need to accept a 9 or 10 French scope. If the duct is not already large enough for scope insertion, it may be dilated with either mechanical over-the-wire graduated dilators or pneumatic dilators.

In either case a guide wire (0.028 or 0.035 inches) is first inserted through the midclavicular port, through the cystic duct, and into the common duct. If graduated dilators are used, a 9 French size is usually the first to be advanced over the wire into the duct. I have found that if a 9 French dilator does not enter the cystic duct relatively easily, the likelihood of dilation to a large enough diameter, 11 or 12 French, is low. Each succes-

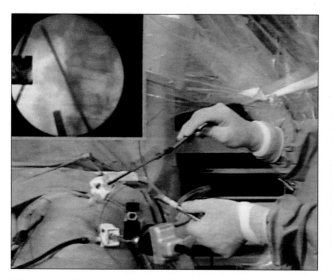

Figure 11. Fluoroscopically guided basket manipulation.

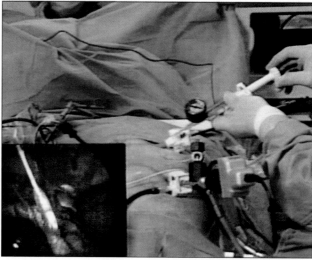

Figure 12. Pneumatic dilation of the cystic duct–Microvasive company dilator (Watertown, MA).

sively larger dilator is advanced over the wire until the duct is patulous enough to accept the scope [1••,15,16].

If a pneumatic dilator is employed, it may also be advanced over the wire into the cystic duct. Then, during observation of both the monitor and the pressure gauge on the screw-type syringe attached to the dilator, the dilatation balloon is filled. It is important to observe closely the physical changes in the duct while dilatation proceeds so that injury to the junction of the cystic and common ducts may be avoided (Fig. 12).

After either of these maneuvers, the guide wire may be removed or left in place for subsequent guidance of the choledochoscope. The dilatation equipment should remain sterile, however, to be available in the uncommon case in which it might be needed again for dilation.

If the cystic duct cannot be dilated enough to accept passage of the scope or the largest common duct stone, or if intrahepatic pathology is suspected, choledochotomy may be necessary. This procedure may be accomplished with a laparoscopic scalpel, scissors, or contact tip laser inserted through the medial epigastric port. A longitudinal incision approximately 1 cm in length, or as long as the largest stone, is sufficient (Fig. 13). This small incision limits the amount of time spent later in closing the choledochotomy. Stay sutures, which are commonly used in open common duct exploration, are not necessary for laparoscopic common duct exploration.

INSERTION AND MANIPULATION OF THE SCOPE

The choledochoscope is inserted through the midclavicular port, with or without wire guidance, into the cystic duct or the choledochotomy. The choledochoscopic and laparoscopic images must be kept in view, either on separate monitors or preferably on the same screen with a video mixer (Fig 14). At the level of the skin, the surgeon initially uses an atraumatic forceps inserted though the medial epigastric port to help guide the scope into the common duct. Saline instillation through the working channel of the scope should be employed at this time to expand the common duct and provide better visualization. When a sufficient length of the choledochoscope is inside the common duct, the forceps is withdrawn. Further manipulations usually require the surgeon to use both hands on the scope. One hand controls torquing maneuvers on the body of the scope at the cannula site; the other holds the scope head and directs the tip of the scope with the deflection lever located there.

As the common duct is negotiated, stones, debris, or other pathology become visible. The distal portion of the common bile duct is usually the easiest to inspect and treat. If a cystic duct approach is employed, access to the proximal ductal system is usually not possible unless the cystic duct is very short or patulous and oriented at 90° to the common duct. If a choledochotomy has been prepared, the scope may be directed into either the proximal system or the distal bile duct.

If the surgeon experiences difficulty in traversing the junction of the cystic and common ducts, further dissection along the lateral border of the ducts, or a Kocher maneuver, may be necessary. Occasionally this maneuver will allow the junction to "unwrap," thereby providing a less convoluted path into the common duct.

INSERTION OF THE BASKET AND ENTRAPMENT OF STONES

In most cases stones identified with the choledochoscope require entrapment in a basket for removal through the cystic duct or the choledochotomy. I believe that these are the most difficult maneuvers associated with laparoscopic common duct exploration. They often require the assistance of the scrub nurse or another assistant.

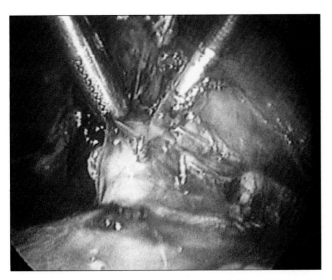

Figure 13. Choledochotomy using a contact tip Nd:YAG laser.

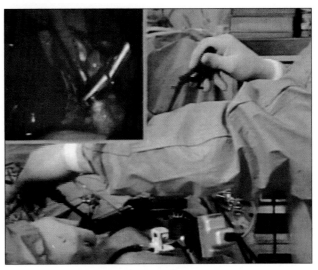

Figure 14. Insertion of the choledochoscope into the cystic duct.

The scope is manipulated by the surgeon so that the stone is in direct view. Control of the body of the scope is then transferred to the assistant, who must provide the same amount of torque on the scope at the level of the midclavicular cannula as the surgeon had applied prior to the transfer (Fig. 15). Although simple in concept, this event can become one of the most frustrating of the entire LCDE. The assistant must understand the importance of keeping the stone in view and must direct undivided attention to the monitor providing the choledochoscopic view. Otherwise the location of the stone will be lost. If this happens after the basket is inserted into the working channel of the scope, it is very difficult to manipulate the scope to find the stone again without removing the basket from the channel. This difficulty occurs because most scopes use the working channel to provide the saline instillation that dilates the duct. With the basket in the channel, very little if any saline is delivered into the duct, and its lumen collapses. This problem becomes compounded when multiple stones are present in the duct because their manipulation and capture usually produce minute debris that "clouds" the fluid in the duct. This cloudiness, combined with loss of the exact location of the stone, makes it nearly impossible to capture the stone. In this case the basket must be removed so that saline instillation may be used to clear the fluid in the duct. Obviously the more inefficient the manipulations performed at this time, the more debris is created, and the likelihood of a successful LCDE becomes remote.

When the stone is in direct view, and after the body of the scope has been transferred to the assistant, the surgeon temporarily interrupts the saline instillation and inserts the basket into the working channel of the scope. Once the basket is located in the channel, the saline may again be allowed to flow, although the amount that actually enters the channel is limited because of the presence of the basket. The basket is then advanced until its tip is seen protruding from the tip of the choledochoscope. The basket is advanced past the stone and then opened. It is withdrawn back to the stone to attempt capture. If this attempt is unsuccessful, as it usually is on the first few passes, the basket must be moved back and forth past the stone until it drops into the interstices. In some cases, this maneuver must be combined with torquing or tip deflection to capture the stone (Fig. 16). The basket is then slowly closed around the stone to secure it. This step usually requires the entire basket ensemble to be advanced as the wires are being closed, because closure usually withdraws the wires toward the scope and may dislodge the stone from its position in the basket.

LITHOTRIPSY

In some cases, the stone may be impacted in the distal portion of the duct. This usually makes basket capture difficult, if not impossible. Here a lithotripter may be of value [8•,11••]. Its probe is inserted through the working channel of the scope and advanced into the appropriate position for application of its energy to the stone. Fragmentation may disrupt the impaction and allow the pieces to be captured and removed with basket techniques. Great care must be taken when using a lithotripter to deliver its energy precisely to the stone and not to the duct wall; otherwise, damage to the duct may occur.

I have also found that application of a pulsatile saline jet (using, *eg*, Waterpik [Teledyne, Fort Collins, CO]) through the working channel of the scope may be useful in freeing debris from the duct wall. Because

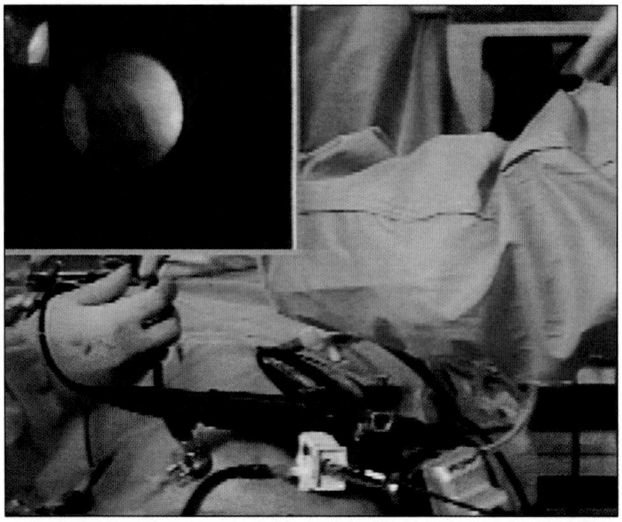

Figure 15. Choledochoscope body control transferred to the assistant.

there are no ready-made adapters to connect such devices to the scope, surgeons must configure their own if they elect to use this modality.

DRAINAGE

In cases in which a drainage procedure appears to be indicated, concomitant sphincterotomy may be performed. Some surgeons have employed endoscopic retrograde sphincterotomy at the same time as the LCDE [27•]. DePaula [28•] in Brazil has shown that antegrade sphincterotomy through the choledochoscope is safe and effective. In his method the procedure is monitored from within the common duct by the choledochoscope, and from within the duodenum by a side-viewing endoscope. This method obviously requires another physician to pass the duodenoscope. If this combined procedure is attempted, it is important for the endoscopist to avoid excessive air instillation into the gastrointestinal tract; otherwise, the dilated gut will obscure the view of the porta hepatis.

T-TUBE PLACEMENT

If a choledochotomy has been used to gain access to the common duct, it is usually chosen over a T-tube after the ductal exploration is complete (Fig. 17). A 14 French T-tube is prepared by removing the back wall of the T-portion. It is then loaded into an 8-mm cylinder and delivered through the 10-mm medial epigastric port into the peritoneal cavity. The entire T-tube is placed into the abdomen and the T is inserted into the common duct. This maneuver usually requires some effort, but it is not much more difficult than in open surgery. After the tube is in the duct, the outlying portion is temporarily occluded at its tip with a hemoclip or ligature to prevent bile drainage into the peritoneal cavity while the remainder of the cholecystectomy is completed. This clip is removed just prior to delivery of the tube through the abdominal wall.

The choledochotomy is closed with a 4-0 or 5-0 Vicryl (Ethicon, Somerville, NJ) suture [1••]. Either interrupted or continuous suture may be used, although the former is usually easier for the novice to complete. The magnification afforded by the laparoscope and camera allows more precise placement of the sutures than is possible in open surgery. The suture is secured with intracorporeal ligation rather than extracorporeal techniques because of the fragility of the duct. The closure may be tested for watertightness by temporarily advancing the end of the tube out of one of the 5-mm portals and injecting saline in the same fashion as would be done in open surgery. It is usually necessary to replace the tube into the peritoneal cavity until the cholecystectomy is completed so that the portal is available for retracting forceps, and so that the tube itself does not limit access to the porta hepatis. While the tube is completely inside the peritoneal cavity, its tip should remain occluded with a clip or ligature.

COMPLETION CHOLANGIOGRAPHY

After the common duct exploration has been completed, cholangiograms should be repeated to ensure that the duct is cleared. If a transcystic duct LCDE approach has been used, the cholangiogram catheter is reinserted into the cystic duct and the films are repeated. If choledochotomy has been performed, the cholangiograms may be obtained through the T-tube. If for some reason the duct is still not cleared, the surgeon must decide whether to proceed with LCDE, convert to open common duct exploration and choledocholithotomy, or leave the stone in place for subsequent treatment with ERC±S.

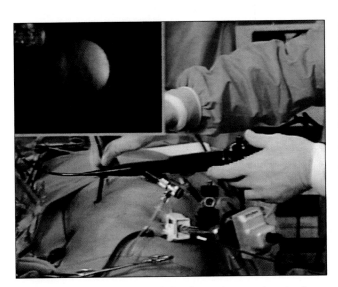

Figure 16. Choledochoscopic basket entrapment and extraction of common bile duct stone.

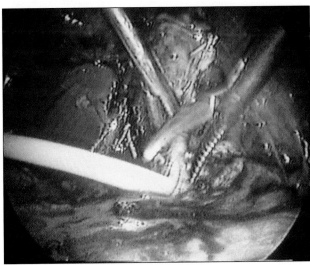

Figure 17. T-tube placement.

COMPLETION OF THE CHOLECYSTECTOMY

The cystic duct stump must be occluded with clips, ligatures, or sutures. If the cystic duct is dilated more than 6 mm, or if subsequent ERC±S is contemplated, it is wise to use a ligature in addition to clips to secure the stump. In these instances the ligature should be applied before the clips to decrease the likelihood of a stump leak.

The remainder of the cholecystectomy is performed in standard laparoscopic fashion. If a T-tube has been inserted, it should be advanced out through the abdominal wall, either through one of the existing 5-mm portals or through a new site if necessary, prior to removal of the gallbladder from the peritoneal cavity. A closed-system drain is usually inserted, at least temporarily, through one of the 5-mm portals into the region of dissection. The gallbladder is then removed from the umbilical site, the remaining ports are removed, and the fascia at all 10-mm sites is closed with 0-Vicryl. The skin is closed with subcuticular suture of 4-0 Vicryl.

REFERENCES

Papers of particular interest, published within the period of review, have been highlighted as:
• Of special interest
•• Of outstanding interest

1.•• Petelin J: Laparoscopic Approach to Common Duct Pathology. *Surg Laparosc Endosc* 1991, 1:33–41.

A comprehensive laparoscopic approach to biliary tract disease is presented. Multiple techniques are described. Heavily illustrated.

2.• Hunter J: Laparoscopic Trancystic Common Bile Duct Exploration. *Am J Surg* 1992, 163:53–58.

Fluoroscopically guided laparoscopic basket extraction of common duct stones is described in detail here. This technique is a significant addition to the armamentarium of the biliary tract surgeon. Especially useful in cases of small diameter cystic and common bile ducts.

3.• Carroll BJ, Phillips EH, Daykhovsky L, Grundfest WS, Gersham A, Fallas M, Chandra M: Laparoscopic Choledochoscopy: an Effective Approach to the Common Duct. *J Laparoendosc Surg* 1992, 2:15–21.

These authors, leaders in the field of laparoscopic common bile duct exploration, review their techniques and early results.

4. Sackier JM, Berci G, Pas-Partlow M: Laparoscopic Trancystic Choledochotomy as an Adjunct to Laparoscopic Cholecystectomy. *Am Surgeon* 1991, 57:323–326.

5. Jacobs M, VCerdeja JC, Goldstein HS: Laparoscopic choledocholithotomy. *J Laparoendosc Surg* 1991, 1:79–82.

6. Quattlebaum JK, Flanders HD: Laparoscopic Treatment of Common Bile Duct Stones. *Surg Laparosc Endosc* 1991, 1:26–32.

7.• Appel S, Krebs H, Fern D: Techniques for Laparoscopic Cholangiography and Removal of Common Duct Stones. *Surg Endosc* 1992, 6:134–137.

Another comprehensive overview of various methods useful in clearing the common duct of stones.

8.• Birkett D: Technique of Cholangiography and Cystic-Duct Choledochoscopy at the Time of Laparoscopic Cholecystectomy for Laser Lithotripsy. Surg Endosc 1992, 6:252–254.

An alternative technique for introduction of the flexible choledochoscope into the common duct via a transabdominal- transcystic sheath is described. The authors report that the method is easier than others and avoids damage to the scope.

9. Fletcher D, Jones RM, O'Riordan B, Hardy KJ: Laparoscopic Cholecystectomy for Complicated Gallstone Disease. *Surg Endosc* 1992, 6:179–182.

10. Dion YM, Morin J, Dionne G, Dejoie C: Laparoscopic Cholecystectomy and Choledocholithiasis. *Can J Surg* 1992, 35:67–74.

11.•• Arregui M, Davis CJ, Arkush AM, Nagan RF: Laparoscopic Cholecystectomy Combined With Endoscopic Sphincterotomy and Stone Extraction or Laparoscopic Choledochoscopy and Electrohydraulic Lithotripsy for Management of Cholelithiais With Choledocholithiasis. *Surg Endosc* 1992, 6:10–15.

An excellent overview of the evolving ERC±S, laparoscopic cholecystectomy, and common duct exploration. The authors review the literature regarding ERC±S and laparoscopic common duct exploration, present their results, and anticipate their movement away from ERC±S as laparoscopic common duct exploration techniques improve.

12. Cotton PB: Endoscopic Management of Bile Duct Stones (Apples and Oranges). *Gut* 1984, 25:587–597.

13. Carr-Locke DL: Acute Gallstone Pancreatitis and Endoscopic Therapy. *Endoscopy* 1990, 22:180–183.

14. Vitale GC, Larson GM, Wieman TJ, Cheadle WG, Miller FB: The Use of ERCP in the Management of Common Bile Duct Stones in Patients Undergoing Laparoscopic Cholecystectomy. *Surg Endosc* 1993, 7:9–11.

15. Petelin J: Laparoscopic Approach to Common Duct Pathology. *Am J Surg* 1992, in press.

16. Petelin J: Clinical Results of Common Bile Duct Exploration. *In* Endoscopic Surgery and Allied Technologies. *Edited by Buess G. Stuttgart, New York:Gerog Thieme Verlag; 1993, [in press].*

17. Petelin J: The Argument for Contact Laser Laparoscopic Cholecystectomy. *Clin Laser Monthly* 1990, 71–74.

18. • Petelin J: Laparoscopic Common Duct Exploration. *American College of Surgeons Motion Picture Library*, Chicago, 1992.

Sixteen-minute comprehensive video presented at American College of Surgeons meeting October 1992 and selected for addition to the library of the college.

19. • Shimi S, Banting Fracs S, Cuschieri A: Transcystic Drainage after Laparoscopic Exploration of Common Bile Duct. *Minimally Invasive Ther* 1992, 1:273–276.

A simple method of providing common duct decompression after laparoscopic common duct exploration using a transcystic duct catheter. The authors report that this technique avoids the need for T-tube placement.

20. Kitano S, Iso Y, Moriyama M, Sugimachi K: A Rapid and Simple Technique for Insertion of a T-Tube into the Minimally Incised Common Bile Duct at Laparoscopic Surgery. Surg Endosc 1993, 7:104–105.

21. Mooney MJ, Deyo G, O'Reilly MJ: T-Tube Placement During Laparoscopic Cholecystectomy. Surg Endosc 1992, 6:32.

22. Reddick EJ, Olsen DO, Daniell JF, Saye WB, McKernan B, Miller W, Hoback M: Laparoscopic Laser Cholecystectomy. Laser Med Surg News Adv 1989, 38–40.

23. Klaiber C, Metzger A, Petelin J: Laparoscopic Cholecystectomy. In Manual of Laparoscopic Surgery. Bern: Hogrefe & Huber; 1993:97–148.

24. Ferzli GS, Massaad A, Ozuner G, Worth MH: Laparoscopic Exploration of the Common Bile Duct. Surg Gynecol Obstet 1992, 174:419–421.

25. Franklin ME, Pharand D: Laparoscopic Common Bile Duct Exploration. In Proceedings, Third International Congress of Laparoscopic Surgery. Brazil: Grafica e Editorial Bandeirante. 1993:100–103.

26. Stoker ME, Leveillee RJ, McCann JC, Maini BS: Laparoscopic Common Bile Duct Exploration. J Laparoendosc Surg 1991, 1:5:287–293.

27. • Gagner M, Deslandres E, Pomp A, Rheault M, Potvin C, Leduc R: Double Endoscopy: the Role of Intraoperative ERCP During Laparoscopic Cholecystectomy for Choledocholithiais. In Proceedings, Third International Congress of Laparoscopic Surgery. Brazil: Grafica e Editorial Bandeirante. 1993:126–127.

Simultaneous choledochoscopy and side-viewing duodenoscopy are used to perform ERCP at the time of laparoscopic cholecystectomy in cases in which a drainage procedure is indicated. Avoids the need for a second procedure.

28. • DePaula AL, Hashiba K, Bafutto M, Zago R, Machado M: Laparoscopic Antegrade Sphinecterotomy. *Surg Laparosc Endosc* 1993, 3:157–160.

In cases in which a biliary drainage procedure is indicated, the authors perform antegrade sphincterotomy via the choledochoscope at the time of the laparoscopic common duct exploration, while the procedure is monitored with a side-viewing duodenoscope. This technique should avoid the potential problems of pancreatitis that can be induced from cannulation of the pancreatic duct during ERCP.

Chapter 8

Complications of Laparoscopic Cholecystectomy

Bruce D. Schirmer

Laparoscopic cholecystectomy, first performed in 1985 by Mühe [1] but commonly attributed to Mouret [2], has recently gained acceptance as the treatment of choice for symptomatic cholelithiasis. The rapidity of this change is unprecedented in modern surgical history. The reasons are multifactorial and include the obvious benefits of the procedure to the patient, a patient-driven demand for the procedure fueled by media and mass communication, and industry-driven publicity and efforts to establish the procedure. The surgical community has been quick to adopt it to provide a better service to patients, but probably also in part because of some of these other factors.

The pressure to incorporate this new technology into the practice of general surgery may have led to performance of laparoscopic cholecystectomy by some ill-prepared surgeons. This occurred despite guidelines issued by the Society of American Gastrointestinal Endoscopic Surgeons (SAGES) and other groups for both training, performing, and credentialing for laparoscopic cholecystectomy [3,4•,5].

Although this ill-prepared group was doubtless a small minority of general surgeons, it is possible their actions may have contributed to what was reported as an alarming rate of severe complications by the New York State Health Authority [6•]. During the same period, concern and attention increased in both the literature and the lay press regarding the higher incidence of serious complications associated with laparoscopic cholecystectomy, the most prevalent of which were bile duct injuries. In this chapter, complications associated with laparoscopic cholecystectomy are reviewed on the basis of the data available in the literature.

OVERALL COMPLICATIONS OF LAPAROSCOPIC CHOLECYSTECTOMY

Laparoscopic cholecystectomy is now the most commonly performed procedure for the surgical treatment of cholelithiasis. It is also the most commonly performed laparoscopic general surgical procedure. The benefits of laparoscopic cholecystectomy, namely, less postoperative pain, shorter hospitalization, and a more rapid return to work, have been extensively documented in many reports [7••–10••,11,12•,13•,14,15•]. These reports also emphasized the safety and relatively low complication rates associated with laparoscopic cholecystectomy.

The overall complication rate for laparoscopic cholecystectomy has been documented as being between 1% and 9% in large series in the literature [7••–10••,11,12•,13•,14,15•,16,17••]. A recent National Institutes of Health consensus conference on laparoscopic cholecystectomy showed the aggregate complication rate of a review of data based on over 100,000 cases to be between 2% and 5% [18••]. The conference noted, however, that these numbers reflected the characteristics of particular patients and the way in which complications were defined more than they did the procedure.

COMPLICATIONS OF PNEUMOPERITONEUM

The creation of a pneumoperitoneum and the performance of laparoscopy itself are associated with a low incidence of morbidity and mortality. In the gynecologic literature, which has analyzed large surveys of cases, the incidence of major complications arising from laparoscopy is from 0.3% to 2.3%. Minor complications occur in 1.1% to 5.1% of cases. Mortality is extremely rare, occurring at a rate of 0.005% to 0.05% [19–21]. These complications can be divided into those associated with the establishment of the pneumoperitoneum and those associated with invasive diagnostic or therapeutic maneuvers. The incidence and seriousness of complications increase in proportion to the increasingly complex therapeutic nature of the procedure.

Veress needle insertion is associated with a low but defined incidence of complications. These include the potential for injury to underlying abdominal organs. Insertion is performed most safely at the umbilical ring, where the abdominal wall is thinnest. Aspiration is performed through the needle after insertion. Evidence of blood or intestinal fluid is a sign that injury has occurred until proven otherwise. Laparoscopic examination of the injury is then indicated if possible. The injury should be treated appropriately on the basis of its size and the patient's clinical course.

The presence of a previous abdominal incision, particularly one involving the midline near the umbilicus, is a contraindication to blind Veress needle placement in the umbilical area. Instead most surgeons use an open laparoscopy approach in this situation. Direct dissection through the abdominal wall layers is followed by insertion under direct vision of a Hasson-type trocar into the peritoneal cavity. Open laparoscopy has its advocates as the procedure of choice for initiating all laparoscopic procedures (de la Torre *et al.*, Paper presented at the Third World Congress of Endoscopic Surgery, Bordeaux, France, 1992). Selective use of this technique can result in a complication rate for laparoscopic cholecystectomy in patients with previous abdominal incisions that is not significantly different from patients without such incisions [22].

An alternative to open laparoscopy in patients with previous incisions is placement of the Veress needle in an alternate site—the abdominal quadrant least likely to have intra-abdominal adhesions. Preoperative ultrasonography has also been successfully used in patients with previous abdominal incisions to evaluate the likelihood of bowel adhering to the anterior abdominal wall at the proposed site of insufflation (Wayabashi *et al.*, Paper presented to Society of American Gastrointestinal Surgeons, Phoenix, AZ, 1993).

Obesity creates added difficulty to infraumbilical Veress needle insertion. Using the technique of insertion of the needle in a 45° angle toward the pelvis, the severely obese patient's abdominal wall may be penetrated with the needle tip, and preperitoneal insufflation can occur (Fig. 1.).

Some surgeons advocate direct insertion of the trocar itself into the abdominal cavity through a small infraumbilical incision, foregoing use of the Veress needle. According to their studies the complication rate of this technique is comparable to that of Veress needle insertion [23]. However, it has been our observation that the most severe complications associated with general surgical laparoscopic procedures are a result of trocar rather than Veress needle insertion injuries. Most gynecologists and general surgeons use a Veress needle approach to create a pneumoperitoneum prior to trocar insertion [24].

Insufflation of gas into an improper tissue plane or space can occur during laparoscopy. Most therapeutic laparoscopic procedures are performed using carbon dioxide gas. Fortunately carbon dioxide is rapidly absorbed in tissues, and its insufflation in improper tissue planes may often be only a transient problem. Inadvertent carbon dioxide insufflation into the subcutaneous tissues, resulting in subcutaneous emphysema, is the most common event in this group of complications. The incidence of subcutaneous emphysema is approximately 0.43% to 2% [25]. We have observed that subcutaneous emphysema is more common in thin, elderly patients. The loose subcutaneous tissues in such patients may allow easier dissection of the gas through tissue planes.

Small amounts of subcutaneous emphysema from carbon dioxide are usually well tolerated. Subcutaneous emphysema is generally readily apparent on examination, but usually the first sign of its occurrence is a rise in the end-tidal carbon dioxide content as monitored by the anesthesiologist. The anesthesiologist must be aware of the need for increased ventilation to increase the exchange of carbon dioxide. This measure alone usually suffices to treat the problem, as do measures to limit further escape of gas into the tissues. Arterial blood gases to measure pH should be obtained because pH falls with carbon dioxide absorption. Administration of sodium bicarbonate as a measure to correct the pH instead is to be avoided because alkalosis can easily result once the carbon dioxide is absorbed. If the amount of emphysema is small, the patient's cardiovascular system sound, and the plasma pH not excessively lowered, the operation may proceed. However, if not, it may be necessary to deflate the pneumoperitoneum and convert the operation to an open laparotomy. Rapid absorption of subcutaneous emphysema is the rule; patients usually have few signs remaining on physical examination after only several hours in the postoperative recovery suite. Although subcutaneous emphysema is the most common result of misdirected carbon dioxide insufflation, the risks for pneumomediastinum, pneumothorax, pneumopericardium, and omental and mesenteric emphysema as an effect of gas insufflation are all known complications of laparoscopy as well [26].

The most serious complication of gas insufflation into an inappropriate location is gas embolism. Fortunately this complication is rare, occurring in only about 0.016% of laparoscopies [27]. Gas embolism can be rapidly fatal if not immediately detected or if the bolus of gas is too large. Small amounts of carbon dioxide are better tolerated than other gases, such as air or nitrous oxide. The most common treatment of gas embolism involves immediate cessation of gas insufflation, placing the patient right side down, and right heart catheterization to aspirate the gas.

Cardiac arrest can occasionally occur following the establishment of a pneumoperitoneum. The incidence is about 1 in 2500 cases [28]. The causes of cardiac arrest include air embolism, decreased venous return to the heart, hypercapnia or anoxia from hypoventilation, and a profound vagal response to peritoneal distention. Treatment is prompt deflation of the pneumoperitoneum, with cardiovascular resuscitative and supportive measures.

Cardiac arrhythmias can also result as a consequence of pneumoperitoneum. The mechanisms of such arrhythmias are thought to be the same as those causing cardiac arrest, but on a lesser scale. Arrhythmias are usually self-limited, but may on occasion lead to serious hemodynamic consequences. The incidence of such events is under 1%.

COMPLICATIONS OF TROCAR INSERTION

Trocar insertion during diagnostic or therapeutic laparoscopy can result in the complication of hemorrhage. In the gynecologic literature, the rate of laparotomy during laparoscopy to treat hemorrhage was 0.26% [19]. The incidence of bleeding following laparoscopic cholecystectomy is higher than that seen

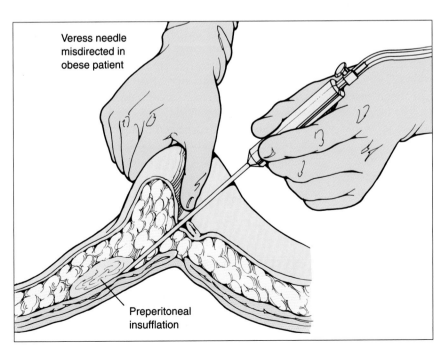

Veress needle
misdirected in
obese patient

Preperitoneal
insufflation

Figure 1. Potential difficulty of inserting a Veress needle correctly through the wall of an obese patient if the standard 45° angle of penetration is used. The thickness of the abdominal wall predisposes to inadvertent preperitoneal insufflation.

following laparoscopy in general. The multicenter study organized by SAGES [7••] reported an incidence of 0.46% to 1.0% complications relating to bleeding, a figure comparable with the results of other large reported series.

With the exception of cardiac arrest, laceration of major blood vessels during trocar insertion is the most immediately life-threatening complication that can occur during laparoscopic cholecystectomy. The New York State Department of Health memorandum reported 13 major vascular perforations [6•]. The literature suggests that the incidence of major vascular injuries from laparoscopic cholecystectomy is approximately 0.1% [7••,17••]. The occurrence of such events is particularly serious because their immediate recognition is necessary if appropriate conversion to open laparotomy and life-saving repair of the vascular injury are to be performed. A significant proportion of the reported mortality related to laparoscopic cholecystectomy has been secondary to this complication.

Trocar insertion can also cause bleeding from the abdominal wall. Such bleeding may be immediately apparent or may present in the postoperative period as an abdominal wall hematoma. The loss of blood from such an event can be significant, requiring transfusion. Surveillance for bleeding at trocar sites should accompany the insertion and removal of the trocar. Trocar site bleeding can be treated in several ways. Enlarging the incision for better exposure of the vessel is one option. Another is use of a full-thickness abdominal wall suture externally tied over a pledget. Direct pressure using the inflated balloon of a Foley catheter may also provide effective tamponade at the bleeding site.

Visceral injury can result from trocar insertion. Few data exist as to the percentage of visceral injuries during laparoscopy resulting from trocar insertion injuries versus injuries resulting from the remainder of the operative procedure. In one past survey of gynecologic laparoscopy, the overall injury rate to the bowel was 0.18%, the injury rate to the urinary tract 0.02%, and the rate of bowel mesentery injury was 0.11% [24]. Such injuries were correlated to the difficulty of trocar insertion as well as the training of the surgeon. The incidence of bowel injury from laparoscopic cholecystectomy has been reported as being in the 0.1 to 0.3% as well.

The small intestine is at highest risk for perforation during trocar insertion for laparoscopic cholecystectomy (Fig. 2A). Such injuries can be minimized by appropriate technique, in particular, an open laparoscopy approach when this procedure is performed in patients with any previous intra-abdominal surgery. Morbidity from intestinal injuries that do occur can be minimized only if the injury is recognized. Unrecognized injury leads to postoperative sepsis, intra-abdominal abscess formation, and not infrequently death.

The consequences of unrecognized visceral injury are major contributors to the morbidity and mortality of both diagnostic and therapeutic laparoscopy. In one large multicenter series of laparoscopic cholecystectomies, unrecognized bowel perforation was responsible for virtually all the rare mortalities reported [7••]. Wolfe *et al.* [16] reported two fatal unrecognized intestinal injuries following laparoscopic cholecystectomy in a series of 381 patients.

COMPLICATIONS OF ELECTROCAUTERY OR LASER

Included in unrecognized injuries at the time of laparoscopy are those secondary to electrocautery or laser. During laparoscopic cholecystectomy, inadvertent cautery or laser injury can occur during dissection. Cautery injury can be unrecognized and frequently presents as delayed perforations following surgery if the bowel is the organ involved. The duodenum is the intestinal structure most frequently injured (Fig. 2B). The incidence of such injuries is probably on the order of 0.1% to 0.5%. Cautery injury to hilar structures is also known; stricture of the common bile duct can result from cautery or laser injury. Touching the metal clips applied to the divided cystic duct with the cautery can transmit a burn injury to the bile duct (Fig. 2C). If the cystic duct alone is injured, postoperative tissue necrosis may cause leakage of the cystic duct stump.

It is unclear whether the use of laser has been responsible for a higher percentage of inadvertent intraabdominal organ injuries than monopolar cautery. Contact lasers probably have not been responsible for any higher percentage of injury than cautery, but free beam lasers may have been. Popularity for the use of laser as part of laparoscopic cholecystectomy is declining after studies have shown that it has no significant advantage but is costly [29•].

The gynecologic literature has devoted much attention in the past to the theory that some of these delayed or unrecognized intestinal injuries during laparoscopy were from arc injuries due to monopolar cautery [30]. Although in theory monopolar cautery arc injuries may certainly have occurred, the subsequent proliferation of laparoscopic use by general surgeons has failed to substantiate this rate of suspected conduction injuries from electrocautery. In addition, laboratory studies in animals suggest that such a mechanism is unlikely [31].

OTHER NONBILIARY COMPLICATIONS OF LAPAROSCOPIC CHOLECYSTECTOMY

Inadvertent injury to other organs can result whenever the laparoscopic telescope is not focused on the surgeon's instruments. An example of such an injury is shown in Figure 2D, where suture ligation of the cystic duct is being performed and the needle, off the videotelescopic screen, has lacerated the undersurface of the liver.

The incidence of infection following laparoscopic cholecystectomy is lower than that seen following open cholecystectomy. This difference is particularly notable in wound infections. Wound infections following laparoscopic cholecystectomy occur at an incidence consistent with clean or clean-contaminated type operations. Management of operative port site wound infection is easier than that of traditional wound infection due to the small size of the wound. Omphalitis at the umbilical port site can be an annoying problem, but its incidence can be markedly decreased through careful preoperative cleansing of the umbilicus. Less common but reported infectious complications include abscess

formation from retained gallstones not removed at the time of laparoscopic cholecystectomy for acute cholecystitis [32].

Other complications of laparoscopic cholecystectomy are those related to the performance of any surgical extirpative procedure. They include missed diagnosis, with return of the patient for readmission to the hospital due to abdominal pain of other etiology; postoperative fever; and urinary tract infection or urinary retention. The incidence of significant pulmonary atelectasis and postoperative ileus are both significantly lower with laparoscopic cholecystectomy than with open cholecystectomy [7••]. Gastric emptying of solid food may be delayed for up to 24 hours following laparoscopic cholecystectomy, although this is often not strikingly mani-

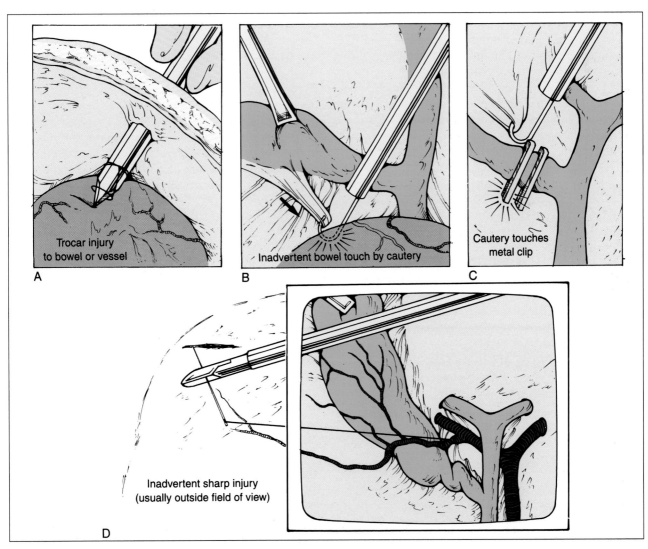

Figure 2. Injuries that may occur during laparoscopic cholecystectomy. **A,** Trocar injury to the jejunum, ileum, or a vascular structure is possible on initial insertion. **B,** Inadvertent cautery injury of the duodenum during dissection of the hilar structures is particularly likely to occur with dense adhesions in the area of the infundibulum of the gallbladder. Unrecognized injury can result in postoperative perforation, peritoni-

tis,and life-threatening sepsis. **C,** Touching the cystic duct clips with the electrocautery can result in postoperative necrosis of the duct, clip dislodgement, and bile leak. **D,** Failure to keep the working instruments on the field of view of the videotelescope can result in off-telescope injury, such as laceration of the liver with a needle.

fested clinically (Schmieg and Schirmer, Paper presented to American Motility Society, Lake Tahoe, NV, 1992). The incidence of bowel obstruction after laparoscopic cholecystectomy has been rarely reported. As with open cholecystectomy, cardiovascular complications make up a significant percentage of the nontechnical life-threatening complications in the elderly population [17••,33].

Postoperative nausea and vomiting, although relatively minor threats to the patient's health, are frequently seen after both laparoscopic procedures in general and laparoscopic cholecystectomy. Their duration is virtually always less than 24 hours and frequently only 6 to 12 hours. Postoperative nausea and vomiting following laparoscopy are more common in women and are related to the time of menstrual cycle in premenopausal women [34•].

One postoperative symptom peculiar to patients undergoing laparoscopic cholecystectomy that is not seen with open cholecystectomy is shoulder pain. This symptom is a result of diaphragmatic stretching during the duration of pneumoperitoneum. Such symptoms rarely last more than a few days and rarely require narcotic analgesics. In fact, almost one third of patients undergoing laparoscopic cholecystectomy require no narcotic medications of any type once leaving the recovery suite [12•].

BILE DUCT INJURIES

There has been significant attention in the surgical literature in 1992 to the rising numbers of bile duct injuries and other complications resulting from laparoscopic cholecystectomy [35••,36–38]. Controversy still exists as to whether these reports identify a true Achilles heel of this procedure, and whether laparoscopic cholecystectomy is a potential threat to the safe treatment of

patients suffering from cholelithiasis, as could be believed from the State of New York Department of Health memorandum [6•]. It is possible that the significant attention in the literature arose from the fact the operation itself had been so widely publicized. As Larson *et al.* [8••] pointed out, the incidence of bile duct injuries in the large reported series of laparoscopic cholecystectomies may not be greatly different from the rate reported in previous large series of open cholecystectomies. However, Dezeil *et al.* [17••] showed a 0.6% incidence of bile duct injury using a survey questionnaire, where the reported incidence of complications might be assumed to underestimate the true incidence of the problem due to the reporting system.

Bile duct injuries are the main source of procedure-specific morbidity for laparoscopic cholecystectomy. The incidence of injuries to the common bile duct during open cholecystectomy was also somewhat controversial. On the basis of large series in the literature, the incidence can be estimated at approximately 0.1% to 0.4% [33,39]. The incidence may have been as high as 0.5% in actuality, because published series probably underestimated the true incidence of ductal injuries in general practice.

The incidence of bile duct injuries in the published literature related to laparoscopic cholecystectomy is slightly higher than that of open cholecystectomy. Most large series of experiences with laparoscopic cholecystectomy have reported the bile duct injury rate to be between 0.1% and 0.7% [7••,8••,11,14,15•,17••, 18••,40]. In smaller series, which usually represented the early phase of experience with the procedure at any one institution, the incidence of ductal injury was often reported as higher [41,42]. In certain reports that focused on laparoscopic bile duct injuries, higher incidences were also noted [37].

Reported series of biliary complications following laparoscopic cholecystectomy have shown that these complications can be grouped into certain general categories (Table 1). Bile leaks are more common than bile duct injuries. Deziel *et al.* [17••] reported an incidence of 0.29% of bile leak following laparoscopic cholecystectomy, making it the most common technical complication related to the procedure. The cystic duct stump is the most common site of leakage, followed by the gallbladder bed. Actual injury to the bile duct occurs most often at the common bile duct, with hepatic duct injury being the next most common.

A type of bile duct injury that seems unique to laparoscopic cholecystectomy has been described by Davidoff *et al.* [35••]. In their experience, the most common type of bile duct injury following laparoscopic cholecystectomy involved the mistaken identification of the common hepatic duct as the cystic duct, resulting in a removal of a portion of the common hepatic duct and transection of the common bile duct (Fig. 3). This injury has now come to be referred to as the "classic injury."

Table 1. Types of biliary tract injuries associated with laparoscopic cholecystectomy

Bile duct leak

Dislodgment of cystic duct clip

Traction injury of cystic/common duct junction

Incomplete removal of gallbladder

Injury of accessory duct in liver bed

Patent duct of Luschka

Bile duct injury

Common bile duct injury/occlusion

"Classic" type injury with resection of portion of duct

Common hepatic duct injury/occlusion

Aberrant bile duct injury

Right hepatic duct injury

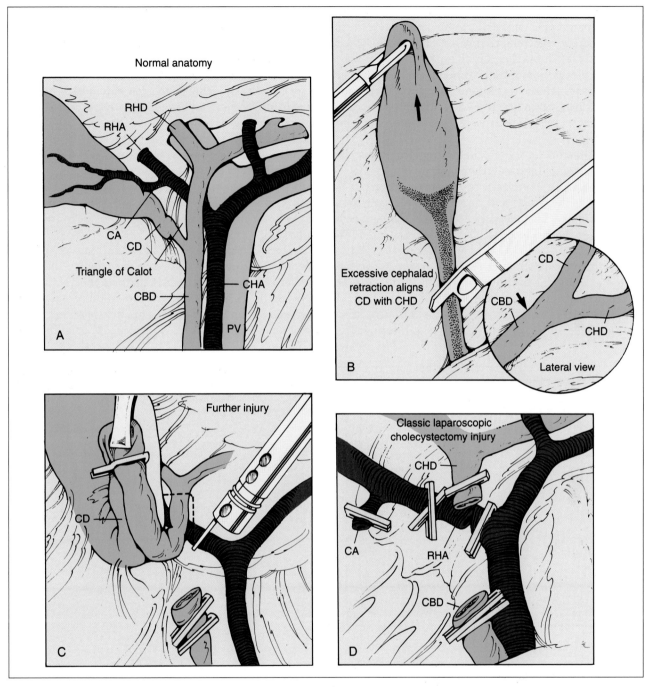

Figure 3. The "classic injury" to the biliary tree during laparoscopic cholecystectomy. **A**, The "normal" or most common, anatomic configuration of the hilar structures. **B**, Excessive cephalad retraction of the gallbladder tends to align the cystic duct, particularly when short, with the underlying common hepatic duct. The common bile duct is mistaken for the distal cystic duct and clipped. **C**, Division of the common bile duct is followed by dissection along the common hepatic duct, mistaken for the cystic duct, until a bile duct division occurs. Bifurcation of the common hepatic duct can be mistaken for the cystic duct/common duct intersection. Simultaneous injury to the right hepatic artery may occur, obscuring the visualization with hemorrhage. **D**, The resulting anatomy once the gallbladder and resected portion of the biliary tree have been removed. (CA-cystic artery; CD-cystic duct; CHA-common hepatic artery; CHD-common hepatic duct; PV-portal vein; RHA- right hepatic artery; RHD-right hepatic duct)

Other injuries to the biliary tree that have occurred during laparoscopic cholecystectomy include placement of clips across the common bile or right hepatic duct, particularly when bleeding or inflammation are present. The partial occlusion of the common duct lumen by clip placement too close to the junction of the cystic and common ducts, an injury also known from open cholecystectomy, is seen with laparoscopic cholecystectomy as well (Fig. 4).

Several factors have been cited as important contributors to bile duct injuries during laparoscopic cholecystectomy. Lack of experience by the surgeon appears to stand out as the single most important risk factor for a bile duct injury. In the experience of the Southern Surgeons Club, the incidence of bile duct injuries was 1.7% for surgeons in their first 13 cases, but dropped to 0.17% in subsequent cases (Meyers *et al.*, Paper presented at National Institutes of Health Conference on "Gallstones and Laparoscopic Cholecystectomy," Bethesda, MD, 1992). In that study the operative experience of the surgeon was the only significant factor found to correlate positively with the rate of bile duct injury.

Other differences between laparoscopic versus open cholecystectomy may contribute to the incidence of bile duct injuries. The surgeon may initially have visual difficulty in clearly defining the relevant biliary anatomy due to differences in loss of depth perception with laparoscopy. Inexperience in performing dissection of the relevant biliary structures using laparoscopic techniques may also be important. However, videotapes of some bile duct injuries, when reviewed, have often shown that factors not unique to laparoscopic surgery, such as poor surgical technique and suboptimal visualization, are important contributors to these complications [43].

Improper exposure of the cystic duct and the triangle of Calot can predispose to bile duct injury. Improper retraction of the cystic duct distorts the relationship between the cystic duct and common bile ducts so that the surgeon may mistake the common bile duct for the cystic duct (Fig. 3B). This is particularly true if the cys-

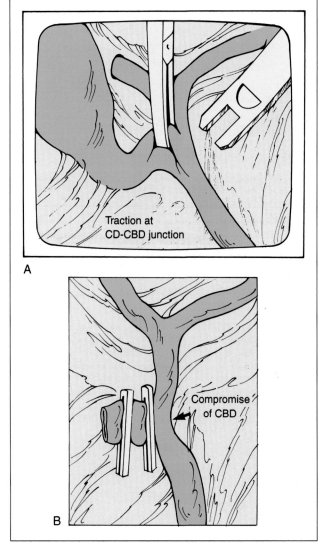

Traction at
CD-CBD junction

A

Compromise
of CBD

B

Figure 4. Traction at the junction of the cystic and common bile ducts distorts the common bile duct, predisposing to partial occlusion from clips placed across what is perceived as the base of the cystic duct.

tic duct is short. Failure to identify the infundibular end of the gallbladder and the takeoff of the cystic duct is a common error in cases of injury to the biliary tree.

Steps that can assist the surgeon in clear identification of the biliary anatomy include retraction of the gallbladder away from the liver bed by the assistant (Fig. 5), allowing maximum exposure of the structures within the triangle of Calot. The peritoneum covering this area should always be removed. Dissection of the cystic duct is more safely performed by beginning on the lateral side of the gallbladder and proceeding medially (Fig. 6). Dissection from the infundibulum of the gallbladder down to the cystic duct is the safest way to delineate the necessary anatomy for performing laparoscopic cholecystectomy. Clear identification of the takeoff of the cystic duct is probably the most important step in preventing bile duct injury.

The role of the first assistant in exposing the triangle

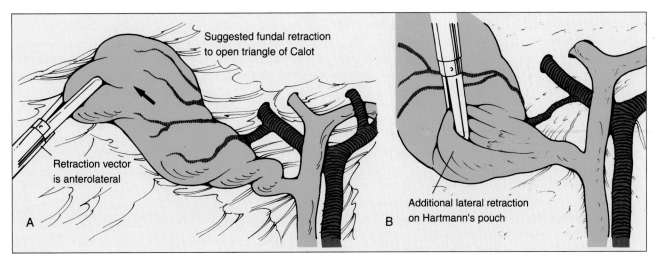

Figure 5. Recommended retraction of the gallbladder by the first assistant during laparoscopic cholecystectomy. **A,** Retraction vector of the fundus of the gallbladder, once cephalad exposure is adequate, is in the anterolateral direction to maximally expose the triangle of Calot. **B,** Additional lateral retraction of Hartmann's pouch will allow further visualization of the cystic duct takeoff, especially if a stone is impacted in the distal gallbladder or the cystic duct is short.

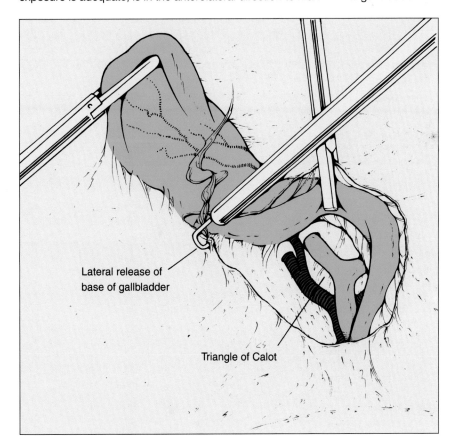

Figure 6. By incision of the lateral peritoneal attachments of the infundibulum of the gallbladder, safe exposure of triangle of Calot is obtained and maximal visualization is achieved before the more variable medial side of the infundibulum is dissected.

of Calot and the infundibular area of the gallbladder is extremely important. Fixed retraction of the gallbladder fundus by the right anterior axillary trocar, at times securing it to the drapes, is to be condemned. The first assistant should instead use a two-handed technique, using the grasping forceps from the right axillary and right midclavicular trocars in the right and left hands, respectively. This technique prevents fixed posterior and cephalad retraction of the gallbladder and allows more lateral retraction of the infundibulum.

Authors have differed in their beliefs about the value of intraoperative cholangiography in preventing bile duct injuries during laparoscopic cholecystectomy. Surgeons who are advocates of routine cholangiography during laparoscopic cholecystectomy include this factor in their argument for routine cholangiography [44•]. They argue that cholangiography can alert the surgeon to anatomic irregularities or misidentification errors already committed, and can clarify questionable biliary anatomy. Surgeons who perform cholangiography selectively are more likely to cite statistics showing that many bile duct injuries have already occurred at the time a cholangiogram is performed, or occur despite an abnormal cholangiogram [8••,37].

Review of series of common bile duct injuries shows that clear identification and dissection of the biliary tree are probably more important than intraoperative cholangiography for preventing bile duct injuries. However, in defense of routine cholangiography, it is true that the procedure clarifies the biliary anatomy in the surgeon's mind if it is properly performed and interpreted. Under these circumstances, it also lessens the severity of bile duct injuries if they have already occurred, and prevents resection of portions of the biliary tree. In addition, it should limit the number of unrecognized bile duct injuries.

Bile duct injury may occur more frequently in the setting of severe scarring or acute cholecystitis. In such situations accurate identification of biliary anatomy is more difficult than in the elective setting with minimal scarring. Surgeons should always adhere to the dictum that open cholecystectomy should be performed whenever laparoscopic visualization is unclear.

Measures that the surgeon and the surgical team may take to avoid injury to the bile duct during laparoscopic cholecystectomy are summarized in Table 2. These are taken from articles in the literature [45••,46•] and our own experience. Essentially all point to the need for surgical experience in both the surgeon and the assistant, excellent visualization of the cystic duct and infundibular area of the gallbladder, and avoidance of placing clips blindly or in situations in which the anatomy is not absolutely clear. Conversion to open cholecystectomy should be a relatively unimportant point in reporting results from laparoscopic cholecystectomy; it is far better to convert a higher percentage of cases to open cholecystectomy than to cause bile duct injuries when the anatomy is unclear.

MANAGEMENT OF BILE DUCT INJURIES

Bile duct injuries are as likely to go unrecognized as to be identified at the time of operation. Reports have shown that approximately 50% of injuries are unrecognized during the operation [17••]. When they are recognized, there is an improved chance for definitive repair, which should be performed immediately if the surgeon is experienced with such procedures. Surgeons inexperienced with biliary reconstruction should refer their patients to someone with experience. Reports are appearing from tertiary care centers, where a significant

---

Table 2. Steps to help avoid bile duct injury

Provision for adequate experience by surgical team

Conversion to open cholecystectomy whenever anatomy unclear

Avoidance of blind clipping or cautery to control bleeding

Careful dissection of cystic duct takeoff from gallbladder

Adequate cephalad retraction of fundus of gallbladder

Lateral retraction of infundibulum of gallbladder

Use of two-handed dynamic retraction by first assistant

Use of 30° telescope to help view hilar structures

Use of intraoperative cholangiography

Cautious interpretation of cholangiograms

Avoidance of excessive traction on cystic/common duct junction

Use of suction and irrigation device to improve visualization

Data from Hunter [45] and Way [46].

percentage of the patients referred for bile duct injuries are seen after a previous biliary reconstruction has been performed unsuccessfully at the referring hospital. Stricture formation after biliary reconstruction can be common, but in experienced hands the success rate for surgical reconstruction is in the 85% to 90% range. In addition, tertiary centers often have better support from invasive radiology teams to assist in cases in which non-surgical treatments suffice.

Patients with unrecognized bile duct injuries generally present with symptoms soon after surgery. Complaints of abdominal pain and tenderness are often present within 24 hours. Jaundice and fever can also be present. Exceptions to this picture of early symptoms are patients with cystic stump leakage, which may not begin until days after surgery, when the injured stump becomes necrotic and the clip falls off. Similarly, patients with cautery or laser injury to the bile duct can present with late stricture formation and jaundice.

Evaluation of patients who present postoperatively with a question of bile duct leakage should include ultrasonography of the abdomen to assess for fluid collection. If a bile fluid collection is documented by ultrasonography and subsequent aspiration, the patient should undergo celiotomy (especially if any sign of peritonitis is present) or further diagnostic evaluation. Patients with jaundice and biliary ductal dilatation on ultrasonography should undergo percutaneous transhepatic cholangiography to accurately diagnose and define the proximal extent of biliary tract injury and obstruction. Patients with bile leakage but no sign of jaundice or extrahepatic bile duct obstruction should undergo endoscopic retrograde cholangiography (ERC) to identify the source of the bile leak and biliary tree injury.

Some authors have recommended the use of radionuclide scans to determine if bile leakage is present [47]. Although this test may confirm that suspicion, an ultrasonogram and fluid aspiration should confirm it as well. Scans are not nearly as helpful as ERC in identifying the location of the bile leak. In addition, when ERC is accomplished, immediate endoscopic sphincterotomy, with or without stent placement or nasobiliary tube drainage, can be performed. After such treatment, small bile leaks may close spontaneously.

Repair of a bile duct injury is based on location and type of injury. Reconstruction using biliary-enteric anastomosis is necessary for all injuries that involve removal of a portion of the bile duct. Such procedures are best performed by surgeons with considerable experience in biliary reconstruction. Simple laceration of the bile duct can be repaired with primary reanastomosis and stenting with a T-tube. The length of time during which the tube should be left in place is not clear, but the significant incidence of stricture following such procedures suggests that a conservative approach is indicated.

Leakage from an incompletely secured cystic duct can be corrected by suture ligation. Depending on the time that has passed since the laparoscopic cholecystectomy and the laparoscopic experience and skill of the surgeon, this procedure may also potentially be done laparoscopically.

In view of the potential long-term morbidity of iatrogenic bile duct injuries, prevention of such injuries should be of paramount importance to the surgeon performing laparoscopic cholecystectomy. The surgeon who follows the principles outlined above for prevention of such injuries will minimize the incidence of bile duct injury.

REFERENCES

Papers of particular interest, published within the period of review, have been highlighted as:
• Of special interest
•• Of outstanding interest

1.   Mühe E: *Langenbecks Arch Chir* 1986, 369:804.

2.   Dubois F, Icard P, Berthelot G, Levard H: Coelioscopic Cholecystectomy: Preliminary Report of 36 Cases. *Ann Surg* 1990, 211:60–62.

3.   Society of American Gastrointestinal Endoscopic Surgeons: The Role of laparoscopic cholecystectomy (LC), Guidelines for Clinical Application. Los Angeles: Society of American Gastrointestinal Endoscopic Surgeons, 1990. [SAGES Publication No. 6 (1990).] SAGES, 11701 Texas Avenue, Suite 101, Los Angeles, CA 90025.

4.•   Society of American Gastrointestinal Endoscopic Surgeons: Granting of Privileges for Laparoscopic General Surgery. *Am J Surg* 1991, 161:324–325.

The best document for recommendations for granting of privileges as put forth by the society that has taken the leadership role in surgical laparoscopy.

5.   Society for Surgery of the Alimentary Tract. Guidelines for Credentialing and Privileging for Laparoscopic Cholecystectomy.

6.•   Hartman TW: Laparoscopic Cholecystectomy. Albany, NY: State of New York Department of Health Memorandum; 1992.

This document is important simply because of the massive interest and media attention that accompanied its release. Its figures lack significant meaning without a denominator of numbers of cases.

7.•• Airan M, Appel M, Berci G, *et al.*: Retrospective and Prospective Multi-Institutional Laparoscopic Cholecystectomy Study Organized by the Society of American Gastrointestinal Endoscopic Surgeons. *Surg Endosc* 1992, 6:169–176.

The largest multicenter experience reported in the United States that set the early standards for expected complication rates following laparoscopic cholecystectomy.

8.•• Larson GM, Vitale GC, Casey J, *et al.*: Multipractice Analysis of Laparoscopic Cholecystectomy in 1983 Patients. *Am J Surg* 1992, 163:221–226.

A very large multipractice series reporting excellent results with laparoscopic cholecystectomy. The discussion regarding the role of cholangiography and the incidence of bile duct injury is particularly well done.

9.•• Cushieri A, Dubois F, Mouiel J, *et al.*: The European Experience with Laparoscopic Cholecystectomy. *Am J Surg* 1991, 161:385–387.

A brief but outstanding article summarizing the results of laparoscopic cholecystectomy as performed by some of the best-known laparoscopic surgeons in Europe.

10.•• The Southern Surgeons Club: A Prospective Analysis of 1,518 Laparoscopic Cholecystectomies Performed by Southern U.S. Surgeons. *N Engl J Med* 1991, 324:1073–1078.

The most widely quoted and read early large US multicenter experience with laparoscopic cholecystectomy. It pointed out very early the importance of surgical experience with relation to bile duct injury.

11 Davis CJ, Arregui ME, Nagan RF, Shaar C: Laparoscopic Cholecystectomy: The St. Vincent Experience. *Surg Laparosc Endosc* 1992, 2:64–68.

12.• Schirmer BD, Edge SB, Dix J, *et al.*: Laparoscopic Cholecystectomy: Treatment of Choice for Symptomatic Cholelithiasis. *Ann Surg* 1991, 213:665–677.

An early series with comprehensive data on postoperative use of analgesics, factors influencing operative time, and conversion rate to open cholecystectomy.

13. Soper NJ, Stockmann PT, Dunnigan DL, Ashley SW: Laparoscopic Cholecystectomy: the New "Gold Standard"? *Arch Surg* 1992, 127:917–923.

Widely read article that documented the rationale for laparoscopic cholecystectomy's becoming the new standard for treatment of symptomatic cholelithiasis.

14. Baird DR, Wilson JP, Mason EM, *et al.*: An Early Review of 800 Laparoscopic Cholecystectomies at a University-Affiliated Community Teaching Hospital. *Am Surg* 1992, 58:206–210.

15.• Spaw AT, Reddick EJ, Olsen DO: Laparoscopic Laser Cholecystectomy: Analysis of 500 Procedures. *Surg Laparosc Endosc* 1991, 1:2–7.

A series by the group who first achieved renown for the performance of laparoscopic cholecystectomy in the United States, and who still have one of the lowest published complication rates.

16. Wolfe BM, Gardiner BN, Leary BF, Frey CF: Endoscopic Cholecystectomy: an Analysis of Complications. *Arch Surg* 1991, 126:1192–1198.

17.•• Dezeil DJ, Millikan KW, Airan MC, *et al*: Complications of Laparoscopic Cholecystectomy: Results of a National Survey of 4,292 Hospitals and Analysis of 77,604 Cases. *Am J Surg* 1993, 165:9–14.

An outstanding compilation of a huge number of cases of laparoscopic cholecystectomy. By far the largest retrospective review of this operation.

18.•• National Institutes of Health: NIH Consensus Conference: Gallstones and Laparoscopic Cholecystectomy. *JAMA* 1993, 269:1018–1024.

A concise summary statement of data presented over two days of hearings that substantiated the important role of laparoscopic cholecystectomy as a safe and improved treatment for gallstones.

19. Peterson HB, Hulka JF, Phillips JM: American Association of Gynecologic Laparoscopists' 1988 Membership Survey on Operative Laparoscopy. *J Reprod Med* 1990, 35:587–589.

20. Bruhl W: Complications of Laparoscopy and Liver Biopsy Under Vision: the Results of a Survey. *German Med Monthly* 1967, 12:31–32.

21. Kane MG, Krejs GJ: Complications of Diagnostic Laparoscopy in Dallas: a 7-Year Prospective Study. *Gastrointst Endosc* 1984, 30:237.

22. Schirmer BD, Dix J, Schmieg RE, Aguilar M: Laparoscopic Cholecystectomy in Patients with Previous Abdominal Surgery. *Surg Endosc* 1992, 6:107.

23. Borgatta L, Gruss L, Barad D, Kaali SG: Direct Trocar Insertion vs. Veress Needle Use for Laparoscopic Sterilization. *J Reprod Med* 1990, 35:891–894.

24. Yuzpe AA: Pneumoperitoneum Needle and Trocar Injuries in Laparoscopy: a Survey on Possible Contributing Factors and Prevention. *J Reprod Med* 1990, 35:485–490.

25. Kalhan SB, Reaney JA, Collins RL: *Cleve Clin J Med* 1990, 57:639–642.

26. Nord HJ, Boyd WP: Diagnostic Laparoscopy. *Endoscopy* 1992, 24:133–137.

27. Phillips J, Keith D, Hulka J, Keith L: Gynaecological Laparoscopy in 1975. *J Reprod Med* 1976, 16:205–217.

28. Shifren JL, Adlestein L, Finkler NJ: Asystolic Cardiac Arrest: a Rare Complication of Laparoscopy. *Obstet Gynecol* 1992, 79:840–841.

29.• Voyles CR, Petro AB, Meena AL, Haick AJ, Koury AM: A Practical Approach to Laparoscopic Cholecystectomy. *Am J Surg* 1991, 161:365–370.

This article contains an interesting discussion on the aspects of laser versus electrocautery use in laparoscopic cholecystectomy, as well as other aspects of the costs of the operation.

30. Thompson BH, Wheeless CR: Gastrointestinal Complications of Laparoscopy Sterilization. *Obstet Gynecol* 1973, 41:669—674.

31. DiGiovanni M, Vasilenko P, Belsky D: Laparoscopic Tubal Sterilization: the Potential for Thermal Bowel Injury. *J Reprod Med* 1990, 35:951–954.

32. Campbell WB, McGarity WC: An Unusual Complication of Laparoscopic Cholecystectomy. *Am Surgeon* 1992, 54:641–642.

33. McSherry CK: Cholecystectomy: the Gold Standard. *Am J Surg* 1989, 158:174–178.

34.• Beattie WS, Lindblade T, Buckley DN, Forrest JB: The Incidence of Postoperative Nausea and Vomiting in Women Undergoing Laparoscopy Is Influenced by the Day of Menstrual Cycle. *Can J Anaesth* 1991, 38:298–302.

An interesting article that should provide food for thought for all surgeons electively scheduling laparoscopic cholecystectomies for their female patients.

35.•• Davidoff AM, Pappas TN, Murray EA, *et al*.: Mechanisms of Major Biliary Injury During Laparoscopic Cholecystectomy. *Ann Surg* 1992, 215:196–202.

One of the earliest and best-written articles describing the "classic" injury to the bile ducts seen with laparoscopic cholecystectomy.

36. Moosa AR, Easter DW, Vansonnenberg E, *et al*: Laparoscopic Injuries to the Bile Duct: a Cause for Concern. *Ann Surg* 1992, 215:203–208.

37. Ferguson CM, Rattner DW, Warshaw AL: Bile Duct Injury in Laparoscopic Cholecystectomy. *Surg Laparosc Endosc* 1992, 1:1–7.

38. Wooton FT, Hoffman BJ, Marsh WH, Cunningham JT: Biliary Complications Following Laparoscopic Cholecystectomy. *Gastrointest Endosc* 1992, 38:183–185.

39. Gilliland TM, Traverso LW: Modern Standards for Comparison of Cholecystectomy with Alternative Treatments for Symptomatic Cholelithiasis with Emphasis on Long Term Relief of Symptoms. *Surg Gynecol Obstet* 1990, 170:39–44.

40. Graffis R: Laparoscopic Cholecystectomy: the Methodist Hospital Experience. *J Laparoendosc Surg* 1992, 1:69–73.

41. Zucker KA, Bailey RW, Gadacz TR, Imbembo AL: Laparoscopic Cholecystectomy: a Plea for Cautious Enthusiasm. *Am J Surg* 1991, 161:36–44.

42. Graber JN, Schultz LS, Pietrafitta JJ, Hickok DF: Complications of Laparoscoic Cholecystectomy: a Prospective Review of an Initial 100 Consecutive Cases. *Lasers Surg Med* 1992, 12:92–97.

43. Branum G, Schmitt C, Baille J, *et al*: Management of Major Biliary Complications After Laparoscopic Cholecystectomy. *Ann Surg* [in press].

44.• Sackier JM, Berci G, Phillips E, *et al*.: The Role of Cholangiography in Laparoscopic Cholecystectomy. *Arch Surg* 1991, 126:1021–1026.

An article outlining the case for performing routine intraoperative cholangiography during laparoscopic cholecystectomy.

45.•• Hunter JG: Avoidance of Bile Duct Injury During Laparoscopic Cholecystectomy. *Am J Surg* 1991, 161:71–76.

An excellent discussion of the technical aspects important in avoiding injury to the bile ducts during laparoscopic cholecystectomy.

46.• Way LW: Bile Duct Injury During Laparoscopic Cholecystectomy [Editorial]. *Ann Surg* 1992, 215:195.

Offers helpful suggestions for avoiding injury to the bile ducts during laparoscopic cholecystectomy.

47. Walker AT, Shapiro AW, Brooks DC, *et al*.: Bile Duct Disruption and Biloma After Laparoscopic Cholecystectomy: Imaging Evaluation. *AJR Am J Roentgenol* 1992, 158:785–789.

Chapter 9

Laparoscopic Treatment of Peptic Ulcer Disease

Namir Katkhouda
Jean Mouiel

Because of previous experience gained in basic laparoscopic procedures, the treatment of duodenal ulcer disease is now possible in elective cases by laparoscopic vagotomy. All types of vagotomy can be performed, *eg*, truncal vagotomy by an abdominal or thoracic approach or more selective procedures such as highly selective vagotomy, posterior truncal vagotomy together with highly selective anterior vagotomy, and posterior vagotomy together with anterior seromyotomy. In general, we recommend two laparoscopic procedures depending on the experience of the surgeon: total truncal vagotomy by laparoscopy or thoracoscopy as the more simple procedure, and posterior truncal vagotomy with anterior seromyotomy as described by Taylor as the more advanced procedure. Both techniques are rapid, reliable, and efficacious in our personal experience. The results obtained are comparable to those of these techniques when performed as conventional open surgery [1••,2•,3••]. Our technique of choice for an indicated surgical treatment of an intractable duodenal ulcer (2% to 5% of the ulcer patient population) is posterior vagotomy and anterior lesser curve seromyotomy.

TECHNIQUES

The preoperative evaluation of the patient, the use of general anesthesia with endotracheal intubation, and the perioperative management are all the same as in open surgery. We emphasize here the issues specific to laparoscopic or thoracoscopic procedures.

TOTAL TRUNCAL VAGOTOMY WITH ENDOSCOPIC PYLORIC DILATATION

Laparoscopic total vagotomy

Patient positioning and trocar insertion

The patient is placed in a supine position with legs spread apart. The operating surgeon stands between the patient legs. The pneumoperitoneum is created by insufflation of carbon dioxide, and a pressure of 14 mm Hg is maintained electronically. Once the abdominal wall is raised off the viscera, five trocars are introduced into the upper part of the abdomen, one for the video laparoscope (30°), one for the operating instruments, two for the grasping forceps, and one for the retractor or irrigator (Fig. 1).

Exploration

The abdominal cavity is explored as soon as the video laparoscope is inserted. The surgeon should be sure that the planned operation is feasible, and particularly that the liver can be retracted so that the operating area is visible. Associated lesions amenable to laparoscopic surgery are noted (*eg*, adhesions, appendicitis, cholecystitis, biliary cyst). If the operation is impossible or seems dangerous or difficult, *ie,* if the liver is cirrhotic, conversion to open surgery is preferred. The patient should be informed of this possibility beforehand. Through pre-

cise preoperative patient selection, we did not have to convert any case in our series.

Approaching the hiatus

The left lobe of the liver is retracted using a xiphoid palpation probe. The pars flaccida is seized on the right and left sides with grasping forceps, and the surgeon incises this membrane with the hook coagulator and enters the lesser sac above the hepatic branch of the anterior vagus nerve. The dissection is continued to the level of the right crus of the diaphragm. A coronary hepatic vein or accessory left hepatic artery may be encountered and have to be divided between two clips.

Posterior truncal vagotomy

The two landmarks for a posterior truncal vagotomy (Figs. 2 and 3) are the caudate lobe and the right crus of the diaphragm. The right crus is seized with the right grasping forceps and retracted to the right to expose the pre-esophageal peritoneum. The peritoneum is incised along the length of the border of the right crus, allowing the separation of the abdominal esophagus outward and to the left and permitting access to its posterior wall and mesoesophagus. Within the depths of this angle is located the white cord of the posterior vagus, easily recognized by its pearly aspect. It is grasped with retraction forceps, while its vasa vasorum is stripped with the hook coagulator. The nerve is transected

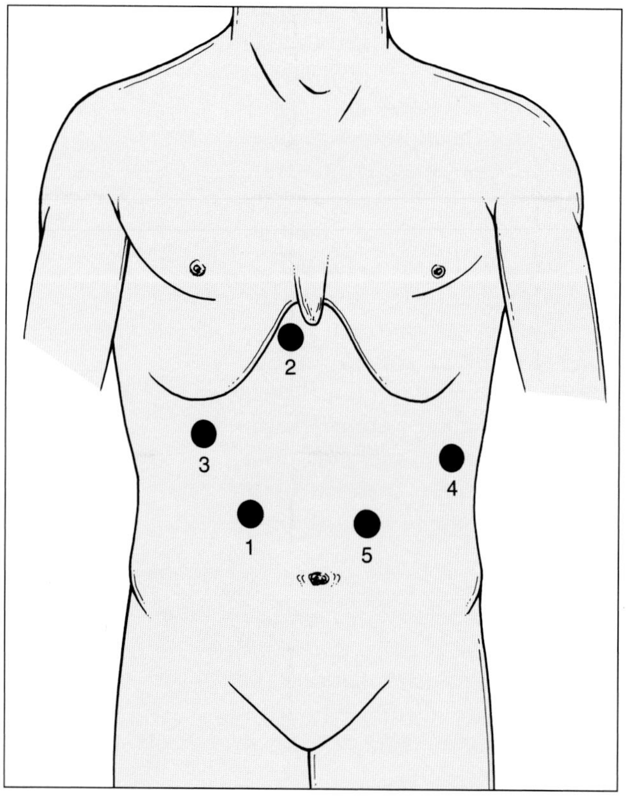

Figure 1. Laparoscopic approaches; trocar placement. **1**, videolaparoscopy trocar port (11 mm); **2**, palpator or irrigation-suction trocar port (5 mm); **3**, right grasping forceps port (10 mm), **4**, left grasping forceps port (10 mm); **5**, operating port (11 mm).

between two clips, and a 1 cm section is removed for histologic confirmation.

Anterior truncal vagotomy

This type of vagotomy consists of sectioning several trunks on the anterior esophagus. They are recognized by their cylindrical appearance and their vertical orientation under the pre-esophageal peritoneum, which is sectioned on the anterior wall of the abdominal esophagus. The transection of these fibers is easy because of their position over the muscular fibers of the esophagus. The only difficulty occurs on the left edge of the esophagus, where there is the possibility of overlooking some branches, even large ones (criminal branch of Grassi).

With the use of a traction forceps and a palpation probe, the esophagus can "roll" to the right so that the left edge is exposed, just as in open surgery to cut the "criminal nerves."

Pyloric dilatation

The dilatation is performed first using an upper fiberoptic endoscope during the same operative period. Two types of dilatation balloons can be used [4,5]. One type is a "through-the-scope" pyloric dilatation balloon of 15 mm that is inflated under manometric control to 45 psi for 10 minutes after ascertaining the correct position using endoscopy and laparoscopy. We prefer the use of the other type: an "over-the-wire" dilatator of 20 mm

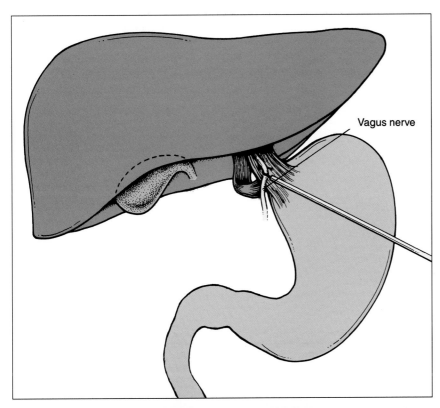

Vagus nerve

Figure 2. The posterior trunk of the vagus nerve is "hooked" in the angle formed by the right crus and the esophagus. Note the two landmarks of posterior truncal vagotomy: the caudate lobe and the right crus.

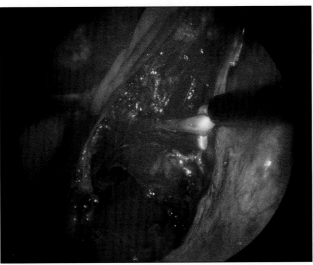

Figure 3. Right vagotomy by laparoscopy.

(inflated to 60 psi) or 30 mm (inflated to 90 psi) to avoid recurrence of pyloric spasm. Nevertheless, the dilatation may have to be repeated intraoperatively or postoperatively. This dilatation, however, is necessary in only 10% to 15% of all patients treated by total truncal vagotomy.

TOTAL TRUNCAL VAGOTOMY BY THORACOSCOPY

This new procedure according to the experience of Dubois [6••] is promising, but its place in the treatment of ulcer has yet to be assessed.

Positioning of the patient and trocar insertion

General anesthesia is carried out with a double endotracheal tube to permit collapse of the left lung. The patient is placed in a right lateral position as for a left semiposterior lateral thoracotomy. Four trocars are inserted; they are for the thoracoscope (at 30°), the irrigator, and the surgical instruments (Fig. 4). In thorascoscopy, carbon dioxide insufflation is not necessary, but if used should be at minimum flow and a pressure of 6 mm Hg

to obtain better collapse of the left lung and avoid a pulmonary embolism or the hazardous effects of electrosurgery. Safe cardiovascular monitoring is necessary to prevent side effects, especially cardiac arrhythmia.

Total vagotomy

The landmark of the procedure is the inferior pulmonary ligament, which is divided so that the left lung is retracted safely in a cephalad direction. The esophagus is identified in the space between the pericardium and the aorta, and the mediastinal pleura is divided using scissors or a hook coagulator. The esophagus could be manipulated with grasping forceps, dissected, and rolled out of its position, thereby avoiding right pleural effusion.

The first step is to expose the left side of the esophagus. Three or four trunks of the plexic anterior nerve are recognized. They are divided between clips, and a segment is removed for histologic examination. The posterior side is exposed in the second step. Usually the right nerve has a larger trunk. It is divided between clips, and a segment is resected for control (Fig. 5).

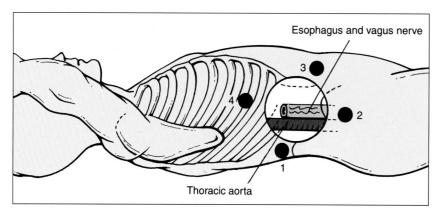

Esophagus and vagus nerve

Thoracic aorta

Figure 4. Thoracoscopic approaches; trocar placement. **1**, video thoracoscopy trocar port (10 mm); **2**, operating port (10 mm); **3**, palpator or irrigation-suction trocar port (5 mm); **4**, grasping forceps port (5 mm).

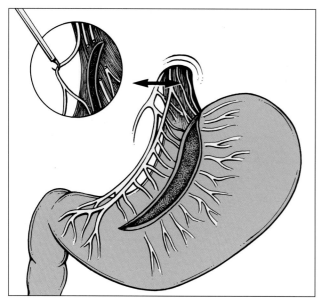

Figure 5. Anterior seromyotomy begins at the esogastric junction, courses parallel to the lesser curvature 1.5 cm from its border, and stops at the "crow's foot," respecting the two last branches. The highlighted portion depicts Taylor's technique.

Exsufflation

After the quality of hemostasis is checked by irrigating the area with warm isotonic saline, the lung is inflated, the trocars are withdrawn, and the incisions sutured without using a chest drain.

Pyloric dilatation

This dilatation is not performed at the same time and is done only if necessary 3 weeks after the initial procedure in the case of pylorospasm.

TECHNIQUE OF POSTERIOR TRUNCAL VAGOTOMY WITH ANTERIOR VAGOTOMY ACCORDING TO TAYLOR'S PROCEDURE

Patient positioning and trocar insertion are the same as for truncal vagotomy. The procedure takes place in three steps: approaching the hiatus, performing the posterior truncal vagotomy, and performing the anterior seromyotomy. The first two steps have been described; therefore, we now describe the anterior seromyotomy (Fig. 5).

Anterior seromyotomy

The anterior surface of the stomach is stretched with the right and left grasping forceps. The outline of the seromyotomy is marked with the hook coagulator, beginning exactly 1 cm from the lesser curvature at the level of the gastroesophageal junction. This distance is maintained parallel to the lesser curvature to a point that is 5 to 7 cm from the pylorus at the level of the trifurcation of the "crow's foot," respecting the integrity of the two inferior branches (Fig. 6). The seromyotomy is performed with the electric hook coagulator, using monopolar current and a setting of half section–half coagulation, and using medium force. The hook successively cuts through the serosa, the oblique puscular layers, and the superficial circular muscular layers. The two grasping forceps hold the edges and help stretch the deep circular fibers, which eventually split as a result of the combined effect of mechanical traction and hook coagulation. After these last muscular fibers are split, the bluish mucosa emerges, and verifying its integrity is easy because of the magnification provided by the video laparoscope, just as in microsurgery (Fig. 7). The seromyotomy is continued in the same fashion. During this part of the procedure, one may encounter three to five short vessels; three vessels should be transected after hemostasis. Several approaches can be used. As described by Taylor in his early cases, the vessels can be isolated in the seromuscularis by passing a hook beneath them and clipping and transecting them. Alternatively, one can use sutures with the aid of a Semm needle holder. All details of the exact anatomic location of the seromyotomy and hemostasis must be observed rigorously or the seromyotomy will be ineffective. Once the seromyotomy is achieved, it appears as a slice of 7- to 8-mm width. The integrity of the mucosa is carefully verified, if necessary, by inflating the stomach with methylene blue through the nasogastric tube. The seromyotomy is closed with a continuous suture in an overlap fashion and stopped with knots. This step completes the hemostasis and allows closure without drainage (Fig. 8). It will also prevent visceral adhesions on the seromyotomy.

A new procedure using the stapling device has been described recently and seems to offer more ease and speed in performing the anterior seromyotomy by anterior linear gastrectomy [7••] (Fig. 9). It has the inconvenience of transforming a benign functional operation into a gastric resection.

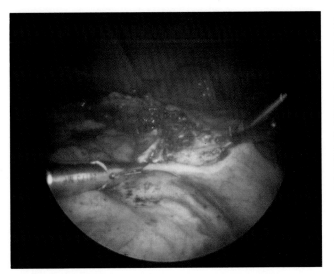

Figure 6. Two graspers hold the edges of the stomach, and the seromyotomy is achieved by combining spreading of tissues and cutting with the hook.

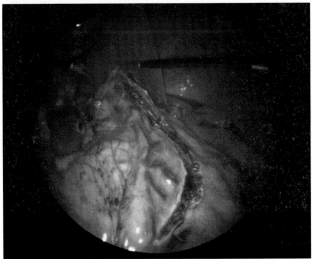

Figure 7. The seromyotomy begins at the cardiac incisura; the blue color of the gastric mucosa attests to the completion of the seromyotomy.

LAPAROSCOPIC TRUNCAL VAGOTOMY AND GASTROJEJUNOSTOMY

This operation (Fig. 10) is indicated for a complicated intractable duodenal ulcer such as gastric outlet obstruction by a chronic ulcer. To the truncal vagotomy described above and performed via a thoracoscopic approach or an abdominal approach, we can add a bypass operation (laparoscopic gastrojejunostomy). Ideally, the procedure should follow the "gold standards" of open gastrojejunostomy. The bypass should be 8 cm long, on the posterior aspect of the greater curvature, and close to the pylorus (6 cm away). This position is realized by opening a window in the transverse mesocolon just behind the colic arcade by using electrical scissors. The first intestinal loop is then exposed, and the second loop of jejunum is brought across the window. A gastrotomy and a small enterotomy are performed using an electrical hook. The linear cutter (60 mm) is introduced through the openings and fired. The internal aspect of the anastomosis is inspected and the hemostasis checked. The enterotomies and gastrotomies are finally closed with a second shot of the linear cutter, perpendicular to the first staple line.

OBSERVATIONS

By December 1992, we had performed 73 elective laparoscopic vagotomy procedures in 13 women and 50 men with a mean age of 33 years (range 19–62). These surgeries consisted of 70 Taylor's procedures, two total laparoscopic vagotomies with pyloric dilatation, and one thoracoscopic total vagotomy.

The selection of patients for laparoscopic surgery is similar to that of open surgery, and the same relative and absolute contraindications apply. For elective surgery, the surgical indications are those of patients with chronic duodenal ulcer disease resistant to optimal medical management. Fifty-two patients had had their disease for at least 4 years, and they all had an average of 2.8 recurrences under medical management. Among them, five patients presented with antecedent gastrointestinal bleeding. In five patients, the operation was done earlier in the disease because of problems of compliance to treatment or follow-up for geographic or socioeconomic reasons.

As for elective open surgery, preoperative work-up includes evaluation of risk factors as well as endoscopy and secretory studies. For all selected patients, endoscopy reveals a persistent duodenal ulcer that is usually linear and without associated stenosis or active bleeding. Secretory studies include complete acidity analysis, including the basal acid output and maximum acid output after pentagastrin stimulation. These tests are necessary to determine the degree of hyperacidity in these patients resistant to medical therapy as well as to provide a preoperative measurement to judge the effectiveness of subsequent surgical treatment by measuring postoperative acidity.

As in all uncomplicated laparoscopic surgery, the postoperative period is relatively calm. Pain is reduced because of minimal parietal trauma and the use of local anesthesic infiltration around the puncture points; systemic analgesics are unnecessary. The patients are ambulatory much sooner because of the lack of invasive

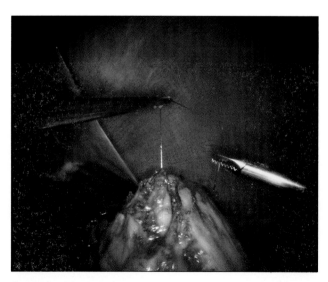

Figure 8. Closure of the seromyotomy by overlap running suture.

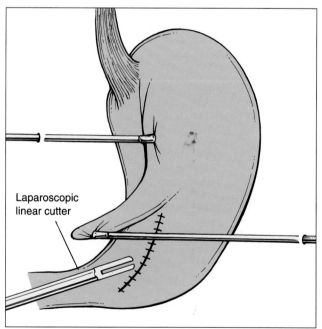

Laparoscopic linear cutter

Figure 9. Anterior linear gastrectomy.

postoperative care. A nasogastric tube is left in place for 24 hours, and oral fluids are resumed after the tube's removal. Unlike for open surgery, the patient is discharged between the third and fifth postoperative days, and we think this length my be shortened further.

In our experience, these laparoscopic procedures yield the same results as open surgery without mortality and with low morbidity. In the follow-up of Taylor's procedure patients, no bloating, diarrhea, or dumping were observed. Two patients developed a sensation of abdominal swelling caused by delayed gastric emptying 2 months postoperatively. The endoscopic control examinations showed in each case a bezoar, which was successfully treated. A third patient developed gastroesophageal reflux without hiatal hernia that was resistant to medical treatment including omeprazole and Cisapride. The patient underwent surgical correction 2 months later. In this patient, who had a history of treated nervous depression, the reflux was probably underevaluated before operation, but the final outcome was successful. In one of the two patients who underwent the total truncal vagotomy, a recurrent duodenal spasm occurred but resolved with redilatation. Retrospectively, we believe the duration of the first dilatation was probably too brief in this patient, who had had a preoperative spasmodic stenosis.

Postoperative upper endoscopic control examinations proved the complete healing of the duodenal ulcer in 67 cases without pain and a residual scar in three. The postoperative secretory control measurements revealed a decrease in the basal acid output value of 78.4% and maximum acid output of 82.7% at follow-up of 2 to 18 months. To this date, two recurrences were observed 2 years after a Taylor's procedure, but of course the follow-up period of the survey is as yet too short to be considered conclusive.

DISCUSSION

The fact that vagotomy heals duodenal ulcers by reducing acid secretion is well known [8]. Total truncal vagotomy leads to an almost total reduction of gastric acid secretion, which is accompanied by pyloric spasm and leads to gastric stasis [7••]. Therefore, this procedure is usually done in conjunction with a drainage procedure, such as pyloroplasty or gastrojejunostomy. The pylorospasm is not constant, however. Its frequency is approximately 20% as assessed by esophagal resection that leads to total vagotomy [9•]. With laparoscopic surgery, an extramucosal pylorotomy should be possible, similar to the pediatric surgery, but at this time such a procedure is still experimental. Thus, we recommend dilatation of the pylorus as a simple and effective procedure that can be repeated in the event of failure and that assures satisfactory drainage of the stomach [2•,5]. Laparoscopic truncal vagotomy with balloon pyloric dilatation via an abdominal approach is a rapid, reproducible procedure with few side effects. The side effects of this procedure are the same as for open surgery in terms of postoperative morbidity: diarrhea, gastric stasis, and dumping. Dubois [6••] recently described the laparoscopic thoracic truncal vagotomy approach for treatment of chronic duodenal ulcer. Pyloric dilatation is performed after 3 weeks for pylorospasm. Recently we became interested in this procedure because of a patient who had been operated upon several times before, and

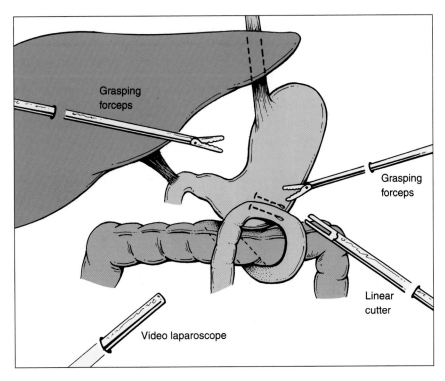

Figure 10. Laparoscopic gastrojejunostomy. **1**, video laparoscope; **2**, linear cutter; **3**, grasping forceps.

Grasping forceps

Grasping forceps

Linear cutter

Video laparoscope

for whom the abdominal approach would be difficult. The ideal indication for thoracic truncal vagotomy is a peptic ulcer after a B-II gastric resection, resistant to a thorough medical treatment.

The posterior truncal vagotomy associated with anterior seromyotomy represents a true advance and an ideal operation [9•]. Acid production is reduced and, by preserving the antropyloric branches of the anterior nerve of Latarget, motility of the antropyloric pump is conserved. This situation avoids pylorospasm and assures the physiologic emptying of the stomach, making drainage procedures unnecessary. This ultraselective anterior vagotomy is rapidly and easily performed by means of a seromyotomy that parallels the lesser curvature from the gastroesophageal junction to the crow's foot. This seromyotomy interrupts the intraparietal tracts and branches of the anterior Latarjet nerve, which accompany short blood vessels entering the gastric wall obliquely. To be efficacious, the seromyotomy must be carried out exactly 1 cm from the lesser curvature, thus respecting the antropyloric branches [8,10••,11••,12]. This requirement has been experimentally established by Daniel and Sarna [12], who showed that the antropyloric branches of the anterior Latarget nerve are sufficient to assure gastric emptying because of vasovagal reflex arcs.

Over the past few years, multicenter controlled clinical studies have shown these two procedures to be effective in healing ulcers, with practically no morbidity or mortality. The recurrence rate is comparable to the open procedure, ranging from 3% to 6% at 5 years. The side effects of diarrhea and dumping syndrome are more common with total truncal vagotomy. Taylor's procedure causes virtually no disturbance of gastric emptying. In the case of delayed gastric emptying, the problem may be overcome by endoscopic dilatation of the pylorus. The rate of patient satisfaction with these procedures with respect to recovery and return to normal activities is 70% for total truncal vagotomy and 90% for Taylor's procedure [2•,11••,14,15].

Our laparoscopic experience is comparable to our experience with open surgery. It was achieved in a straightforward fashion, and we have never had to interrupt a laparoscopy, even at the beginning of our experience. In our experience, the procedure lasts from 55 to 190 minutes (mean 60 minutes). Three technical points merit emphasis. First, the initial exposure of the esophagus in the first cases was facilitated by transillumination via a gastroscope, which allowed us to identify the landmarks for the posterior vagotomy. Second, the seromyotomy was performed in the same fashion as in open surgery for several years, using the method of Kahwaji and Grange [16], which begins at the level of the gastroesophageal junction and parallels the lesser curvature until the crow's foot area. This technique contrasts with that of Taylor, who starts at the anterior aspect of the esophagus. With the Taylor approach, one encounters three to five short blood vessels, and hemostasis is achieved according to the above-described technique. With meticulous care, we have never had a hemorrhagic complication nor gastric necrosis. Third, we recommend performing the overlap suture with a straight 20-mm needle and monofilament thread. This method avoids the rotations of a curved needle and facilitates formation of interrupted knots.

The results of this initial experience are promising and comparable to our results with open surgery as well as those in the literature [15,17–19]. Naturally, these results need to be confirmed by multicenter, controlled prospective studies with a follow-up period of at least 5 years. Other highly selective vagotomy procedures have been performed [6••]. By the opinion of experienced laparoscopic surgeons, however, these procedures are tedious, lasting several hours. Recently, Bailey and coworkers [20••] published a combined laparoscopic cholecystectomy and selective vagotomy according to the procedure of Hill and Barker [21]. This procedure consists of a posterior truncal vagotomy and anterior highly selective vagotomy, and initial results are good. The technical danger of this procedure is the possibility of bleeding that could lead to a hematoma of the lesser sac and cause the procedure to be difficult to pursue. Also, multicenter studies of the open, conventional surgery are necessary to assess the value of the technique before proposing it be done on a large scale by laparoscopy.

CONCLUSION

Duodenal ulcer is a common disease. More than 100,000 new cases occur annually in France (prevalence of the disease). Despite the large number of effective medical treatments available, the recurrence rate of ulcers treated medically is on the order of 90% at 1 year, regardless of which medication is used if medical treatment is discontinued after the initial treatment. Furthermore, the widespread use of these agents over the past 10 years has not diminished the mortality caused by complications of ulcer disease, particularly in the elderly [19]. A minimally invasive, effective vagotomy performed by laparoscopy has a place in the management of patients with intractable chronic duodenal ulcer, and this treatment can be offered to 2% to 5% of ulcer patients. Multicenter prospective studies are needed to assess the early results. Thorough experimental training is an unquestionable condition before a surgeon should perform this procedure on patients.

REFERENCES

Papers of particular interest, published within the period of review, have been highlighted as:
• Of special interest
•• Of outstanding interest

1.•• Katkhouda N, Mouiel J: Laparoscopic Treatment of Peptic Ulcer Disease. In *Minimal Invasive Surgery*. Edited by Hunter J, Sackier J. New York: McGraw Hill; 1993:123–130.

Description of the laparoscopic procedures for treatment of peptic ulcer disease, focusing on posterior vagotomy and anterior seromyotomy.

2.• Mouiel J, Katkhouda N: Laparoscopic Truncal and Selective Vagotomy. In *Surgical Laparoscopy*. Edited by Zucker KA. St. Louis: Quality Medical Publishing; 1991:263–279.

Description of initial experience with drawings.

3.•• Katkhouda N, Mouiel J: Laparoscopic Treatment of Peritonitis. In *Update in Surgical Laparoscopy*. Edited by Zucker KA. St. Louis: Quality Medical Publishing; 1992, 8:287–300.

Description of treatment of perforated ulcer.

4. Taylor TV: Experience with the Lunderquist Ownman Dilator in the Upper Gastro-Intestinal Tract. *Br J Surg* 1983, 710:445.

5. Craig PI, Gillespie PE: Through the Endoscope Balloon Dilatation of Benign Gastric Outlet Obstruction. *Br Med J* 1988, 297:396.

6.•• Dubois F: La Chirurgie de l'Ulcére Duodénal. In *La Chirurgie Digestive par Voie Coelioscopique*. Edited by Testas P, Delaitre B. Paris: Maloine; 1991:127–136.

Dubois' experience with truncal vagotomy and initial highly selective vagotomy.

7.•• Hannon JK, Snow LL, Weinstein SL: Endoscopic Staple Assisted Anterior Highly Selective Vagotomy Combined with Posterior Truncal Vagotomy for Treatment of Peptic Ulcer Disease. *Surg Laparosc Endosc* 1992, 2, 3:254–257.

The first published case report on stapled linear gastrectomy with posterior vagotomy.

8. Dragstedt LR: Section of the Vagus Nerves to the Stomach in the Treatment of Peptic Ulcer. *Ann Surg* 1947, 126:687–708.

9.• Bemelman WA, Brummelkamp WH, Bartelsman JFWM: Endoscopic Balloon Dilation of the Pylorus After Esophagogastrectomy Without a Drainage Procedure. *Surg Gynecol Obstet* 1990, 170:424–426.

Proof of unnecessary pyloroplasty after esophagogastrectomy.

10.•• Taylor TV, Lythgoe JP, McFarland JB, *et al.*: Anterior Lesser Curve Seromyotomy and Posterior Truncal Vagotomy Versus Truncal Vagotomy and Pyloroplasty in the Treatment of Chronic Duodenal Ulcer. *Br J Surg* 1990, 77:1007–1009.

Recent paper on Taylor's experience in open surgery.

11.•• Katkhouda N, Mouiel J: A New Surgical Technique of Treatment of Chronic Duodenal Ulcer Without Laparotomy by Videocelioscopy. *Am J Surg* 1991, 161:361–364.

First publication worldwide on laparoscopic vagotomy.

12. Taylor TV: Lesser Curve Superficial Seromyotomy: An Operation for Chronic Duodenal Ulcer. *Br J Surg* 1979, 66:733–737.

13. Daniel EE, Sarna SK: Distribution of Excitatory Vagal Fibers in Canine Gastric Wall to Central Motility. *Gastroenterology* 1976, 71:608–612.

14. Hoffman J, Jensen HE, Christiansen J, *et al.*: Prospective Controlled Vagotomy Trial for Duodenal Ulcer. Results After 11–15 Years. *Ann Surg* 1989, 209:40–45.

15. Pringle R, Irving AD, Longrigg JN, Wisbey M: Randomized Trial of Truncal Vagotomy With Either Pyloroplasty or Pyloric Dilatation in the Surgical Management of Chronic Duodenal Ulcer. *Br J Surg* 1983, 70:482.

16. Kahwaji F, Grange D: Ulcére Duodénal Chronique. Traitement par Séromyotomie Fundique Antérieure avec Vagotomie Tronculaire Postérieure. *Presse Médicale* 1987, 16(1):28–30.

17. Triboulet JP: Progrés dans le Traitement de l'Ulcére Duodénal: La Séromyotomie avec Vagotomie. In *Actualités Digestives Médico-Chirurgicales*, vol 10. Edited by Mouiel J. Paris: Masson; 1989, 15–22.

18. Oost Vogel HJM, Van Vroonhoven TJMV: Anterior Seromyotomy and Posterior Truncal Vagotomy. Technic and Early Results of a Randomized Trial. *Neth J Surg* 1985, 37:69–74.

19. Taylor TV, Gunn AA, MacLeod DAD, *et al.*: Morbidity and Mortality After Anterior Lesser Curve Seromyotomy and Posterior Truncal Vagotomy for Duodenal Ulcer. *Br J Surg* 1985, 72:950.

20.•• Bailey RW, Flowers JL, Graham SM, Zucker KA: Combined Laparoscopic Cholecystectomy and Selective Vagotomy. *Surg Laparosc Endosc* 1991, 1:45–49.

Open surgery experience on a few patients by anterior highly selective vagotomy and posterior truncal vagotomy.

21. Hill GL, Barker MCJ: Anterior Highly Selective Vagotomy with Posterior Truncal Vagotomy: A Simple Technique for Denervating the Parietal Cell Mass. *Br J Surg* 1978, 65:702–705.

Chapter 10

Laparoscopic Management of Gastroesophageal Reflux Disease

Bernard Dallemagne
Joseph M. Weerts
Constant Jehaes
Serge Markiewicz

Gastroesophageal reflux is often considered synonymous with hiatal hernia but is not. Although symptoms of reflux are most commonly associated with hiatal hernia (80%), reflux can occur in the absence of hernia, and hernias are often symptom-free. Gastroesophageal reflux disease (GERD) is produced by increased esophageal exposure to gastric juice, which induces esophagitis, esophageal ulceration with hemorrhage or perforation, stricture, and Barrett metaplasia [1].

One cause of increased esophageal exposure to gastric juice is a mechanically defective lower esophageal sphincter, which accounts for approximately 60% of GERD [2]. Other causes are inefficient esophageal clearance of refluxed gastric juice and an abnormality of the gastric reservoir that augments physiologic reflux [3,4,5••,6]. The goal of antireflux operations is to increase the efficacy of the lower esophageal sphincter and the cardia.

A rational, stepwise approach is thus necessary to determine the cause of abnormal exposure to gastric juice and the specific therapy needed to correct the abnormality. The most appropriate way of proving pathologic exposure of the esophagus to gastric juice is by 24-hour pH metry. Gastroesophageal manometry is the most valuable tool available to detect an insufficient valve mechanism at the lower esophageal sphincter. A complete assessment of GERD includes endoscopy, an upper gastrointestinal series, manometry, and 24-hour pH metry. As mentioned, hiatal hernia can be responsible for GERD. By itself, hiatal hernia can cause symptoms without evidence of GERD [7].

TREATMENT

Treatment of gastroesophageal reflux is first medical: diet, prokinetic agents, anti-H2 blockers, and omeprazole. A mechanically defective lower esophageal sphincter that causes GERD will not be treated successfully by medical treatment, however, and esophageal-mucosa injuries will recur as soon as the therapy is discontinued. The presence of gastric juice contaminated with duodenal contents explains why some patients fail medical therapy that aimed only at suppression of acid secretion. Other noxious ingredients of gastric juice, such as pepsin, trypsin, and bile salts, maintain the mucosal injury [5••]. Complications of GERD are particularly frequent and severe in patients with the combination of a defective lower esophageal sphincter and increased esophageal acid and alkaline exposure.

Surgical treatment must be considered if medical therapy fails. Numerous surgical antireflux techniques have been developed; these procedures include reconstruction of the angle of Hiss, angulation of the cardioesophageal junction with the ligamentum teres, and anterior, posterior, or complete valvuloplasty. The most effective procedures to date, however, appear to be the modified Nissen and Belsey Mark IV procedures [8].

With the development of laparoscopic procedures and the success of laparoscopic cholecystectomy, a variety of different laparoscopic approaches to gastroesophageal reflux have been described, including Nissen fundoplication, cardiopexy using the ligamentum teres, insertion of an Angelchik prosthesis, Toupet or Lind fundoplication, Thal fundoplication, and the Belsey Mark IV procedure.

PATIENT SELECTION

Once a patient has undergone a failed attempt to control symptomatic GERD with medical therapy, the indication to proceed with antireflux surgery is documentation of a mechanically defective lower esophageal sphincter and increased exposure to gastric juice [6]. Patients with significant complications, such as Barrett esophagus, deep ulceration with bleeding, recurrent aspiration, or esophageal stricture, should be evaluated individually to determine the appropriate timing of surgical intervention.

Some patients have large paraesophageal hiatal hernias or small hiatal hernias with a Schatzki ring. They complain mainly of dysphagia, chest pain, and sometimes heartburn. The lower esophageal sphincter is often normal. Surgical repair will relieve the symptoms but must be done with an antireflux procedure because of the potential destruction of the competency of the cardioesophageal junction during the reduction of the hernia [7]. Criteria for acceptability for surgery are the same as for all abdominal surgery. A standard preanesthetic work-up is done.

TYPES OF ANTIREFLUX OPERATIONS
Laparoscopic ligamentum teres cardiopexy

This procedure has been described by Nathanson and coworkers [9]. They adapted a technique described by Narbona-Arnau and coworkers [10] in 1965 in which

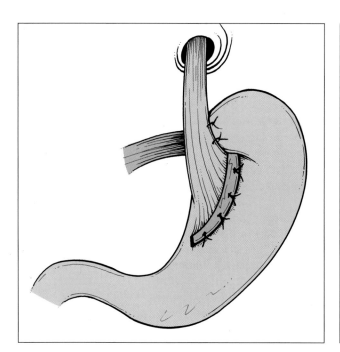

Figure 1. Ligamentum teres cardiopexy.

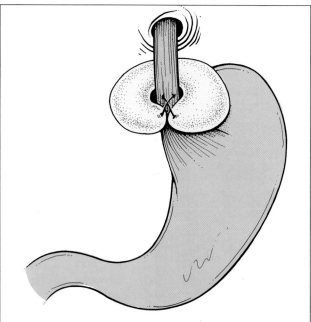

Figure 2. Placement of the Angelchik prosthesis.

the ligamentum teres is used to lengthen the intraab-dominal segment of the esophagus and to increase the high-pressure zone at the lower esophageal sphincter.

Technique

A five-puncture technique is used. The procedure consists of three sequential parts: mobilization of the ligamentum teres and preservation of its blood supply, mobilization of the abdominal esophagus, and cardiopexy using a ligamentum teres sling (Fig. 1). The degree of traction on the ligamentum influences both the length of the intraabdominal segment of the esophagus and the pressure within the lower esophageal sphincter. The degree of traction is adjusted by esophageal manometry to achieve a pressure increment of 15 to 20 mm Hg.

Early (1 to 6 month) postoperative results published [9] were satisfactory, but after an initial report of five operations, they do not use this technique any more. The main problem encountered in this procedure is the progressive fibrosis of the ligamentum teres. In conventional surgery, however, Narbonna and coworkers reported up to 94% good results (Narbonna, Personal communication).

Laparoscopic placement of Angelchik prosthesis

In 1979, Angelchik and Cohen [11] published encouraging preliminary results from a study of the use of a prosthesis in 46 patients with GERD. The device is a silicone ring that is secured around the distal esophagus to restore lower esophageal sphincter function (Fig. 2). Since the original report, an estimated 30,000 antireflux prostheses have been placed, with a published success rate of 80% to 90% [12]. Multiple prospective clinical trials comparing the Angelchik procedure with conventional antireflux operations have demonstrated the efficacy of the technique in controlling symptomatic gastroesophageal reflux.

Those results have been overshadowed, however, by reports of migration or disruption of the prosthesis, sepsis, persistent dysphagia, and erosion into the stomach or esophagus. Thus, the prosthesis has been redesigned to avoid migration and disruption. In 1991 Berguer and coworkers [13] reported experience with laparoscopic placement of Angelchik prostheses in pigs. Controversies still exist with the Angelchik prosthesis, and the investigators have begun new clinical trials.

Laparoscopic Nissen fundoplication

Nissen's technique [14] initially consisted of the invagination of the esophagus into a sleeve of the gastric wall obtained from the upper portion of the stomach. The gastrosplenic vessels and the diaphragmatic hiatus were untouched. Numerous adaptations were subsequently applied to the original technique; these adaptations included closure of the hiatal orifice, more or less exten-sive mobilization of the fundus, modifications of the valve, and variations of the length of the valve [15,16].

Two types of laparoscopic Nissen's procedures have been described to date. We [17•] started with the Nissen fundoplication in January 1991, and Geagea [18•] described the Nissen-Rosetti adaptation the same year. Geagea's adaptation eliminates the need to take down the short gastric vessels. A different part of the fundus is used for the fundoplication. Our approach is based on a previous study by DeMeester and coworkers [16] that compared different types of fundoplication and their results. They concluded that a short wrap (1 cm) is associated with a lower rate of postoperative dysphagia. The fundoplication is constructed with the mobilized gastric fundus to ensure complete relaxation of the reconstructed cardia.

Technique

The operative technique has been described previously [19]. The patient is positioned in a modified lithotomy position and the surgeon works between the spread legs of the patient with an assistant on each side. A five-trocar approach is used. Figure 3 shows the placement of the trocars. The laparoscope is introduced through trocar number one. Trocars three and two are used by the surgeon's left hand (dissecting forceps) and right hand (scissors, clip-applier, needle holder), respectively. Trocar number four is used for the liver retractor, and trocar number five is used by the assistant on the right side (grasping forceps).

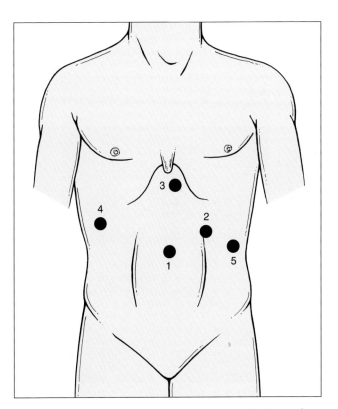

Figure 3. Positioning of the laparoscopic ports for the performance of a Nissen fundoplication (personal technique).

The usual steps of the Nissen fundoplication are successively performed:

1. Mobilization of the distal esophagus by opening the hiatus and blunt dissecting along the right and left crura (Fig. 4)
2. Dissection of the posterior aspect of the esophagus including identification of the posterior vagus nerve and retroesophageal channel, which will admit the wrap (Fig. 5)
3. Crural repair by using posterior stitches on the crural muscles (Fig. 6)
4. Mobilization of the gastric fundus by taking down the short gastric vessels
5. Passage of the gastric fundus around the esophagus to create the wrap (Fig. 7)
6. Calibration of the wrap with a 50-F bougie

7. Fixation of the wrap (1–2 cm long) using three interrupted or running nonabsorbable sutures, while the esophagogastric junction is being calibrated with a 50-F bougie (Fig. 8)

We use the Nissen-Rosetti variation in two types of situations. In large, sliding hiatal hernias, the short gastric vessels are not short any more, and we can create a wrap without any tension. When we perform antireflux repairs associated with highly selective vagotomy, we prefer to preserve the gastrosplenic ligament to avoid necrosis of the gastric wall. For both indications, a short wrap is constructed.

No nasogastric tube is left in place, and the patient is allowed to drink on the first evening. At the latest, an intravenous line is left in place until the morning of the first postoperative day. On the second postoperative

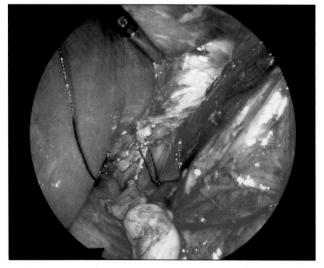

Figure 4. Dissection of the hiatal orifice and elongation of the intraabdominal esophagus.

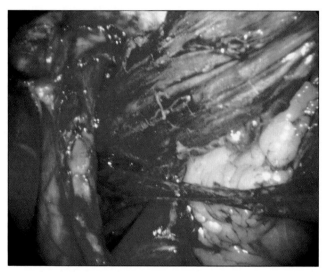

Figure 5. Dissection of the retroesophageal channel. This step includes identification of posterior vagus nerve, both crura, and esophagus.

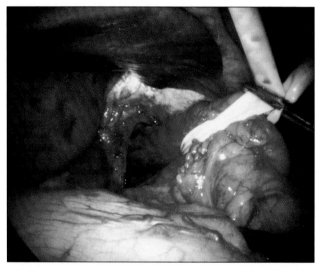

Figure 6. Crural repair, showing separated stitches.

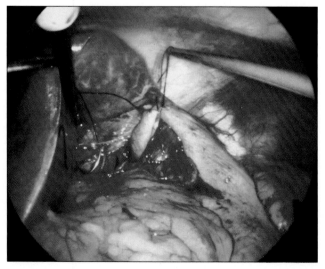

Figure 7. Wrapping of the gastric fundus around the esophagus, showing the first stitch in place.

day, a barium upper gastrointestinal series is performed to verify the position and proper functioning of the antireflux valve. The patient is discharged after this examination. Dietary instructions are given to avoid the risk of food impaction in the distal esophagus during the early postoperative period.

Geagea [18•] uses similar trocar positioning. Retraction of the liver is done trough the subxiphoid trocar. He uses a 60-F bougie and performs a 1- to 2-cm short wrap without taking down the short gastric vessels.

Cuschieri and coworkers [20•] reported their experience of laparoscopic treatment of large hiatal hernia in eight patients. They place the patient in the supine position, and the surgeon stands on the left side. A five-trocar approach is used that is different from the previously described techniques. Figure 9 shows their placement of trocars. They use a left-crus approach to the esophagus. Most of the dissection starts from the left side as in the dissection of the retroesophageal channel. They perform a crural repair. The short gastric vessels are kept intact, and they fix the wrap to the anterior margin of the hiatus and the anterior wall of the esophagus.

Laparoscopic Toupet and Lind techniques

The Toupet [21] and Lind [22] techniques differ from the Nissen technique in that the wrap does not go entirely around the esophagus. In both techniques, the wrap stops at left and right anterior margins of the esophagus, thus creating a 270° wrap in the Lind procedure and a 180° wrap in the Toupet operation (Fig. 10).

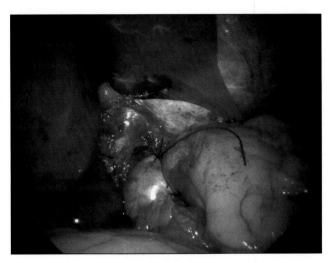

Figure 8. Nissen fundoplication: short (2-cm) wrap.

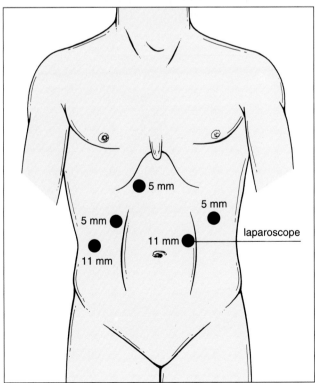

Figure 9. Positioning of the trocars for a left-sided surgical technique.

Technique

The placement of the trocars and the procedures for esophageal mobilization are the same as for the Nissen fundoplication, except for the division of the gastrosplenic ligament and the type of the wrap. The wrap (180° or 270° is fixed on both sides of the esophagus with running or separated nonabsorbable sutures. The postoperative outcome is identical to that of the Nissen procedure. In our experience, these operations are best performed in reflux patients with poor esophageal peristalsis or small fundi.

Other antireflux procedures

The Belsey Mark IV operation and intrathoracic Nissen fundoplication have been performed thoracoscopically. No results are available. We performed two antireflux repairs as described by Watson and coworkers [23] with good results.

RESULTS OF LAPAROSCOPIC ANTIREFLUX SURGERY

Since our initial report [17•] in 1991, we have performed in our department 246 laparoscopic antireflux operations. These operations include:

187 Nissen fundoplications
51 Nissen-Rosetti fundoplications
6 Toupet operations
2 Watson's techniques
0 ligamentum teres cardiopexies
0 Angelchik prosthesis procedures
0 intrathoracic procedures

Our mortality was 0% and morbidity was 2%. Conversion to conventional laparotomy was required in five patients (2%). The most frequent (three patients) reason was inaccessibility to the hiatal region because of a large left liver lobe. Mean duration of the operation was 142.5 minutes (range 60–300) in 1991 and 82.5 minutes (range 32–200) in 1992. Mean hospital stay was 2.8 days (range 1–8).

At the third postoperative month, 118 patients agreed to be reassessed by the gastroenterologist. Ninety-two patients were symptom-free; 17 patients described occasional dysphagia. Three patients experienced persistent dysphagia that required endoscopic dilatation, successfully done in two patients; unsuccessfully in the other. This latter woman was reoperated on 7 months after the initial laparoscopic procedure. Three patients described recurrent heartburn: endoscopic examination was normal in two patients and demonstrated esophagitis stage 1 in one patient. Twenty-four-hour pH metry results were normal in one patient not yet performed in the other two patients. Six patients complained of transient abdominal discomfort because of gas. No patients exhibited dumping syndrome or diarrhea.

Endoscopy demonstrated healing of previous esophagitis in 94 of 95 patients. It showed stricture of the esophagus at the site of the Nissen procedure in three patients. The gastroesophageal manometry performed pre- and postoperatively in 65 patients showed a mean lower esophageal sphincter pressure of 24.8 mm Hg compared with a preoperative value of 4.4 mm Hg.

The same physiologic approach and surgical procedure were used by de Paula (Paper presented at Second Gastrointestinal Tract International Meeting, Belgium, 1992) and Hinder and Filipi (Paper presented at Second Annual International Minimal Access Surgery Sympo-

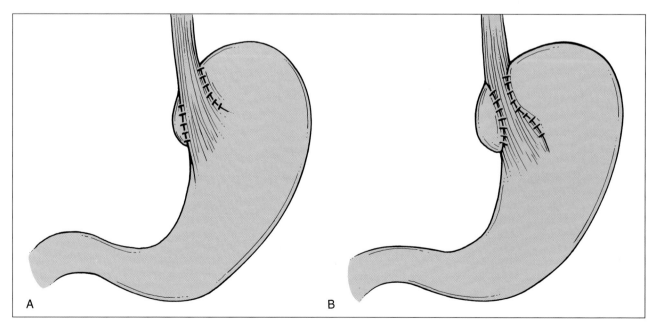

A

B

Figure 10. Wrapping of the gastric fundus according to the techniques described by Toupet (**A**) and Lind (**B**).

sium, Kansas City, 1992). Hinder and Filipi reported an initial series of 60 patients. Follow-up after 1 to 4 months showed 80% of patients to be symptom-free, 14% to have mild dysphagia, and 4% to have heartburn. They reported one recurrence of GERD and one reoperation for stricture.

De Paula reported experience with a series of 111 patients. His group performed 69 modified Nissen operations and 42 Lind operations. The average length of the operation was longer for the Lind procedure (160 minutes) than for the Nissen procedure. He reported a very short hospital stay: 22 to 25 hours. Mortality was 0%. Of 79 postoperative gastroscopies, 72 showed normal findings. Only one patient (after a Lind operation) out of 52 who were submitted to postoperative 24-hour pH metry still experienced abnormal acid exposure. One patient had persistent dysphagia 3 months after surgery and underwent successful endoscopic dilatation. Two patients presented with gas-bloat syndrome. All of the patients had remission from their preoperative heartburn. Four patients still complained of epigastric pain. Postoperative manometric studies demonstrated a rise in the pressure of the lower esophageal sphincter; this value was significantly higher in the Nissen group.

CONCLUSIONS

Recent advances in laparoscopic techniques have prompted several teams throughout the world to inves-

tigate possibilities for minimal-access surgery to treat gastroesophageal reflux disease. For the past 30 years, this disease has been the subject of many reports and publications regarding different techniques and results. In the past few years, the number of antireflux surgeries being performed has decreased. The reason is the higher comfort level of patients treated with hydrogen blockers and proton pump inhibitors as compared with patients treated surgically.

A surgical antireflux procedure is, however, currently the most effective way to reconstruct a defective antireflux mechanism at the gastroesophageal junction and effectively abolish gastroesophageal reflux. Recent studies have proved the superiority of surgery in the treatment of patients with well-documented reflux [24••].

Laparoscopic surgery has the theoretical potential to reduce the failings of conventional surgery, but practitioners must adhere to the principles of antireflux surgery. Actually, there is no place for unproved techniques that would discredit the laparoscopic approach in these patients. Well-documented techniques must be used by well-experienced surgeons aware of the principles of this surgery. Up to now, the abdominal Nissen fundoplication has been the most-appreciated procedure, but excellent results have been achieved by surgeons performing Lind or Toupet operations. In the future, the proponents of the Belsey procedure will probably defend the use of the Belsey technique in the surgical treatment of patients with GERD.

REFERENCES

Papers of particular interest, published within the period of review, have been highlighted as:
• Of special interest
•• Of outstanding interest

1. Spechler SJ: Barrett Esophagus. *N Engl J Med* 1986, 362–371.

2. Stein HJ, DeMeester TR, Naspetti R, *et al.*: Three-Dimensional Imaging of the Lower Esophageal Sphincter in Gastroesophageal Reflux Disease. *Ann Surg* 1991, 214:374– 384.

3. Little AG, DeMeester TR, Kirchner PT: Pathogenesis of Esophagitis in Patients with Gastroesophageal Reflux. *Surgery* 1980, 88:101–107.

4. Skinner BD: Pathophysiology of Gastroesophageal Reflux. *Ann Surg* 1985, 206:546–556.

5.•• Stein HJ, Barlow AP, DeMeester TR, Hinder RA: Complications of Gastroesophageal Reflux Disease. *Ann Surg* 1992, 216:35–43.
Paper explaining the causes of failures of medical treatment of GERD and value of antireflux surgery.

6. DeMeester TR, Stein HJ: Surgical Treatment of Gastroesophageal Reflux Disease. In *The Esophagus*. Edited by Castell DO. Boston: Little, Brown; 1992:579–625.

7. Kaul BK, DeMeester TR, Oka M: The Cause of Dysphagia in Uncomplicated Sliding Hiatal Hernia and its Relief by Hiatal Herniorraphy: A Roentgenographic, Manometric and Clinical Study. *Ann Surg* 1990, 211:410–415.

8. DeMeester TR, Johnson LF, Kent AH: Evaluation of Current Operations for the Prevention of Gastroesophageal reflux. *Ann Surg* 1974, 180:511–522.

9. Nathanson LK, Shimi S, Cuschieri A: Laparoscopic Ligamentum Teres (Round Ligament) Cardiopexy. *Br J Surg* 1991, 78:947–951.

10. Narbona-Arnau B, Molina E, Ancho-Fornos S, *et al.*: Hernia Diaphragmatica Hiatal: Pexia Cardio-gastrica con el Ligamento Redondo. *Medicina de Espana* 1965, 2:25.

11. Angelchik JP, Cohen R: A new surgical procedure for the treatment of gastroesophageal reflux and hiatal hernia. *Surg Gynecol Obstet* 1979, 14:246–249.

12. Angelchik PD, Angelchik JP: The Antireflux Prosthesis: Simple, Effective Therapy for Gastroesophageal Reflux. In *Debates in Clinical Surgery*. vol 2. Edited by Simmons RU. St Louis: Mosby 1991:98–110,130–133.

13. Berguer R, Stiegmann GV, Yamamoto M, *et al.*: Minimal Access Surgery for Gastroesophageal Reflux: Laparoscopic Placement of the Angelchik Prosthesis in Pigs. *Surg Endosc* 1991, 5:123–126.

14. Nissen R: Eine Einfache Operation zur Beeinflussung der Refluxoesophagitis. *Schweiz Med Wochenschr* 1956, 86:590–592.

15. Rosetti M, Hell K: Fundoplication for the Treatment of Gastroesophageal Reflux in Hiatal Hernia. *World J Surg* 1977, 1:439–444.

16. DeMeester TR, Bonavina L, Albertucci M: Nissen Fundoplication for Gastroesophageal Reflux Disease: Evaluation of Primary Repair in 100 Consecutive Patients. *Ann Surg* 1986, 204:9–20.

17.• Dallemagne B, Weerts JM, Jehaes C, *et al.*: Laparoscopic Nissen Fundoplication: Preliminary Report. *Surg Laparosc Endosc* 1991, 1:138–143.

Initial description of the laparoscopic fundoplication including the division of short gastric vessels.

18.• Geagea T: Laparoscopic Nissen's Fundoplication: Preliminary Report on Ten Cases. *Surg Endosc* 1991, 5:170–173.

Initial description of the laparscopic fundoplication without taking down the short gastric vessels.

19. Dallemagne B, Weerts JM, Jehaes C, *et al.*: Laparoscopic Management of Gastroesophageal Reflux. In *Surgical Laparoscopic Update.* Edited by Zucker KA. St. Louis: Quality Medical; 1993:217–239.

20.• Cuschieri A; Shimi S, Nathanson LK: Laparoscopic Reduction, Crural Repair, and Fundoplication of Large Hiatal Hernia. *Am J Surg* 1992, 163:425–430.

Description of an alternative surgical technique for laparoscopic Nissen fundoplication.

21. Toupet A: Technique d'Oesophago-Gastroplastie avec Phrenogastropexie Appliquee dans la Cure Radicale des Hernies Hiatales et Comme Complement de l'Operation de Heller dans les Cardiospasmes. *Mem Acad Chir* 1963, 89:394–396.

22. Lind JF, Burns CM, MacDougall JT: Physiologic Repair for Hiatus Hernia: Manometric Study. *Arch Surg* 1965, 91:233–237.

23. Watson A, Jenkinson LR, Ball CS, *et al.*: A More Physiological Alternative to Total Fundoplication for the Surgical Correction of Resistant Gastro-oesophageal Reflux. *Br J Surg* 78:1088–1094.

24.•• Spechler SJ, Williford WO: Comparison of Medical and Surgical Treatment for Complicated Gastroesophageal Reflux Disease in Veterans. *N Engl J Med* 1992, 326:786–792.

Important medical prospective study comparing medical and surgical treatment of GERD.

Chapter 11

Laparoscopic Staging and Investigation of Intra-abdominal Malignancy

Frederick L. Greene
Douglas Dorsay

The revolutionary acceptance of therapeutic laparoscopy by general surgeons has enabled this technique to reemerge as an important adjunct in the preoperative staging of abdominal malignancy. During the early 1990s, the medical and surgical literature were replete with reports of laparoscopic staging of esophageal and gastric carcinoma, hepatocellular tumors, gallbladder carcinoma, metastatic disease of the liver, retroperitoneal nodal disease, and abdominal lymphoma.

Because imaging studies such as ultrasonography, computed tomography, and magnetic resonance imaging have traditionally played seminal roles in diagnosis and staging of abdominal malignancy, comparing laparoscopy to these techniques is appropriate. Recent studies indicate a significant advantage in sensitivity, specificity, and accuracy for laparoscopy as compared with these modalities in the assessment of esophageal and gastric carcinoma [1]. Similarly, the use of the laparoscope to direct biopsies of diffuse and focal liver lesions has been compared favorably [2] and unfavorably [3] with conventional imaging studies. Leuschner and Leuschner of Frankfurt [3] conducted prospective studies using laparoscopy for liver biopsy and found no significant value of laparoscopy in directing biopsies of diffuse hepatic disease. Laparoscopic-directed biopsy was more beneficial than ultrasound, however, in the histologic confirmation of focal hepatic lesions. These authors further suggested that, in fact, there is a "decreasing need for diagnostic laparoscopy" because of the availability of new imaging techniques. The Ger-of the availability of new imaging techniques. The German workers agree, however, that laparoscopy has a role in identifying small, superficial hepatic lesions and should be performed when conventional imaging techniques give "normal" results.

Computed tomography and ultrasound cannot reveal lesions smaller than 1 cm in diameter. Small lesions on the peritoneal surface and omentum may be undetected by these imaging techniques (Fig. 1). The false-negative rate for computed tomography has been supported by three prospective studies [4–6] that showed false-negative rates ranging from 21% to 48% for laparoscopic evaluation performed in patients with abdominal malignancy. The benefit of laparoscopic staging is especially clear in pancreatic cancer that involves the body or tail, which is associated with increased risk of unresectability.

Other abdominal malignancies, such as primary liver cancer, gallbladder carcinoma, and neoplasms of the upper gastrointestinal tract, may be appropriate for laparoscopic staging (Fig. 2). Laparoscopy is particularly helpful in assessing the degree of cirrhosis associated with hepatocellular cancer and in determining the extent of hepatic resection necessary (Fig. 3). Laparoscopic-directed biopsy also aids in avoiding large, superficial varices that may be present in the cirrhotic patient. Multiple biopsies may be performed safely if there is concern about multiple focal lesions of hepatocellular tumor, as reported in a majority of patients.

The opportunity to diagnose gallbladder carcinoma using laparoscopy is especially helpful if celiotomy can be avoided in patients with advanced unresectable disease. Isolated reports of finding gallbladder cancer at the time of laparoscopic cholecystectomy indicate that celiotomy should be performed to achieve resection of the gallbladder bed and regional nodes in these patients

[7]. If gallbladder carcinoma is suspected at the time of laparoscopic cholecystectomy, conversion to open celiotomy should be made.

Laparoscopic staging may be applied reasonably to carcinomas of the esophagus and gastric cardia. Studies by Lightdale [8•], Sotnikov and Litvinov [9], Shandall and Johnson [10], Kriplani and Kapur [11], and Dagnini and coworkers [12] reported advanced regional or metastatic disease, undetected by conventional imaging studies, that was found laparoscopically in 15% to 58% of patients. The advantage of preoperative laparoscopy is to aid in decision-making regarding operative extirpation or nonoperative palliative techniques. Palliation, using stents, high-dose-rate brachytherapy, laser ablation with or without porphyrin derivatives, or chemotherapy, will play a major role in esophageal and proximal gastric carcinomas during the 1990s, suggesting an even more prominent role for laparoscopic assessment of these lesions. Laparoscopy has less of a role currently in preoperative assessment of colonic and rectal lesions because resection continues to offer the best palliation. A study reported approximately 20 years ago by Atanov and Gallinger [13] suggested a role for laparoscopy in detecting incurable rectal carcinoma. These findings may have more timely interest since palliative resection, ablation, and radiation techniques may play prominent roles in patients with evidence of advanced regional or metastatic rectal cancer not detected by conventional imaging studies.

Since the early 1950s, the concept of routine "second look" has been advocated for management of gastrointestinal tract cancer [14]. Because of poor long-term outcome and the limited ability to render the abdominal cavity tumor-free, this concept has generally been lim-

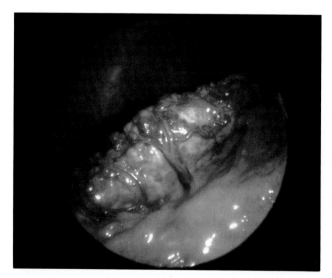

Figure 1. Small peritoneal nodules, not identified on computed tomography scan, representing metastatic pancreatic carcinoma on surface of gallbladder and edge of right lobe of liver. (Courtesy of Jonathan Sackier, MD, University of California, San Diego.)

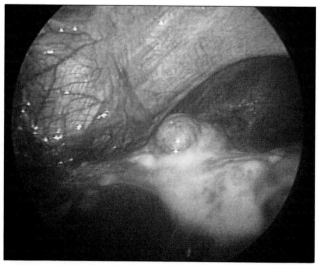

Figure 2. Exophytic hepatocellular carcinoma with nodular component in right lobe of liver. (Courtesy of Jonathan Sackier, MD, University of California, San Diego.)

ited to patients with increased tumor-marker levels (carcinoembryonic antigen) or imaging studies suggestive of recurrent and limited disease. Using laparoscopy, the potential revitalization of the second-look concept, especially in the management of colorectal cancer, may occur. Clinical trials and parameters for patient inclusion are currently being considered to assess laparoscopy as a second-look tool.

Despite resection for cure, approximately one half of all colorectal carcinomas will recur, most frequently within 2 years of operation [15]. Patterns of recurrence differ markedly between colon and rectal carcinomas after "curative" resection. Willett and coworkers [16] discussed recurrence patterns 5 years after supposedly curative resection of colon malignancies with a typical distribution of stages. Of 533 patients, 163 (31%) developed recurrence during that period, with metastatic disease in 25% and local disease in 19%. Six percent had local disease only, and 71 patients (13%) had extra-abdominal metastases. We now recognized that, if identified early, aggressive resection of recurrent local disease, as well as of limited metastatic disease, may result in long-term survival. The key word is "early," leading to the discussion as to what constitutes ideal follow-up.

In 1987, Sugarbaker and coworkers [17] published the results of a prospective study begun in 1978 that examined the concept that early recognition and management of local or residual colorectal carcinoma in the abdomen could lead to appropriate salvage through second-look laparotomy. They studied 66 patients deemed high risk on the basis of stage (Dukes' C/TNM stage III), perforation, invasion of adjacent organs, locally recurrent disease, or age less than 30 years. All underwent resection with no apparent residual disease and were followed for a median of 4 years with all modalities available at that time. Follow-up included a review of symptoms and physical examination at every visit, monthly carcinoembryonic antigen assays, abdomino-pelvic computed tomography scanning, complete lung tomograms, and liver-spleen scintigraphy every 4 months, with intravenous pyelography, barium enema, and bone scintigraphy every year. Thirty-one patients (47%) developed recurrences. A serial increase in carcinoembryonic antigen levels was the first indication in 22 (67%), whereas symptoms or examination results provided the first indication in seven (21%). Abdominal computed tomography uncovered two recurrences and corroborated disease in 17 of 20 cases; however, this record is marred by a 50% false-positive rate. The other studies were useful only for corroboration and localization of relapse.

Even in the best of circumstances and with thorough preoperative staging, many patients are found to be unresectable at second-look laparotomy. Laparoscopy may be used to reduce this number, and may, in the future, offer therapeutic benefit as well. Remember that a normal examination in no way rules out recurrence and, therefore, may be followed by celiotomy.

Second-look laparoscopy has been reported in the gynecologic literature. In 1984, Xygakis and coworkers [18] reported on 46 asymptomatic women who underwent laparoscopy 10 to 18 months after surgical, radiation, or chemical therapy for ovarian cancer. Findings in 20 patients obviated laparotomy, and 16 of the remainder underwent exploration, at which time three were found to have recurrence. They reported no major morbidity. Marti-Vicente and coworkers [19] performed 44 second-look and 28 third-look laparoscopies in 52 women with ovarian cancer in clinical remission.

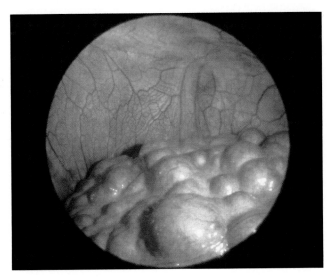

Figure 3. Macronodular cirrhosis of liver associated with hepatocellular carcinoma.

Nearly 50% of these examinations demonstrated recurrent tumor; yet there was a 31% false-negative rate discovered at laparotomy. Neither of these studies addresses the benefits of surgical debulking in the treatment of this disease.

Currently, the indications and opportunities for second-look laparoscopy remain limited. If recurrence is suggested on the grounds of a rising carcinoembryonic antigen level or clinical findings, evidence of unresectable disease should be sought using roentgenography, computed tomography, ultrasound, magnetic resonance imaging, and possibly scintigraphy using radiolabeled monoclonal antibodies. The presence of distant metastases, if unresectable, would make further evaluation unnecessary except for histologic confirmation. The extent of locally recurrent disease is difficult to appraise using noninvasive imaging studies because of scar formation, alteration of the normal anatomy, and possible reactive lymphadenopathy. Therefore, the suggestion of recurrence by history, examination, or rising carcinoembryonic antigen levels, as well as a completely negative or equivocal evaluation using imaging studies, would justify invasive evaluation. Laparoscopy may represent the next stage in the evolution of the second-look evaluation with a goal of performing celiotomy only in patients with resectable disease. A major obstacle to this goal is the prevalence of adhesions in the previously operated abdomen. These adhesions are frequently present to such a degree as to severely limit or even prevent inspection by this method. In most patients, however, the careful insertion of trocars, using an open technique, followed by careful adhesiolysis permits laparoscopic examination. Visual examination may be augmented by laparoscopic ultrasound and radioimmunolocalization techniques in the near future. A finding of peritoneal carcinomatosis or unresectable hepatic metastases would obviate further surgical intervention, but other findings may be more difficult to interpret. In general, a finding of potentially resectable recurrence or lack of evidence of unresectable disease would warrant a subsequent celiotomy with aggressive resection of all malignant tissue in the low- or moderate-risk patient.

Laparoscopy may have a therapeutic role in the near future as well. Several recent studies have demonstrated prolonged remission in up to 22% of patients with multiple hepatic metastases from colorectal cancers [20] and 37.5% in patients with unresectable hepatocellular carcinoma [21] after ultrasound-guided hepatic cryosurgery. Instruments are now being developed for the laparoscopic application of this technique.

A further role for laparoscopic staging is in patients with lymphoma, especially Hodgkin's disease. As previously noted in the assessment of intra-abdominal solid tumors, conventional imaging may "understage" lymphoma in the abdomen. Twenty percent of patients with hepatic involvement with Hodgkin's disease have normal laboratory data and imaging studies [8]. Laparoscopy also helps in avoiding "overstaging" because of laboratory or imaging studies that suggest the presence of disease secondary to inflammatory lesions. The focal nature of Hodgkin's disease in the liver is ideal for approaches that add specificity and direction to hepatic biopsy, thereby avoiding the need for blind, percutaneous biopsy techniques that are helpful in the minority of patients (15%) with diffuse hepatic involvement [8].

Laparoscopic nodal and splenic biopsy may be of further help in staging lymphoma patients. Spinelli and DiFelice [22] in Milan report extensive experience with needle biopsy of the spleen and believe that this aspect of laparoscopic staging should be routine. These authors first reported splenic biopsy in 1973 and findings in staging of lymphoma in 1975. An important part of the evaluation of patients with lymphoma is a careful search for accessory splenic tissue, which may occur in 14% to 30% of patients, especially those who require splenectomy for hematologic disease. Unfortunately, the laparoscope shows only a few of the accessory spleens present, but the laparoscopist should look carefully in the greater omentum, hilar area of the spleen, and retroperitoneum for accessory splenic tissue. These small areas may be dissected and divided from the blood supply with silver clips. Small accessory spleens may be delivered easily from the abdominal cavity and may serve as excellent material for histologic assessment in the staging of lymphoma.

The spleen itself is best evaluated once the patient is turned in the reverse Trendelenburg position and rotated into a right semilateral decubitus position. At times, the omentum may need to be teased from the left upper quadrant and, in fact, a portion of it may need to be removed from the greater curvature to facilitate full assessment of the spleen. Visual inspection of the convex surface of the spleen and proper assessment of splenic size should be performed routinely. Spinelli and DiFelice [22] recommend that when splenic biopsy is performed, the needle should be introduced in the direction the spleen moves with respiration. This direction is downward from a cephalad to caudad position and posterior to anterior when the diaphragm pushes the organ secondary to respiration. By placing the needle along this axis, Spinelli has reported no complications over a 15-year period. The benefit of retroperitoneal nodal biopsy is in the ability to obtain adequate quantities of nodal tissue for histologic and immunochemical studies for complete characterization of the lymphoma. Laparoscopy may also be helpful in follow-up staging of patients who show evidence of relapse after therapy or who are at significant risk of relapse.

The natural progression from laparoscopic diagnosis and staging is to apply the technique to curative and palliative resection [23], bypass, or application of additional therapies. The laparoscope does provide success-

and therapeutic techniques to be applied in the management of our patients with abdominal malignancy [24].

PATIENT PREPARATION AND TECHNICAL CONSIDERATIONS

Considering that laparoscopic evaluation for staging or diagnosis in the abdomen is performed using general anesthesia, in our practice, the patient is prepared for diagnostic laparoscopy as vigorously as for any other major abdominal procedure [25•]. The major considerations are to assure that coagulation studies are assessed and that any coagulation defects are corrected before the procedure. In addition, full evaluation for the possibility of metastatic disease in the chest, bone, or other sites is mandated, especially if biopsy of other accessible areas is indicated. This evaluation also includes careful assessment of node-bearing areas and the skin. We prefer general anesthesia for our examination because of the discomfort that occurs with abdominal distension and the need for sufficient time for full diagnostic evaluation of the abdomen. Although some recommendations suggest that local infiltration of the abdominal wall and intravenous sedation may be adequate for diagnostic laparoscopy [22], the benefits of general anesthesia for abdominal staging of tumors outweigh the possible risks.

The choice of insertion site for creation of the pneumoperitoneum camera and accessory trocar placement (Fig. 4) depends on the presence of healed abdominal incisions, abdominal masses, organomegaly, or ascites. Although the Veress needle is used in the majority of patients to create the pneumoperitoneum, we prefer an open technique using the Hasson cannula for patients with previously operated abdomens. The periumbilical approach is usually selected, but prior evaluation of the abdomen with ultrasound may indicate the presence of adhesions, which suggest the use of an alternate site to create the pneumoperitoneum. If ascites is present, the classical Trendelenburg position for establishment of pneumoperitoneum must be changed to allow for safer abdominal wall puncture and introduction of intraperitoneal gas. Using the reverse Trendelenburg position instead allows the gastrointestinal contents to "float" in a cephalad position on the surface of the ascitic fluid, thereby giving a safe cushion of fluid for introduction of any needle into the pelvis. In addition, carbon dioxide should be instilled above the level of ascitic fluid to reduce the troublesome presence of bubbles throughout the abdomen as would occur if carbon dioxide were introduced directly into the ascitic collection. In the presence of ascites, the best approach is to completely drain the peritoneal cavity before introducing carbon dioxide.

As in any laparoscopic procedure, careful inspection is the first part of an adequately performed diagnostic laparoscopic examination for malignancy. This inspec-

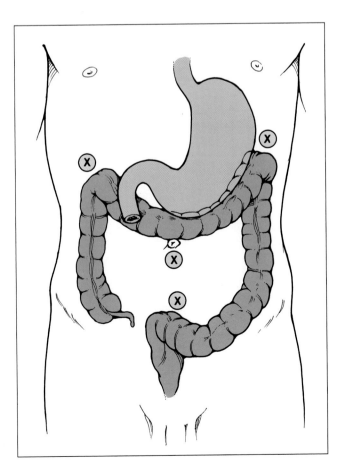

Figure 4. Trocar placement for staging laparoscopy denoted by Ⓧ. These sites are appropriate for staging of pancreatic cancer of abdominal lymphoma.

laparoscopic examination for malignancy. This inspection may uncover small lesions on the surface of the gastrointestinal serosa or other organs and may direct the laparoscopist to avoid or perform biopsy of these regions (Figs. 5, 6). By changing the angle of the operating table, the surgeon may reposition the small bowel to allow identification of the spleen, which is extremely helpful in the full characterization of abdominal involvement in lymphoma. The patient may be placed in the right semilateral decubitus position, which allows for complete evaluation of the greater curvature of the stomach, the esophageal hiatus, and the spleen and also

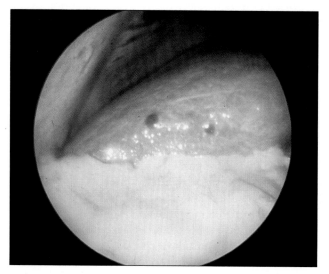

Figure 5. Small implants of metastatic melanoma on right lobe of liver, not identified by routine computed tomography imaging.

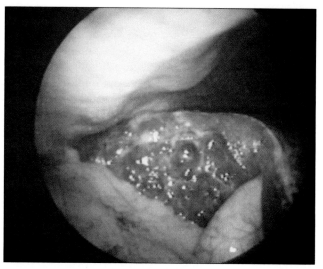

Figure 6. Hemangioma of right lobe of liver identified during intraoperative evaluation for staging. Appropriate interpretation avoids complications of biopsy. (Courtesy of Jonathan Sackier, MD, University of California, San Diego.)

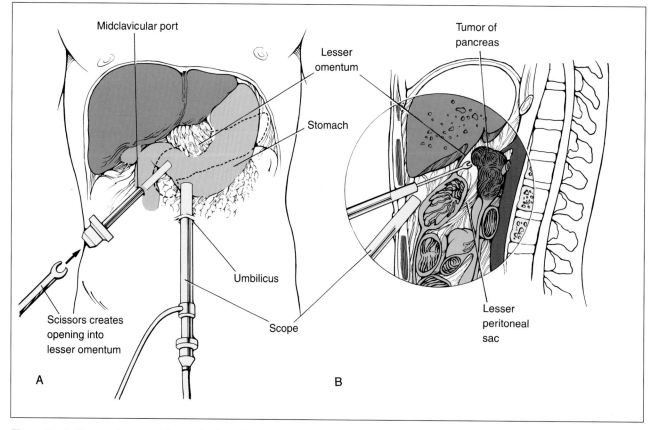

Figure 7. A, Trocar placement for evaluation of pancreas and retrogastric region. **B,** Lateral view shows placement of accessory instruments into lesser omental area.

facilitates approach to the retroperitoneum through the gastrohepatic omentum [26] (Figs. 7,8).

The main indication for laparoscopic intervention may be for retrieval of histologic specimens, especially from the liver. The entire liver must be examined carefully, and the left lateral lobe of the liver must be elevated to assure that the region of the triangular ligament is free of lesions (Fig. 9). Biopsy may be performed routinely through alternate trocar sites or through direct puncture of the abdominal wall using biopsy needles. The "guillotine-

type" needles are very effective for biopsy of liver and other solid organs; they may be passed directly through the abdominal wall and positioned over the organ to allow for safe and focally directed biopsies. Similarly cytologic specimens may be taken of nodal tissue or solid organs using a needle and syringe for further characterization in the histology laboratory. In patients with cirrhosis, careful assessment of the liver surface to determine safe biopsy is mandatory. Many patients with cirrhosis have surface varices that would create signifi-

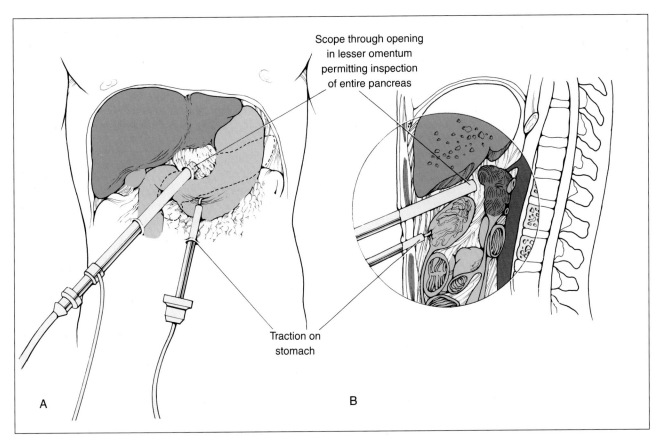

Scope through opening
in lesser omentum
permitting inspection
of entire pancreas

Traction on
stomach

A

B

Figure 8. **A**, Alternative camera and trocar position for entry into gastrohepatic omentum. **B**, Lateral view of entry into gas- trohepatic omentum, allowing evaluation of pancreatic head and body.

Figure 9. Technique of identifying lesions beneath left lateral lobe of liver during laparoscopy.

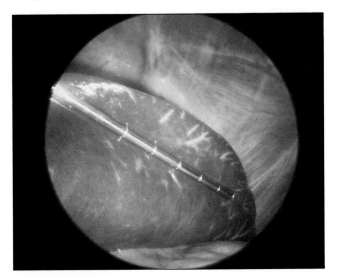

tion to needle biopsy, the use of appropriate cupped forceps allows for adequate biopsies without causing a crush artifact. Peritoneal implants may be approached directly using sharp dissection techniques to allow for large pieces of tissue to be evaluated by the pathologist. Avoiding an overzealous approach is important in using electrocautery in dissecting these peritoneal implants because cautery artifact may interfere with full evaluation.

If no lesions are noted on routine laparoscopic intervention, lavage and aspiration for cytologic specimens may in fact give useful data if no abnormal solid lesions are found. The instillation of 500 mL of saline into the abdomen with a change in patient position facilitates proper lavage. This fluid may be totally aspirated from the pelvis as the patient is placed in reverse Trendelenburg position. Separate aliquots of fluid may be introduced in selected areas if one suspects isolated regions of tumor involvement. Two hundred to 300 mL of fluid may be placed in the upper abdomen and aspirated followed by a similar amount of fluid placed in the pelvis with subsequent retrieval. In addition, brush biopsies may be obtained from various organ surfaces and peritoneal lesions by introducing appropriate-size brushes into the laparoscopic trocar.

The morbidity and mortality of diagnostic laparoscopy, even when associated with aggressive biopsy, is quite low. Mortality of 0.1% and morbidity of less than 2% have been reported. As in any procedure, the risk of complications is directly related to the skill of the operator, and the morbidity of diagnostic laparoscopy generally relies on safe introduction of the initial pneumoperitoneum and biopsy techniques. During the initial assessment of the patient, cardiac and pulmonary disease should be recognized because the establishment of pneumoperitoneum reduces cardiac output and creates hypercarbic conditions that may lead to significant cardiac arrhythmia or other sequelae [27]. Mon-

itoring of the patient during and after laparoscopic intervention should be routine and similar to that for patients undergoing general anesthesia for open surgery. Performing routine diagnostic laparoscopy on an outpatient basis is certainly reasonable when the patient's overall cardiac, pulmonary, and metabolic evaluation suggests no need for in-hospital monitoring.

COMPLICATIONS

Although uncommon, the development of abdominal-wall metastases may occur as a consequence of introducing the laparoscope in patients with peritoneal implants or malignant ascites. Cava and coworkers [28] report a subcutaneous metastasis from gastric carcinoma after laparoscopy. Implantation in the presence of ovarian malignancy has also occurred. Keate and Shaffer [29] recently reported seeding of hepatocellular carcinoma in a laparoscopic trocar site. Such seeding has been recognized as a complication of percutaneous liver biopsy and fine-needle aspiration biopsy. In their report, Keate and Shaffer noted the patient had a painful area in the laparoscopic insertion site 5 months after the procedure. The obvious source of seeding is from biopsy instrumentation or the trocar itself as it becomes contaminated with tumor cells following biopsy. As the trocar is removed, these tumor cells are transplanted into the abdominal wall to later manifest as tumor nodules. In patients who develop ascites after laparoscopic evaluation, ascitic fluid may also play a role in transporting tumor cells to areas of the abdominal wall that are fertile for implantation, *ie*, healing percutaneous needle or laparoscopic trocar sites. The rare occurrence of transplantation of tumor cells to the abdominal wall should not deter the use of laparoscopy in the assessment of abdominal tumors.

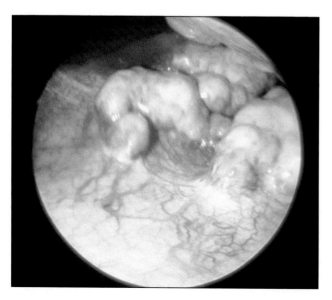

Figure 10. Significant venous varices of peritoneum and surface of liver associated with portal hypertension.

REFERENCES

Papers of particular interest, published within the period of review, have been highlighted as:
• Of special interest
•• Of outstanding interest

1. Watt I, Stewart I, Anderson D, *et al.*: Laparoscopy, Ultrasound, and Computed Tomography in Cancer of the Oesophagus and Gastric Cardia: A Prospective Comparison for Detecting Intra-Abdominal Metastases. *Br J Surg* 1989, 76:1036–1039.

2. Boyce HW: Diagnostic Laparoscopy in Liver and Biliary Disease. *Endoscopy* 1992, 24:676–681.

3. Leuschner M, Leuschner U: Diagnostic Laparoscopy in Focal Parenchymal Disease of the Liver. *Endoscopy* 1992, 24:689–692.

4. Brady PG, Goldschmid S, Chappel G, *et al.*: A Comparison of Biopsy Techniques in Suspected Focal Liver Disease. *Gastrointest Endosc* 1987, 33:289–292.

5. Brady PG, Pebbles M, Goldschmid S: Role of Laparoscopy in the Evaluation of Patients with Suspected Hepatic or Peritoneal Malignancy. *Gastrointest Endosc* 1991, 37:27–30.

6. Warshaw AL, Tepper JE, Shipley WV: Laparoscopy in Staging and Planning of Therapy for Pancreatic Cancer. *Am J Surg* 1986, 151:76–80.

7. Swaroop VS, Udwadia TE: Laparoscopic Cholecystectomy for Gallbladder Cancer. *Am J Gastroenterol* 1992, 87:1522–1523.

8. • Lightdale C: Laparoscopy for Cancer Staging. *Endoscopy* 1992, 24:682–686.
This article is a well-done review that covers all aspects of laparoscopy in the diagnosis and staging of cancer, especially from the view of the gastroenterologist.

9. Sotnikov VN, Litvinov SS: The Diagnoses of Intra-Abdominal Metastases of Esophageal Cancer by Laparoscopy. *Vopr Onkol* 1973, 19:35–37.

10. Shandall A, Johnson C: Laparoscopy or Scanning in Esophageal and Gastric Carcinoma. *Br J Surg* 1985, 22:449–453.

11. Kriplani AK, Kapur ML: Laparoscopy for Pre-Operative Staging and Assessment of Operability in Gastric Carcinoma. *Gastrointest Endosc* 1991, 37:441–443.

12. Dagnini G, Caldroni MW, Marin G: Laparoscopy in Abdominal Staging of Esophageal Carcinoma. *Gastrointest Endosc* 1986, 32:400–402.

13. Atanov IP, Gallinger I: Laparoscopy in the Diagnosis of Several Abdominal Tumors. *Sov Med* 1972, 35:93–95.

14. Wagensteen O, Lewis FJ, Tongen LA: The "Second Look" in Cancer Surgery. *Lancet* 1951, 71:303–307.

15. Beahrs OH: Staging and Prognostic Features of Cancer in the Colon and Rectum. In *Colorectal Tumors*. Edited by Beahrs OH, Higgins GA, Weinstein JJ. Philadelphia: Lippincott; 1986:115.

16. Willett CG, Tepper JE, Cohen AM, *et al.*: Failure Patterns Following Curative Resection of Colonic Carcinoma. *Ann Surg* 1984, 200:685–690.

17. Sugarbaker PH, Gianola FJ, Dwyer A, Neuman NR: A Simplified Plan for Follow-Up of Patients with Colon and Rectal Cancer Supported by Prospective Studies of Laboratory and Radiologic Test Results. *Surgery* 1987, 102:79–87.

18. Xygakis AM, Politis GS, Michalas SP, Kaskarelis DB: Second-Look Laparoscopy in Ovarian Cancer. *J Reprod Med* 1984, 29:583–585.

19. Marti-Vicente A, Sainz S, Soriano G, *et al.*: Utilida de la Laparoscopia como Metodo de Second-Look en las Noplasias del Ovario. *Rev Esp Enferm Dig* 1990, 77:275–278.

20. Onik G, Rubinsky B, Zemel R, *et al.*: Ultrasound-Guided Hepatic Cryosurgery in the Treatment of Metastatic Colon Carcinoma. *Cancer* 1991, 67:901–906.

21. Zhou X-D, Tang Z-Y, Yu Y-Q, Ma Z-C: Clinical Evaluation of Cryosurgery in the Treatment of Primary Liver Cancer: Report of 60 Cases. *Cancer* 1988, 61:1889–1894.

22. Spinelli P, DiFelice G: Laparoscopy in Abdominal Malignancies. *Prob Gen Surg* 1991, 8:329–347.

23. Cuschieri A, Berci G: Laparoscopic Management of Pancreatic Cancer. In *Laparoscopic Biliary Surgery*, 2nd ed. Oxford: Blackwell Scientific; 1992:170–182.

24. Cuesta MA, Meijer S, Borgstein PJ: Laparoscopy and Assessment of Digestive Tract Cancer. *Br J Surg* 1992, 79:486–487.

25. • Greene FL: Laparoscopy in Malignant Disease. *Surg Clin N Am* 1992, 72:1125–1137.
This paper reviews the historical aspects as well as specific findings at diagnostic laparoscopy. In-depth discussion of future considerations and uses of the laparoscope as a vehicle for further therapy is included.

26. Cuschieri A, Berci G: Diagnostic Laparoscopy, Tissue Diagnosis and Other Procedures. In *Laparoscopic Biliary Surgery*, 2nd ed. Oxford: Blackwell Scientific; 1992:183–194.

27. Ho SH, Gunther R, Wolfe B: Intraperitoneal Carbon Dioxide Insufflation and Cardiopulmonary Functions. *Arch Surg* 1992, 127:928–933.

28. Cava A, Roman J, Quintela AG, *et al.*: Subcutaneous Metastasis Following Laparoscopy in Gastric Adenocarcinoma. *Eur J Surg Oncol* 1990, 16:63–67.

29. Keate RF, Shaffer R: Seeding of Hepatocellular Carcinoma to Peritoneoscopy Insertion Site [letter]. *Gastrointest* 1992, 38:203.

Chapter 12

Laparoscopic Biliary and Gastric Bypass for Unresectable Disease

David R. Fletcher

PALLIATION OF MALIGNANCY

The principle in surgically palliating malignancy must be to relieve symptoms rapidly at least risk to the patient and to maintain the patient symptom free until his or her inevitable death. The most common symptom to relieve is obstruction, and the most frequent example is carcinoma of the pancreas with bile duct obstruction. Ten percent to 20% of these patients also develop duodenal obstruction [1]. Other circumstances in which palliative bypass might be used include distal carcinoma of the stomach (gastroenterostomy), secondary malignant obstruction of the small intestine (enteroenterostomy), and primary unresectable malignant obstruction of the colon (entero- or colocolostomy). The minimal invasive approach in providing this palliation, however, must not compromise the potential for the occasional cure by surgical resection. This point is particularly important in malignant obstructive jaundice [1,2], and the role of laparoscopy and investigation in determining resectability is referred to in Chapter 11 by Greene and Dorsay. In this chapter, I discuss the indications for and techniques of laparoscopic biliary and gastric bypass in nonresectable malignant disease.

THERAPEUTIC OPTIONS

Once investigations have confirmed nonresectability in malignant jaundice, the two options have been either surgical bypass or stent, the latter either percutaneous or endoscopic. The stents have the advantage of an initial short hospital stay and perhaps lesser morbidity and mortality, but in the longer term they have a high readmission rate because of recurrent obstruction-cholangitis and duodenal obstruction [3••,4•]. This requirement of stents for retreatment robs these unfortunate patients of their independence in the twilight days of their lives.

CHOICE OF THERAPY

These treatment options, however, are not competitive or mutually exclusive, as suggested by some endoscopists who believe one or the other should be used to treat all biliary obstruction [5]. The advantages of both approaches, long-term patency of surgery and low initial morbidity and mortality of stent, can be had by careful patient selection on the basis of surgical risk and probable survival time [1,6••]. Patients thought unlikely to survive long enough to develop late complications (stent obstruction) or who have a high risk of surgical complication are best managed by stent. Patients likely to survive more than the four months during which stents usually occlude or who may develop duodenal obstruction are best managed by surgery [6••].

Therapeutic laparoscopy, *ie*, laparoscopic cholecystenterostomy, appropriately chosen, has the potential to fulfill both goals of palliation, the low risk of minimum access of the stent but the longer permanent drainage of the wide stoma of surgery [7–10].

INDICATIONS FOR LAPAROSCOPIC CHOLECYSTENTEROSTOMY

CONFIRMATION OF BILIARY OBSTRUCTION

Liver function tests and ultrasound can confirm that the patient has obstructive jaundice, and in cancer of the pancreas they usually can identify a mass in the head of the pancreas with dilation of the bile duct cephalad of the mass. Pancreatic cancer is rarely resectable [1,2], but this situation requires confirmation preoperatively if possible. Sometimes the ultrasound shows hepatic metastases, but generally computed tomography (CT) is required to show superior mesenteric vein or artery invasion or to show celiac or superior mesenteric node involvement; these findings confirm resection would be either not curative or impossible. The final decision regarding potential cure, however, may be made at the time of laparoscopy, if peritoneal or hepatic metastases are identified.

In selecting patients for laparoscopic cholecystenterostomy, three criteria must be met. First, the gallbladder has to be present and contain no calculi. This fact would have been established by the prior ultrasound. Second, expected survival from the malignancy should be greater than four months, and surgical risk should not be excessive should conversion to laparo-

tomy be required. Evidence for this requirement will come from the staging investigations plus risk factors identified as described by Pitt [11••], *ie*, advanced age, sepsis, anemia, severity and duration of obstruction, renal impairment, and malnourishment. Third, the cystic duct must enter the common hepatic duct at least 1 cm above the tumor, *ie*, it will not be invaded and obstructed by tumor progression in the patient's remaining lifetime. Tumor progression and invasion of the cystic duct has been a major cause of recurrent jaundice and thus of failure of palliation following surgical cholecystenterostomy [1]. It can be prevented only by careful selection of patients, which demands contrast imaging of the biliary tree. Approximately one fourth of patients have a common channel for some distance between the common hepatic duct and cystic duct before the ducts fuse [1], and surgical or even laparoscopic dissection of the region will not adequately identify this anatomy. These patients will be excluded from gallbladder bypass and, if unsuitable for a stent, will require a surgical hepaticodochojejunostomy.

Contrast imaging of the biliary tree can be achieved prior to or during surgery. Prior to surgery, the choices are endoscopic retrograde cholangiopancreatography (ERCP) or percutaneous transhepatic cholangiography (PTC). ERCP is preferable for two reasons. First, if the patient's survival is expected to be short, a stent can be done in the same procedure as the diagnosis is made. Second, the endoscopic examination can show invasion of the duodenum, suggesting later duodenal obstruction and thus allowing for a prophylactic gastroenterostomy to be performed. If ERCP is not available, preoperative upper-gastrointestinal endoscopy can be performed to assess the duodenum and then the biliary tree imaged intraoperatively. With the surgeon using an image intensifier and laparoscopic control, the gallbladder can be needled percutaneously, bile aspirated, and then contrast injected. The advantage of this approach is that it enables laparoscopy to be used as a final step in determining resectability, thereby ensuring no patient misses a potentially curative resective procedure. The disadvantage, however, is that those found unsuitable for gallbladder bypass on anatomic grounds, if also at higher risk for surgery, have to be referred subsequently for ERCP-stent. The cholangiogram of a patient who would be unsuitable for laparoscopic cholecystenterostomy is shown in Figure 1.

TECHNIQUE OF LAPAROSCOPIC CHOLECYSTENTEROSTOMY

The procedure is performed using general anesthesia with the patient supine on the operating table, which has a radiolucent top. The umbilicus and linea alba are infiltrated with 0.5% marcaine and adrenalin, which not only reduces bleeding but minimizes postoperative pain. The umbilicus is incised vertically, and the skin of the umbilical cicatrix is detached from the linea alba. Fat protrudes through the opening in the linea alba following detachment of the cicatrix; this opening is enlarged and a Hasson (Stortz-Tutlingen) cannula is inserted and held in place with stay sutures. The remaining cannulae, as indicated in Figure 2, are placed within laparoscopic view. Because manipulations such as laparoscopic suturing and knot tying are required, for ease of use, these cannulae should have a flap top rather than a trumpet valve and, to prevent dislodgment, should be anchored to the abdominal wall. This requirement generally means the use of disposable cannulae and sutures or screw locks to anchor them. Patients who are particularly cachetic and have thin abdominal walls may have gas leaks. If this problem is thought probable, a disposable cannula with a balloon at its tip might be used. If these supplies are unavailable, an alternative method to prevent gas leak is to insert a nylon suture with circumferential bites down to the muscle layer around the cannula and tie it securely. This suture is removed at the end of the procedure.

A 12-mm cannula is placed inferior to the tip of the xiphisternum (Fig. 2, *position 2*). This cannula is available as an alternate site for the placement of the stapler for cholecystenterostomy, should it be necessary, as well as a principal site for the stapler for gastroenterostomy, should it be required, this latter decision having been made preoperatively. By using either a 5- or 10-mm reducer, this cannula can also be used for needle holders, graspers, and scissors.

With the xiphisternal cannula in place, a grasper can be passed through to handle the viscera. This step allows the surgeon to inspect the peritoneal cavity for evidence of metastasis and estimate the degree of spread, essential if the decision regarding resectability has not already been made. A tissue diagnosis should always be made and can be achieved easily using percutaneous fine-needle aspiration cytology with immediate fixation of the smears and immediate staining and evaluation. This procedure is most easily performed using a long, 23-gauge spinal needle introduced into the abdomen with its central obturator in place. The hard mass can be palpated with a grasper passed via the xiphisternal cannula. The needle obturator is removed and multiple passes of the needle through the tumor are made while negative pressure is maintained on an attached syringe to aspirate tissue fluid and cells.

If intraoperative biliary imaging is required, transcholecystic cholangiography is performed at this point. A long, 19-gauge needle is passed percutaneously into the apex of the fundus of the dilated gallbladder at a position where the final anastomosis is expected to be performed. Approximately 20 mL of bile is aspirated and then replaced with contrast fluid under laparoscopic and roentgenographic-image-intensifier view. By rotating the image intensifier C arm to obtain oblique projections and using the grasper in the xiphisternal cannula (Fig. 2, *position 2*) to manipulate Hartmann's pouch, the surgeon can easily see the anatomy of the junction of the cystic duct and common hepatic duct. A head-up tilt may be required to get the contrast to run to the bottom of the bile duct.

If the decision is made that laparoscopic cholecystenterostomy is appropriate, the remaining two cannulae are inserted. A 10-mm cannula (Fig. 2., *position 3*) is

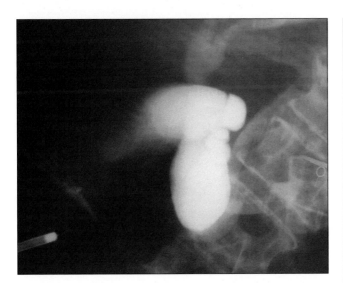

Figure 1. Percutaneous transcholecystic cholangiogram of a patient who would be unsuitable for laparoscopic cholecystenterostomy. The cystic duct can be seen overlying the common hepatic duct, and there is no patent common bile duct below the junction of the two ducts. Early obstruction of the cystic duct by tumor growth could be expected.

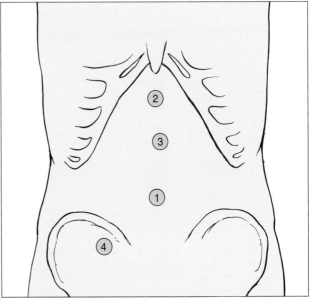

Figure 2. The position of the cannulae showing their size and the order in which they are inserted. Position 1 is 10mm; 2, 12mm; 3, 10mm; 4, 12mm.

placed approximately in the midline between the umbilicus and xiphisternum. This cannula is used for graspers to manipulate the jejunum and gallbladder and to transfer the needle when suturing the gallbladder to the jejunum. Its placement should therefore be such that the needle holder passed through the xiphisternal cannula (Fig. 2, *position 2*) should meet the grasper passing through the midline cannula (Fig. 2, *position 3*) at the fundus of the gallbladder at a little less than a right angle. This positioning makes needle transfer from one instrument to another easier. An infiltration needle passed through the abdominal wall under laparoscopic view helps select the most appropriate site. It also provides an opportunity to infiltrate the muscle and peritoneum with marcaine and adrenalin to reduce postoperative pain. If a gastroenterostomy is also to be performed, this midline cannula (Fig. 2, *position 3*) will be used with a needle holder to suture the jejunum to the stomach; the grasper for the needle transfer is passed via the xiphisternal cannula (Fig. 2, *position 2*). Placement of the midline cannula therefore must take into account dual needs.

Finally, a 12-mm cannula is placed in the right iliac fossa (RIF) (Fig. 2, *position 4*). This cannula must be placed appropriately. Even though the gallbladder does collapse when opened, the cannula must be inserted sufficiently far down in the RIF to allow room between the end of the cannula and the gallbladder such that the ENDO G.I.A 30 stapler (US Surgical Corporation, Norwalk, CT) can be passed into the abdominal cavity and opened clear of the cannula before the tips of the jaws reach the gallbladder and small bowel to be stapled. Second, the line of entry from the abdominal wall to the gallbladder should be in the long axis of the gallbladder to facilitate the passage of the jaws into the open gallbladder and small bowel. Extra manipulation of the viscera at this time can lead to tearing of the bowel or gallbladder, requiring extra suturing or stapling to close the final defects.

The procedure begins with the surgeon standing on the patient's right side and using two Du Val (Stortz-Tutlingen) forceps through the xiphisternal and upper midline cannulae (Fig. 2, *position 2 and 3*), to identify the proximal jejunum. This procedure may be facilitated by elevating the head of the operating table as the assistant passes an instrument through the RIF cannula (Fig. 2, *position 4*) to first displace the omentum onto the patient's right side and then push the transverse colon cephalad. By "walking" the jejunum between the two Du Val forceps, the surgeon identifies the duodeno-jejunal flexure. The jejunum is then approximated to the gallbladder using the Du Val forcep in the midline cannula (Fig. 2, *position 3*). In choosing the segment to be anastomosed, the surgeon must be sure it is suffi-

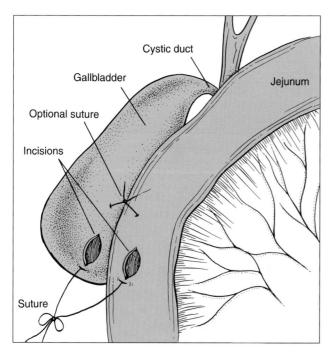

Figure 3. An illustration of a loosely tied anchoring suture at the very apex of the gallbladder and the antimesenteric border of the jejunum. Incisions are made as close to the suture as possible; importantly, the gallbladder incision is made as close as possible to the apex of the gallbladder to facilitate passage of the stapler. An optional anchoring suture is shown tied securely where the distal end of the staple line is expected to be.

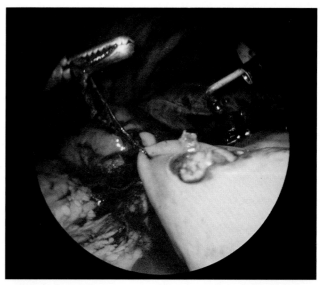

Figure 4. The small bowel in the foreground has been approximated to the gallbladder in the background with a loosely tied silk suture. The suture is being held by a grasper passed via the right iliac fossa cannula. The needle diathermy sucker is seen in the xiphi sternal cannula after it has made incisions in the jejunum and in the gallbladder close to the anchoring suture. White bile can be seen coming from the gallbladder opening and pink mucosa pouting from the jejunal opening.

ciently distant from the duodenojejunal flexure to prevent tension on the subsequent biliary enteric anastomosis. Extra length is required if a gastroenterostomy is also to be performed.

The surgeon then moves to the left side of the patient. The assistant, who is now standing on the patient's right side, passes the grasper through the RIF cannula (Fig.2, *position 4*), regrasps the jejunum, and holds it in proximity to the gallbladder. This positioning allows the forceps in the midline cannula to be removed. A 2-0 silk suture (minimum length 70 cm) on a curved, round-body needle is pushed into the abdominal cavity via the xiphisternal cannula using a 5-mm needle holder and holding the thread behind the needle. A grasper is used in the surgeon's left hand in the midline cannula to hold the tissue and transfer the needle. The grasper first pulls the thread coming down from the xiphisternal cannula into the abdominal cavity and places it in loops on the surface of the liver. Sufficient length is left outside to allow an extracorporeal knot. The needle is then regrasped with the needle holder in the xiphisternal cannula and the needle is passed through the very apex of the gallbladder, ensuring adequate bite. The needle is regrasped and a second bite is taken of the antimesenteric border of the jejunum. The thread is grasped with the needle holder behind the needle, and the needle and thread are withdrawn through the same cannula, *ie*, xiphisternal.

During this process, the surgeon must maintain view of the jejunum and gallbladder to ensure that the thread runs through smoothly and that tissue tearing does not occur. The grasper in the midline cannula may assist with thread transfer. Once the needle is delivered outside, the assistant places a finger over the opening of the cannula to prevent gas leak past the valve. A half-hitch knot is tied and pushed inside using a knot pusher. Again, the tissues are watched carefully to prevent excess tension and tearing. An additional half hitch is pushed in to form a knot approximately 1 cm from the gallbladder-jejunal junction; it is then cut long (Fig. 3). Leaving this suture loose allows it to be held subsequently with a grasper to anchor the viscera while the stapler is inserted; it also still allows sufficient movement for positioning the viscera over the jaws of the stapler.

This loosely tied suture is now held by the assistant using a grasper passed through the RIF cannula. Next, the surgeon uses a grasper in the midline cannula and a needle diathermy-sucker in the xiphisternal cannula to make longitudinal, 5- to 6-mm–long incisions in both the gallbladder and the jejunum. These incisions must be made as close as possible to the anchoring suture (Fig. 3, 4). The grasper in the RIF cannula is removed, and the assistant passes it into the xiphisternal cannula

and grasps the anchoring suture to provide caudad traction while the viscera are fed onto the stapler.

The stapler, containing a 3.5 cartridge, is passed through the RIF cannula and opened; the surgeon uses a grasper through the midline cannula to manipulate the cartridge side of the stapler into the gallbladder. Again using the midline grasper, the surgeon feeds the jejunum over the anvil of the stapler and pushes the stapler its full, 3-cm length into the viscera as the assistant provides counter traction on the anchoring suture through the xiphisternal cannula. When the staple jaws are closed, the staple line is ensured to run along the antimesenteric border of the jejunum. If there is difficulty either in getting the viscera fed or oriented correctly onto the stapler, an optional suture may be placed and tied securely as indicated in Figure 3, *ie*, where the end of the completed staple line is expected to be. The potential disadvantage of this suture is that traction may lead to tearing, particularly of the gallbladder. If this tearing is not incorporated into the staple line, it may result in leakage. The stapler is fired, opened, and removed from the viscera; then, it is reclosed and removed from the abdomen. This technique results in a common opening with anterior and posterior staple lines (Figs. 5, 6). The staple lines should be inspected using a suction probe to palpate the staple line to ensure that they are intact.

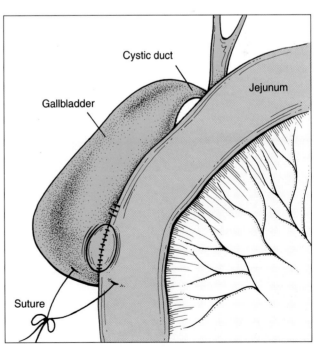

Figure 5. An illustration of the common opening formed between the gallbladder and the jejunum after firing of the stapler. The anterior and posterior staple lines, as formed in a V, are shown.

The combined entry sites into gallbladder and jejunum now remain to be closed. The edges of the incision, *ie*, the jejunum and the gallbladder, are apposed using two to three silk sutures placed via instruments in cannulae 2 and 3 as described previously. These sutures should be tied firmly to tightly close the edges, but once more the ends are left long for later manipulation (Fig. 7). One of the sutures must be placed at the opposite end of the common incision to that of the original anchoring suture to be sure that the second firing of the stapler completely closes the opening (Fig. 8). The stapler is reloaded with a 3.5 cartridge and again introduced into the abdomen via the RIF cannula. The surgeon uses a grasper in the midline cannula and the assistant uses one in the xiphisternal cannula, as they hold the sutures at each end of the common incision

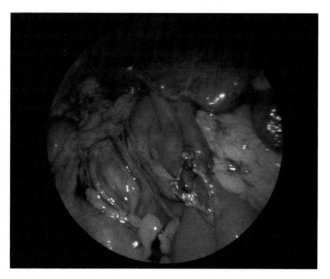

Figure 6. The jejunum in the foreground can be seen stapled to the gallbladder, and a moderate-sized common opening is apparent.

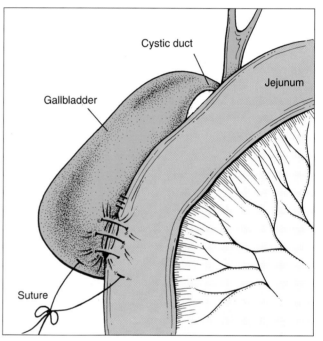

Figure 7. An illustration showing how the sutures are placed to close the common opening. The sutures are cut long and placed such that they incorporate the entire length of the incision. They will be used to pull the adjacent sides of the common opening between the opened jaws of the stapler.

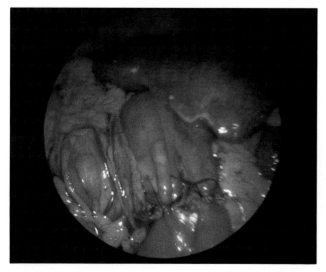

Figure 8. The common opening has been closed by sutures that have been left long.

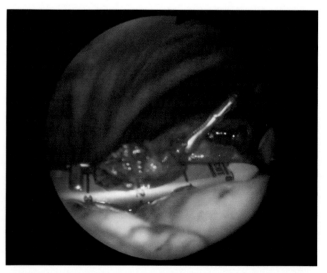

Figure 9. The stapler has been passed via the right iliac fossa cannula, and a grasper manipulating the tissue has been passed via the xiphisternal cannula. Excess tissue must not be gathered between the jaws to avoid narrowing the stoma, but the full length of the common opening needs to be stapled.

and push caudad to slide the viscera between the opened jaws of the stapler. When the jaws of the stapler are closed, excess tissue must not be pulled between them such that the final anastomosis might be narrowed, yet the full length of the common opening as indicated by the sutures must be placed between the markers on the stapler jaws (Fig. 9). If the full length of the incision cannot be encompassed in the stapler jaws, then rather than narrow the opening, a second firing of the stapler may be required to completely close the incision. When a satisfactory position is achieved, the stapler is fired, opened, and removed from the abdomen. The remnant of gallbladder and jejunum that had extended above the jaws of the stapler prior to stapling is now amputated and removed from the abdomen via a grasper in the xiphisternal cannula. If this remnant is not completely amputated, it should be removed with scissors (Fig. 10) and a suture placed at the amputation site. The anastomosis now consists of three staple lines, two in the form of a V from the first firing of the stapler and a third across the base of the V from the second firing.

If a palliative gastroenterostomy is required, it is either performed now or can be done prior to the biliary bypass. This part of the procedure is done with the surgeon on the right side of the operating table and the assistant on the left. If the falciform ligament is bulky from tumor deposits, the cannulae may need to be reintroduced and then pushed through the ligament to get instruments to pass to the left side of the abdomen. A suture is introduced into the abdomen with a needle holder passed via the midline cannula. A proximal loop of jejunum (afferent to the gallbladder if the biliary anastomosis is already done) is loosely sutured to the antrum of the stomach; to transfer the needle, a grasper is held in the surgeon's left hand in the xiphisternal cannula. As for the gallbladder, if there is difficulty maintaining tissue orientation, a more firmly tied suture can be placed between the antrum and the jejunum at the

predicted distal end of the staple line. The risk of this suture's tearing is much lower than in the gallbladder. The stapler is introduced via the xiphisternal cannula into the antrum and then into the jejunum using a grasper in the midline cannula. This process may be assisted if necessary with a grasper passed via the RIF cannula. If the liver is large and bulky from a secondary tumor and the stapler cannot be angled from the xiphisternal cannula into the stomach under the liver, the stapler can be passed via the RIF cannula. The anastomosis is completed as described for the gallbladder but for the following modification [9,10]. Because of the thickness of the gastric wall and because of the solidity of the gastric content, to make large enough stoma the stapled opening has to be extended. This requires a second firing of the stapler before closing the gastrotomy/enterotomy. When performing this second firing, be sure that the reloaded stapler is inserted the full length of the first stapled opening. This can be confirmed when the stapler is closed, and the stomach and jejunum beyond the first staple line are apposed. An alternative is to use a 60 mm stapler, but this does require the use of larger cannulae for its insertion.

OUTCOME, COMPLICATIONS, AND SEQUELAE

Evaluation of laparoscopic cholecystenterostomy and gastroenterostomy is limited; the literature includes a case report by the author [7] now extended to five cases, a series of five cases from Scotland [8], the latter mostly hand sewn, a description of the technique of gastroenterostomy by Fowler [9], and one further case report [10]. As recommended by the authors of two of those papers [7,8], the procedure should not be attempted by the surgeon lacking laparoscopic suturing skills, as this technique is still a major portion of the procedure even though the stapler is used.

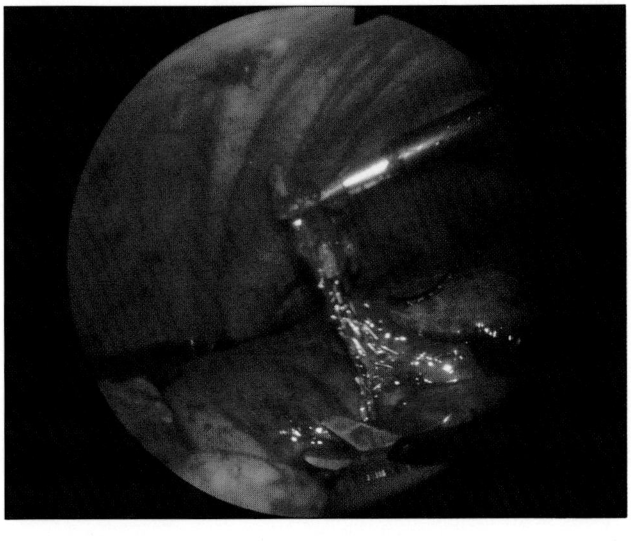

Figure 10. The stapler has been fired and removed. The amputated but stapled excess jejunum and gallbladder is to be trimmed off with scissors. In this circumstance, a reinforcing suture is required.

OPERATIVE PERIOD

For the author, operating time was 200 minutes for the first case but is now 75 minutes, similar to the average 90 minutes reported by Shimi *et al.* [8]. As with laparoscopic cholecystectomy, patient safety comes first. Because these debilitated patients are likely to have only a short survival, to avoid their spending a proportion of that time in the hospital recovering from a complication, conversion to open procedure should be undertaken without hesitation. One procedure on a patient of the author's series was converted to open surgery when adhesions from previous surgery resulted in a tear in the jejunum as the jejunum was being passed to the right side of the abdomen by the assistant using a 5-mm grasper. This instrument is now recognized as being totally inadequate for the purpose.

POSTOPERATIVE PERIOD

As with laparoscopic cholecystectomy, recovery is rapid. The use of marcaine injections at the cannula sites obviates the need for postoperative narcotic injections, often in the first 12 hours and certainly after the first 24 hours unless pain occurs from malignant infiltration. With still limited experience, few complications have been reported. Shimi *et al.* [8] had one patient who required reintervention to clear a clot obstructing the stoma. With the already debilitated patients undergoing these procedures, hospital stays are slightly longer (4–7 days) than for patients who undergo laparoscopic cholecystectomy.

SEQUELAE

Shimi *et al.* [8] had no adverse outcome during the survival of his five patients, an example of first-class palliation. In this author's experience, the longest survivor at nearly 12 months is still symptom free. One patient, however, the first in the series, returned with recurrent jaundice caused by invasion of the cystic duct as well as vomiting resulting from duodenal invasion. This result was despite the initial ERCP showing that the duodenum was not invaded and that the cystic duct was

patent. She required laparotomy and hepatodochojejunostomy as well as gastroenterostomy. She represents the patient population with aggressive tumor growth that is difficult to predict. Another circumstance in which the cystic duct may become occluded is in those expected to have long survival times that would allow more time for the tumor to invade the cystic duct. If this situation appears likely, then the limit of uninvolved duct below the cystic–common hepatic duct junction should be extended beyond the 1 cm recommended for the majority.

CONCLUSION

The laparoscope can be expected to provide a major advance in the palliation of gastrointestinal malignancy, as evidenced by the treatment of malignant bile duct obstruction. Laparoscopic cholecystenterostomy has the advantage of surgery, *ie*, long-term patency of the large surgical stoma (provided the patient is appropriately selected), plus the advantage of stent *ie*, minimal access. It has the added advantage over stenting of allowing palliative gastroenterostomy during the same procedure. Patient selection for the procedure is based on the predicted length of survival and assessment of whether the gallbladder is appropriate for bypass, as evidenced by biliary imaging. This selection process should result in approximately 50% of patients with malignant obstructive jaundice being managed by this relatively simple laparoscopic technique. Further evaluation is required to determine its safety as compared with the established techniques of open surgery and stenting.

ACKNOWLEDGMENTS

The author thanks David Slattery, medical illustrator, for preparation of the illustrations and Gayle Henry for preparation of the manuscript.

REFERENCES

Papers of particular interest, published within the period of review, have been highlighted as:
• Of special interest
•• Of outstanding interest

1. Fletcher DR, Hurley RA, Hardy KJ: The Effect of Selective Therapy on Malignant Obstructive Jaundice. *Med J Aust* 1989, 151:560–564.

2. Huang JF, Little JM: Malignant Jaundice. *Aust N Z J Surg* 1987, 57:905–909.

3.•• Bornman PC, Harries-Jones EP, Tobias R, *et al.*: Prospective Controlled Trial of Transhepatic Biliary Endoprosthesis Versus Bypass Surgery for Incurable Carcinoma of Head of Pancreas. *Lancet* 1986, i:69–71.
One of the first of the clinical trials of surgery versus percutaneous stent, highlighting the lesser morbidity of stent early but higher complications later.

4.• Speer AG, Cotton PB, Russell RCG, *et al.*: Randomised Trial of Endoscopic Versus Percutaneous Stent Insertion in Malignant Obstructive Jaundice. *Lancet* 1987, ii:57–62.

An early control clinical trial of endoscopic versus radiologic stent, showing greater initial safety of endoscopic stent but the same long-term complications.

5. Summerfield JA: Biliary Obstruction is Best Managed by Endoscopists. *Gut* 1988, 29:741–745.

6.•• Little JM, Wong KP: Palliation of Malignant Jaundice. *Aust N Z J Surg* 1991, 61:501–504.

One of the rare publications that attempts to assess the total quality of life over time of the different techniques of managing malignant bile duct obstruction. It recommends a strategy of how the techniques might be best used.

7. Fletcher DR, Jones RM: Laparoscopic Cholecystjejunostomy as Palliation for Obstructive Jaundice in Inoperable Carcinoma of Pancreas. *Surg Endosc* 1992, 6:147–149.

8. Shimi S, Banting S, Raft A: Laparoscopy in the Management of Pancreatic Cancer: Endoscopic Cholecystojejunostomy for Advanced Disease. *Br J Surg* 1992, 79:317–319.

9. Fowler DL: Palliative Surgery in the Upper Digestive Tract—Laparoscopic Gastroenterostomy. In *Minimally Invasive Surgery in Gastrointestinal Cancer.* Edited by Cuesta M., Nagy A. 1993. London: Churchill Livingstone, in press.

10. Wilson RG, Varma JS: Laparoscopic Gastroenterostomy for Malignant Duodenal Obstruction. *Br J Surg* 19??, 79:1348.

11.•• Pitt HA, Cameron JL, Postier RG, Gadacz TR: Factors Affecting Mortality in Biliary Surgery. *Am J Surg* 1981, 141:66–71.

An original description of multivariate analysis of preoperative factors that predict adverse outcome following surgery in obstructive jaundice.

Chapter 13

Laparoscopic Surgery of the Liver and Spleen

Adrian E. Ortega
Jeffrey H. Peters

The application of laparoscopy to the study of liver and spleen afflictions is deeply rooted in the history of this operative approach. Newer diagnostic and therapeutic applications are emerging and offer the same potential benefits as other laparoscopic procedures in which an upper abdominal incision can be obviated (Tables 1 and 2).

HISTORICAL ASPECTS

George Kelling, a surgeon from Dresden, Germany, was the first to describe examination of intra-abdominal viscera with a cystoscope in 1901 [cited in 1••]. He described performance of the technique in a dog and reported his method at the 73rd Congress of German Naturalists and Physicians convened in Hamburg, 1901.

Precisely determining whether or not Kelling was the first to apply this technology to human subjects is difficult. He did, however, comment to the German Surgical Society in 1923 how the dire economic situation of the population in post–World War I Germany had compelled him to make wider use of this diagnostic method because it saved patients the prolonged, costly hospital stay of a nontherapeutic laparotomy. With the aid of laparoscopy, he could determine whether or not a case of carcinoma of the stomach, for instance, was still operable.

Jacobaeus of Stockholm described cystoscopic examination of the pleural, pericardial, and peritoneal cavities in 1910 [cited in 1••]. He referred to his methods as *thoraco-laparoscopy*. Initially, he performed laparoscopy only on patients with ascites. One year following his original publication, Jacobaeus reported 115 examinations on 72 patients. He could distinguish between cirrhosis of the liver, lues, metastatic tumors, tuberculous peritonitis, and several pleural afflictions.

Kalk was the most influential European proponent of peritoneoscopy. He employed a pneumoperitoneum needle and developed a 135° endoscope. He is generally credited with the use of a second puncture [2]. Kalk reported 4000 liver biopsies and published extensively on liver and gallbladder disease.

John C. Ruddock, a physician from Los Angeles, California, was one of the earliest proponents of peritoneoscopy in the United States. He worked primarily on improving the diagnosis of ascites of unknown etiology and reported his work before the Pacific Coast Surgical Association in 1934 [3]. He considered peritoneoscopy superior to diagnostic laparotomy for investigation of the source of tumors, for the operability of intra-abdominal lesions, and for excluding the diagnosis of intra-abdominal metastases. By 1939, Ruddock had performed a series of 900 cases [4]. Among his primary indications for peritoneoscopy, Ruddock included splenomegaly and hepatomegaly.

Except for isolated reports, the focus of laparoscopic applications shifted into the gynecologic realm until the introduction of the computer-chip camera in 1986 [5]. The coupling of the laparoscope to a video system enabled the safe performance of more complex surgical procedures and resulted in the era of therapeutic laparoscopy.

DISEASE OF THE LIVER

DIAGNOSTIC LAPAROSCOPY

Malignant disease and the limitations of current imaging techniques

The modest popularity of laparoscopy for the diagnosis of diseases of the liver waned during the 1970s and 1980s as less-invasive techniques including ultrasound, computed tomography (CT), and magnetic resonance imaging (MRI) emerged. Luning and coworkers [6] published a study comparing MRI, CT, and ultrasound in the diagnosis of focal hepatic lesions. MRI showed the highest accuracy and sensitivity. The positive predictive value was 97% for MRI and CT and 95% for ultrasonography. The negative predictive value was 97% for MRI, 98% for CT, and 93% for ultrasonography. Spinelli and coworkers [7] investigated the accuracy of ultrasonography in the diagnosis of hepatic tumors. They found that sonography was superior in the diagnosis of hemangiomas and malignant primary tumors but inferior in the detection of metastases.

Although these newer imaging techniques have

Table 1. Laparoscopic liver surgery

Diagnostic
Staging of gastrointestinal malignancies
  Gastric carcinoma
  Pancreatic carcinoma
Evaluation of metastatic colon cancer following treatment of the primary lesion (eg, rising CEA with normal endoscopic and radiologic imaging studies)
Staging of Hodgkin's disease (?)
Cirrhosis
Exudative ascites of unknown etiology
  Tuberculosis
  Malignancy
  Trauma
  Infectious processes

Therapeutic
Cystic liver disease
  Hydatid
  Congenital
  Wedge excision of metastatic tumors (?)

Table 2. Laparoscopic surgery of the spleen

Diagnostic
Splenic biopsy for splenomegaly and tumors of unknown etiology trauma

Therapeutic
Splenectomy

undoubtedly resulted in fewer unnecessary exploratory laparotomies, their limitations are also well established. Specifically, the utility of radiologic techniques in assessing focal parenchymal disease is generally limited to lesions more than 1 cm in diameter, and such techniques are particularly poor at visualizing masses on the liver's surface. Autopsy studies show metastatic liver disease, in particular, is evident on the liver's surface in 90% of instances [8]. Based on their own studies and a review of the literature, Leuschner and Leuschner [9•] concluded that laparoscopy is not superior to imaging techniques such as ultrasonography, CT, or MRI in the detection of hepatic masses but seems more sensitive in the detection and characterization of small tumors. For small lesions, laparoscopy had a specificity of 100%.

The comparative value of a normal staging examination in the evaluation of intra-abdominal malignancy is also important. Brady and coworkers [10•] demonstrated the high predictive value for a normal laparoscopy (89%) as compared with a normal CT scan (50%) in patients with suspected liver or peritoneal malignancy.

Based on these observations, a rational approach to the evaluation of hepatic masses and the staging of intra-abdominal malignancy can be formulated. Primary liver lesions can generally be approached via conventional imaging techniques complemented by radiologic-guided biopsy. At present, laparoscopy is limited to lesions that can be seen on the surface. The staging of intra-abdominal malignancies should be individualized, depending on the primary lesion. Colonic, gastric, and pancreatic neoplasms represent the most common gastrointestinal malignancies that metastasize to the liver. Preoperative staging in colon cancer is not as important as for gastric and pancreatic lesions because removal of the primary lesion in the colon is generally desirable. The determination of hepatic involvement in gastric and pancreatic cancers becomes important, as it generally precludes resection. When conventional imaging techniques fail to reveal hepatic metastases in the face of conflicting clinical data, laparoscopy may be considered.

Possik and coworkers [11] examined the discriminatory capacity of laparoscopy for the staging of gastric cancer and detection of liver metastases. Laparoscopy was associated with a 96.5% efficiency (proportion of correct abnormal and normal results) in the detection of hepatic metastases. Warshaw and coworkers [12] investigated the role of laparoscopy in staging and planning of therapy for pancreatic cancer. In this series, laparoscopy yielded an overall accuracy of 93%. The accuracy for a normal examination was 88%. In Warshaw's study, laparoscopy was employed only in patients in whom ultrasonography and CT had shown no evidence of metastases. Seventeen of 40 patients (43%) had metastatic lesions; 14 were found by laparoscopy. All 14 lesions were 1 to 2 mm in diameter.

Overall, laparoscopy and imaging techniques such as ultrasonography, CT, and MRI should be regarded as complementary modalities in the staging of gastrointestinal malignancies and the detection of hepatic metastases.

Laparoscopy may be particularly advantageous, although unstudied, in the evaluation of colorectal carcinomas when a rising carcinoembryonic antigen level is noted in the presence of normal findings at endoscopy of the large bowel and imaging techniques of the liver.

Laparoscopic ultrasonography

A potentially useful adjunct to diagnostic laparoscopy of the liver and other intra-abdominal parenchymal structures is contact sonography. Miles and coworkers [13••] applied this technique to the staging of hepatic neoplasms. In this report, contact hepatic sonography was shown able to establish the presence of unsuspected bilobar metastases as well as tumor thrombus extension into the portal vein. Intracorporeal ultrasound is also useful in the delineation of hepatobiliary anatomy.

Cirrhosis and ascites

The cause of cirrhosis and ascites is often suggested from a patient's history and immunoserologic examination. Liver biopsy is often informative although not uniformly necessary.

Many European centers have advocated the use of laparoscopic-guided liver biopsy in patients with cirrhosis, whereas blind percutaneous or ultrasound-guided techniques have predominated in this country. Proponents of laparoscopic evaluation and biopsy of the liver for cirrhosis argue the superiority of this technique on the basis that more severely affected areas of the liver can be sampled under direct vision with the concomitant ability to obtain hemostasis. Pagliaro and coworkers [14] compared blind percutaneous biopsy and laparoscopic-guided biopsy for the diagnosis of cirrhosis. Percutaneous biopsy was correct in 82% of patients, and the laparoscopic approach was accurate in 100%. Nord's [15] review of six studies comprising 1251 cases that compared macroscopic diagnosis at laparoscopy with direct-vision biopsy demonstrated that the false-negative rate for biopsy diagnosis of cirrhosis ranged from 7% to 51%, with an average of 29%. In contrast, the false-negative rate for diagnosis of macroscopic surface changes at laparoscopy ranged from 4% to 18%, with an average of 9%. Comparison of ultrasound-guided and laparoscopic-guided liver biopsy shows no clear superiority of either method [16].

Other potential advantages of laparoscopy in the evaluation of cirrhosis and chronic hepatitis include the ability to characterize the morphologic changes associated with the process and to detect early evidence of primary hepatocellular carcinoma in high-risk patients.

Characterization of the architectural changes associated with cirrhosis has prognostic utility. Tameda and coworkers [17] looked at cumulative survival rate with respect to the development of regenerating nodules, size of the right hepatic lobe, formation of small lymphatic vessels, and degree of splenomegaly. These observations characterize the stage of evolution in the cirrhotic process and may be of value in determining the correct timing of liver transplantation.

Kameda and Shinji [18] demonstrated that the presence of yellow surface nodules on the liver surface are reliable indicators for the early detection of hepatocellular carcinoma by laparoscopy in cirrhotic patients. These yellow nodules are caused by focal fatty changes.

The diagnosis of ascites is established by a combination of the patient's history and results of physical, laboratory, and radiologic examinations. The characterization of ascites by paracentesis as transudative or exudative narrows the differential diagnosis. Transudation results from an increase in pressure in the portal or systemic venous systems or a lowering of the plasma osmotic pressure. It is often associated with congestive heart failure, pericarditis, cardiomyopathy, or cor pulmonale. Portal hypertension in the presence of either a lower plasma protein level that accompanies cirrhosis or increased hepatic lymphatic pressure that accompanies hepatic vein obstruction in Budd-Chiari syndrome is also associated with transudative ascites. Finally, gross depletion of plasma proteins produced by such conditions as starvation or nephrotic syndrome are associated with transudation as well as generalized anasarca.

Exudative ascites occurs usually in the presence of either tuberculous peritonitis or carcinomatosis peritonei. Paracentesis may in some cases suggest the precise cause of this process but is frequently inconclusive. Manohar and coworkers [19] employed laparoscopy in the evaluation of 145 patients with tuberculous peritonitis. The findings on paracentesis revealed an exudate, with none being positive for acid-fast bacilli. Typical peritoneal tubercles were seen in almost all patients, and a few demonstrated only erythematous patches. Histologic diagnosis was confirmed by the presence of caseating granulomata in all patients, while acid-fast bacilli were seen in 74%. Because conventional imaging techniques are relatively poor in the evaluation of peritoneal disease, diagnostic laparoscopy may be invaluable for evaluation of exudative ascites of undetermined cause.

Staging laparoscopy of Hodgkin's disease

Staging of Hodgkin's disease by laparotomy is not as common a practice today as in the past. There are a variety of reasons for this trend. Although staging laparotomy frequently upstages the disease in 25% to 30% of cases, the converse situation occurs in 10% to 15% [20]. Overall, as more patients are treated with a combination of chemotherapy and radiation, fewer are candidates for exploratory surgery. For instance, stage IIIb and IV patients all receive combination chemo- and radiation therapy. These patients do not benefit from additional surgical staging. Patients with extensive mediastinal and extranodal disease are also increasingly treated with combination therapy because of limited success of single-modality treatment with radiation. Moreover, splenectomy performed as part of staging laparotomy in patients over 40 years of age who receive combination chemotherapy are at increased risk of developing acute leukemia. The indications for surgical staging in Hodgkin's disease continue to evolve. Staging still may be appropriate for the lower clinical stages (IA, IIA, and IIIA).

Classical staging laparotomy consists of a systematic abdominal exploration, splenectomy, liver biopsy, and selective excision of abdominal and retroperitoneal lymph nodes. The selection of lymph node regions for sampling depends on the results of CT scan examination, lymphangiography, and intraoperative findings. Although evaluation of the liver can be done well laparoscopically, splenectomy may present a greater challenge depending on the degree of splenomegaly present. Incision of the lesser omentum with lymph-node sampling in the celiac region is also feasible, as is inspection of the liver hilum and the cystic and common bile duct areas. Lymph nodes from the small bowel mesentery, mesocolon, and iliac regions are also readily accessible laparoscopically. Exposure of paracaval and para-aortic lymph nodes represents a greater challenge but, depending on the size and location of these nodes, may be feasible. Oophoropexy and bone-marrow biopsy complete the staging procedure. Experienced laparoscopists should be able to perform the majority of the maneuvers necessary for the proper staging of Hodgkin's disease. The application of laparoscopy for this purpose is a realistic possibility that deserves further clinical investigation.

Trauma

Laparoscopy for liver trauma is promising. Alterations in mental status in victims with blunt abdominal trauma generally oblige the surgeon to perform either diagnostic peritoneal lavage or abdominal CT to exclude an intra-abdominal injury. Hemoperitoneum secondary to liver, splenic, or arterial injuries is a relatively common finding of diagnosis peritoneal lavage or abdominal CT in this situation. These findings yield a 15% to 20% incidence of nontherapeutic laparotomies because these tests are too sensitive and are relatively nonspecific.

Berci and coworkers [21••] demonstrated the utility of minilaparoscopy performed as a bedside procedure in 150 cases of blunt trauma. In their series, 56% of patients had normal examinations, and none had false-negative results. Another 25% had minimal-to-moderate hemoperitoneum without identifiable injury, or only a small laceration was encountered. These patients were observed in an appropriately monitored setting, and only one patient subsequently required a formal laparotomy. Nineteen percent of patients studied had either a significant hemoperitoneum, defined as the bowel floating in blood upon insufflation, or a hollow viscus perforation and underwent formal laparotomy. This study suggests that patients with mild-to-moderate hemoperitoneum can be safely treated expectantly and that a significant number of nontherapeutic laparotomies for blunt trauma to solid abdominal viscera such as the liver and spleen can be avoided.

Few reports have focused on the role of laparoscopy in the evaluation of penetrating abdominal trauma [22•,23]. The accuracy of laparoscopy in this situation is gaining credibility. A few anecdotal reports [23] describe nontherapeutic laparotomies being obviated after the finding of nonbleeding liver injuries secondary to penetrating trauma. Overall, laparoscopy may be an excellent tool for the evaluation of liver injuries for penetrating and blunt abdominal trauma, but further work in this area is necessary.

Infectious processes

Laparoscopy has been used in the diagnosis of such parasitic diseases as echinococcosis, amebiasis, and schistosomiasis in areas of the world in which those diseases are endemic [24]. Opportunistic infections in immunocompromised patients are also amenable to laparoscopic diagnosis. Specifically, focal hepatic candidiasis diagnosed laparoscopically has been reported [25,26]. These patients typically demonstrate a liver-function profile with disproportionate elevation of alkaline phosphatase as compared to aminotransferases. At laparoscopy, the liver surface reveals multiple white plaques. In the era of acquired immune deficiency syndrome, the utility of this approach for a variety of other infectious processes can be expected to expand.

THERAPEUTIC LAPAROSCOPY

Cystic liver disease

Katkhouda and coworkers [27] published a case report of laser resection of a liver hydatid cyst under videolaparoscopy. The 6-cm lesion was located in the left hepatic lobe. A four-port technique was employed. In addition to the infraumbilical cannula for the videoscope, another 10-mm port was placed to the right of the umbilicus through which an electrical hook, scissors, NdYAG laser fiber, and clip applier were passed. A 5-mm subxiphoid port was used for a suction-irrigation cannula and a palpation probe. The fourth 5-mm port was placed to the right of the umbilicus, through which an atraumatic grasping forceps was inserted. The

pericystectomy required 160 minutes, and the patient made an uneventful recovery. He was discharged home on the third postoperative day and resumed work one week after surgery.

Way (Way, Paper presented at the Scientific Session of the Society of American Gastrointestinal Endoscopic Surgeons, Washington, DC, 1992) reported nine patients with benign simple cysts of the liver treated laparoscopically. Two patients had congenital polycystic disease, five patients had large solitary cysts at the surface of the liver, and two patients had large solitary intrahepatic cysts. He treated the large surface liver cysts by excising 30% to 50% of their surface area and tacking omentum over the residual lining. The intrahepatic cysts were opened and drained by removing a small portion (*eg*, 10%) of their surface area. Omentum was placed within the cavity and tacked in place. The patients with polycystic disease were treated by simple unroofing of as many cysts as possible (*eg*, 50 cysts). His results were excellent in all but the patients with polycystic disease, although the latter patients reported some symptomatic improvement. The remaining seven patients remained asymptomatic. One patient was noted to have a recurrence by CT scan. No complications occurred in this series, and all patients were discharged within 1 to 2 days postoperatively. Way concluded that, overall, results of laparoscopic treatment of liver cysts are equivalent to open surgery, with the salient exception of a shorter hospital stay. He also suggested that laparoscopic therapy may become the treatment of choice in patients with symptomatic liver cysts.

Techniques in diagnostic and therapeutic laparoscopy of the liver

Laparoscopic-guided liver biopsy can often be performed with a single trocar placed infraumbilically for accommodation of the laparoscope. Lesions that appear on the anterior surface of the liver are often accessible percutaneously using a fine needle or a biopsy needle (*eg*, Tru-Cut, Vim-Silverman, Mehghini). Inspection of the undersurface of the liver requires placement of a second port through which a palpation instrument or elevating retractor is inserted (Fig. 1). The authors prefer using a fan-type retractor for this purpose. Moreover, angled-viewing and flexible laparoscopes may represent a genuine advantage for inspection of the entire surface of the liver. If larger samples of tissue are required, standard cup-type biopsy forceps can be inserted through the second trocar with hemostasis accomplished by using cautery or laser energy. Brush biopsies of vascular lesions for cytology can also be obtained safely.

Performance of wedge biopsies, wedge excision of lesions, and cystectomies all require insertion of additional trocars to accommodate suction and irrigation, atraumatic tissue forceps, and some form of electrosurgical energy. Laparoscopic adaptation of the Argon beam laser may be particularly well suited for this purpose. A laparoscopic ultrasonic dissector (ValleyLab, Boulder, CO) is also under development and may play a useful role in laparoscopic liver surgery.

DISEASES OF THE SPLEEN

DIAGNOSTIC LAPAROSCOPY

Because of its position in the posterior subphrenic space, the spleen is difficult to visualize during the course of routine laparoscopic examination of the abdomen. Easy visualization of this organ usually signals a relative-to-moderate degree of splenomegaly. Percutaneous splenic biopsy, at least in theory, poses a risk of bleeding. However, Dagnini and coworkers [28] reported experience with 1243 laparoscopic splenic biopsies. The procedure was applied to the staging and follow-up of malignant lymphomas and to the examination of suspected splenopathy. They concluded that the risk of splenic biopsy is minimal and commented that fears regarding its performance are unjustified.

The role of diagnostic laparoscopy for trauma has

been previously mentioned. Laparoscopy offers advantages over diagnostic peritoneal lavage in that the nature of splenic injuries in otherwise hemodynamically stable patients can be evaluated. The presence of ongoing bleeding, as well as associated injuries, can be excluded. Similar to the situation for liver trauma, abdominal CT has shortcomings with respect to visualization of the traumatized spleen. Not infrequently, a splenic fracture or laceration is observed on CT scan in association with free fluid in the abdominal cavity. This finding may represent hemoperitoneum from the splenic injury, a remote intrabdominal source, or perforation of a hollow viscus. Laparoscopy in this situation allows for the exclusion of other injuries and for a focus on splenic preservation and avoidance of nontherapeutic laparotomy.

LAPAROSCOPIC SPLENECTOMY

Reports of laparoscopic splenectomy emerged in 1992. Carroll and coworkers [29••] reported three cases–two for Hodgkin's disease and one for idiopathic thrombocytopenic purpura. All patients were discharged between 2 and 5 days postoperatively, and there were no complications. Hashizume [30] reported two cases in which laparoscopic splenectomy was performed with

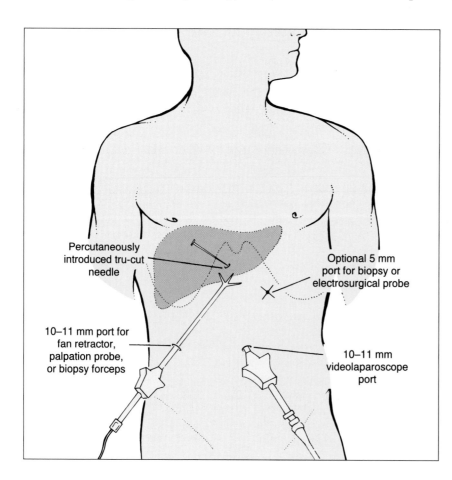

Figure 1. Laparoscopic liver biopsy can occasionally be performed with a single trocar placed infraumbilically, combined with percutaneous passage of a Tru-cut or other needle biopsy technique. Thorough examination of the liver surface requires placement of a second port for placement of a palpation probe or fan-type retractor. Biopsy forceps may also be introduced through the second port. Alternatively, a third port may be added for additional instruments, such as graspers, biopsy forceps, cautery, or laser, as well as suction/irrigation for wedge excision of lesions.

Percutaneously introduced tru-cut needle

Optional 5 mm port for biopsy or electrosurgical probe

10–11 mm port for fan retractor, palpation probe, or biopsy forceps

10–11 mm videolaparoscope port

the aid of an ultrasonic dissector. Both patients had idiopathic thrombocytopenic purpura. Neither patient suffered untoward sequelae, and both were able to discontinue steroid treatment. These reports illustrate the feasibility of laparoscopic splenectomy.

Although a variety of conditions represent absolute versus relative indications for splenectomy (Table 3), the disease processes that seem most amenable to laparoscopic splenectomy are those without massive splenomegaly. Conditions associated with chronic massive splenomegaly include chronic myeloid leukemia, myelofibrosis, polycythemia, portal hypertension, Gaucher's disease, and thalassemia major in children. More moderate degrees of splenomegaly are found in the preceding conditions if discovered at earlier stages. Moderate splenomegaly occurs in chronic lymphocytic leukemia, lymphoma, acute leukemia in its late phases, hemolytic disorders, thalassemia, and some of the hemoglobinopathies. A variety of other conditions are associated with acute splenomegaly, although the enlargement tends to be less significant. These diagnoses include a variety of infectious and granulomatous diseases that do not require splenec-

tomy as well as Felty's syndrome, splenic infarction, splenic vein thrombosis, and a variety of cystic diseases and benign tumors including hydatid disease, dermoids, hemangiomas, lymphangiomas, endothelioma, and polycystic disease.

The conditions in which splenopathy is generally present without massive splenomegaly may be most conducive to laparoscopic splenectomy. These disorders include hereditary spherocytosis, autoimmune anemia, Hodgkins's disease, immune thrombocytopenic purpura, thrombotic thrombocytopenic purpura, symptomatic cysts, and primary splenic tumors, as well as the occasional patient with sickle cell disease and hypersplenism. Splenic abscesses and ruptured spleens from any cause are probably best approached via laparotomy as are those processes associated with significant splenomegaly.

TECHNIQUE OF LAPAROSCOPIC SPLENECTOMY

The operative technique of laparoscopic splenectomy remains to be standardized. Ideally, the surgeon should be in a position to work two-handed (Fig. 2). Because

Table 3. Indications for splenectomy

Absolute	Relative
Splenic tumors	Congential hemolytic anemias
Splenic abscess	Enzyme deficiencies
Hereditary spherocytosis	Glucose-6-phosphate deficiency
Massive trauma	Pyruvate kinase deficiency
Splenic vein thrombosis	Hereditary elliptocytosis
	Thalassemia major
	Sickle cell anemia
	Idiopathic autoimmune hemolytic anemia
	Idiopathic thrombocytopenic purpura
	Thrombotic thrombocytopenic purpura
	Primary hypersplenism
	Agnogenic myeloid metaplasia
	Polycythemia vera
	Myelofibrosis
	Myeoloid leukemia
	Felty's syndrome
	Hodgkin's disease
	Non-Hodgkin's lymphoma

the spleen is in the upper abdomen, the modified lithotomy position may be advantageous (Fig. 3). The insufflation and camera port can be placed infraumbilically if an angled laparoscope (30° or 45°) is employed (Fig. 4). Use of a zero-degree laparoscope generally requires placement of this port in the supraumbilical position; it

may be situated even higher in the midline, depending on the patient's body habitus. Two additional ports are placed laterally at the same level to allow the surgeon to operate with two hands. One to two additional ports may be placed in the right subcostal or subxiphoid positions to facilitate retraction, suction, and

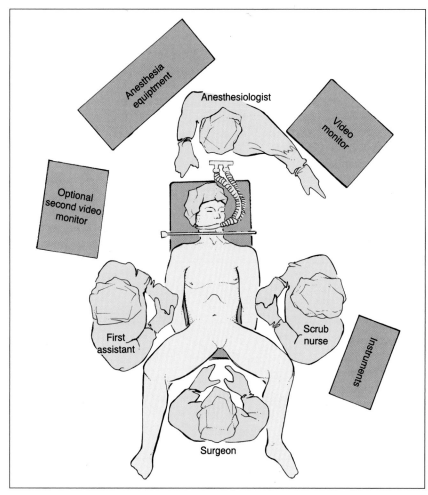

Figure 2. Operating room set up. The assistant(s) and video system should be oriented to optimize the surgeon's capacity to work two-handed in the direction of spleen and associated structures.

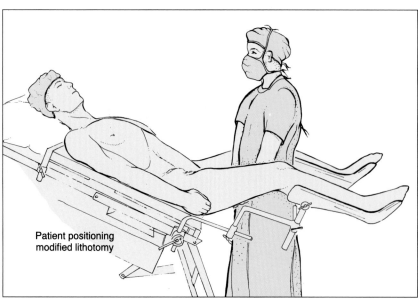

Figure 3. Patient positioning. Modified lithotomy is a convenient position for the dissection of upper abdominal structures. Reverse Trendelenburg position and rotation of the table with the left side up enhances the effect of gravity in exposure of the spleen and its attachments.

irrigation. Because of their greater flexibility for introducing 5- or 10-mm instruments, 10- to 11-mm ports are useful at each of these sites.

As in conventional open splenectomy, the operation is approached by initial ligation of the splenic vessels after opening the lesser sac. Ligating these vessels individually is safer, preferably with extracorporeal knotting techniques. Alternatively, the short gastric vessels can be dissected first and individually clipped (Fig. 5). Their exposure is facilitated by medial retraction and slight anterior elevation of the greater curvature of the stomach. After mobilization of the greater

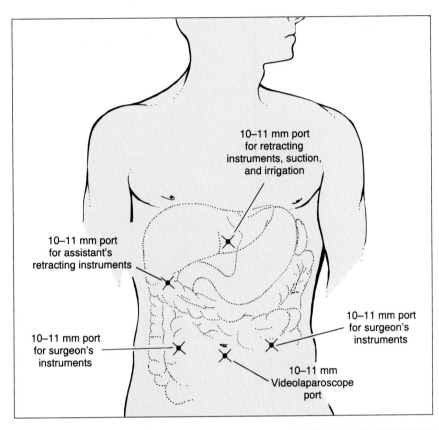

Figure 4. Trocar placement. A five-trocar arrangement is suggested for splenectomy. Body habitus is an important consideration in each individual case.

10–11 mm port for retracting instruments, suction, and irrigation

10–11 mm port for assistant's retracting instruments

10–11 mm port for surgeon's instruments

10–11 mm port for surgeon's instruments

10–11 mm Videolaparoscope port

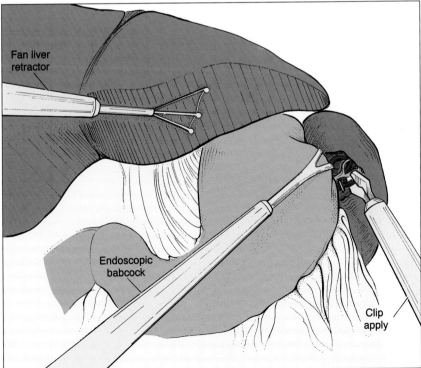

Figure 5. Division of the short gastric vessels. Medial and slight anterior retraction of the stomach facilities exposure of each short gastric vessel. Complete division of the gastrosplenic attachments generally exposes the splenic artery and vein.

Fan liver retractor

Endoscopic babcock

Clip apply

curvature, the splenic artery and vein can be visualized within the hilum (Fig. 6). The remaining ligamentous attachments can be divided by a combination of electrosurgical energy, ligation, or both with extracorporeal knots (Fig. 7). Once mobilized, spleens removed for benign disease can be placed into a plastic bag or other receptacle within the abdominal cavity and morcellated for extraction via the infraumbilical or camera port. Spleens removed for malignancy are best delivered through a small subcostal incision to allow uncompromised histologic and architectural study (Fig. 8).

CONCLUSION

Diagnostic laparoscopy of the liver and spleen occupies an important place in the history of endoscopic surgery. The improved resolution and magnification of today's video endoscopy systems may broaden the applications of laparoscopy in the study of hepatic and splenic afflictions because of greater accuracy than conventional imaging techniques and lower morbidity than laparotomy. Although experience with newer therapeutic applications is limited, laparoscopy for the treatment of these conditions merits serious consideration and careful study.

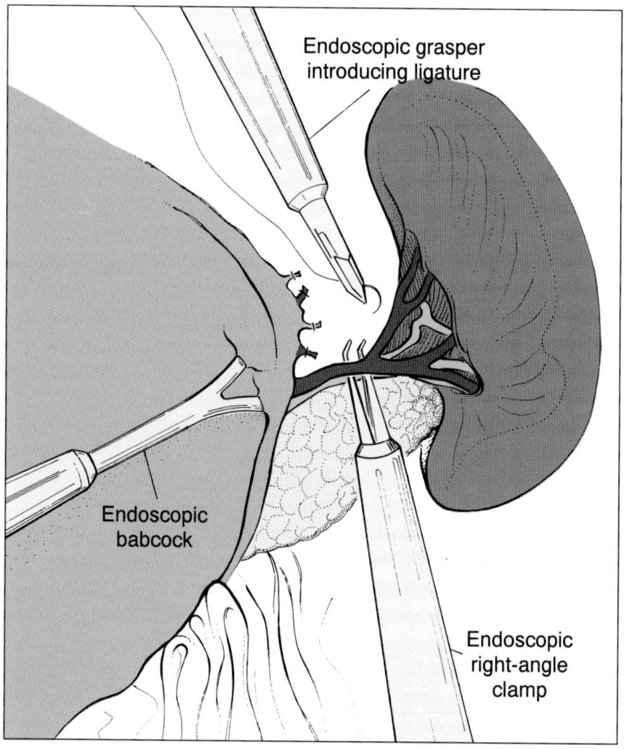

Figure 6. Ligation of the splenic artery and vein is performed with placement of extracorporeally tied ligatures.

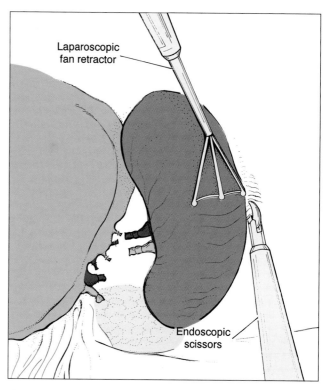

Figure 7. Division of the diaphragmatic, renal, and colon attachments can be performed with electrosurgical energy, ligatures, or linear stapling devises to complete mobilization of the spleen.

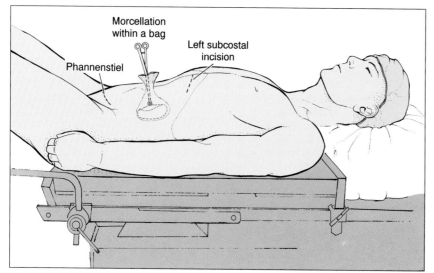

Figure 8. Removal of the spleen. Introduction of a resilient bag into the pelvis with its exteriorization through a trocar wound facilitates morcellization of spleens removed for benign disease. Extraction of spleens with malignant disease can be performed through either a small left upper quadrant or a Pfannenstiel incision.

REFERENCES

Papers of particular interest, published within the period of review, have been highlighted as:
• Of special interest
•• Of outstanding interest

1.•• Nadeau OE, Kampmeier OF: Endoscopy of the Abdomen; Abdominoscopy. *SGO* 1925, 41(3):259.
An excellent description of the early history of laparoscopy and its applications.

2. Gunning JE, Rosenzweig BA: Evolution of Endoscopic Surgery. In *Endoscopic Surgery.* Edited by White RA, Klein SR. St. Louis: Mosby; 1991:3–9.

3. Ruddock JC: Peritoneoscopy. *West J Surg* 1934, 42:392.

4. Ruddock JC: Peritoneoscopy. *SGO* 1937, 65:623.

5. Ortega AE, Peters JH, Ortega AF: Origenes, Presente y Futuro de la Video-Cirugia [The Origins, Present and Future of Video-Assisted Surgery]. *Med Interam* 1992, 11(9):41.

6. Luning M, Koch M, Abel L: Treffsicherheit Bildgebender Verfahren (Sonographie, MRT, CT, Angio-CT, Nuklearmedizin) bei der Charakterisierun von Lebeertmumorenn. *Fortschr Rontgenstr* 1991, 154(4):398.

7. Spinelli P, Dal Fante M, Garbagnati F: Ultrasonography Versus Laparoscopy in the Diagnosis of Hepatic Tumors. *Ital J Surg Sci* 1984, 14:103.

8. Lightdale CJ: Laparoscopy and Biopsy in Malignant Liver Disease. *Cancer* 1982, 50:2672.

9.• Leuschner M, Leuschner U: Diagnostic Laparoscopy in Focal Parenchymal Disease of the Liver. *Endoscopy* 1992, 24:689.
This report places the complimentary role of laparoscopy in the context of the less invasive imaging techniques in the evaluation of focal liver lesions.

10. • Brady PG, Peebles M, Goldschmid ST: Role of Laparoscopy in the Evaluation of Patients with Suspected Hepatic or Peritoneal Malignancy. *Gastrointest Endosc* 1991, 37:27.
This article examines the relative merits of negative CT scans and laparoscopy in patients with suspected liver or peritoneal malignancies.

11. Possik RA, Franco EL, Pires DR, *et al.*: Sensitivity, Specificity, and Predictive Value of Laparoscopy for the Staging of Gastric Cancer and for the Detection of Liver Metastases. *Cancer* 1986, 58:1.

12. Warshaw AL, Tepper JE, Shipley WU: Laparoscopy in the Staging and Planning of Therapy for Pancreatic Cancer. *Am J Surg* 1986, 151:76.

13.•• Miles WFA, Paterson-Brown S, Garden OJ: Laparoscopic Contact Hepatic Ultrasonography. *Br J Surg* 1992, 79:419.
A provocative and futuristic report on the role of intraoperative laparoscopic ultrasound in the evaluation of hepatic neoplasms. This technique may prove superior to conventional imaging techniques and perhaps even palpation during open laparotomy in the staging of hepatic neoplasms.

14. Pagliaro L, Fortunato R, Craxi A: Percutaneous Blind Biopsy Versus Laparoscopy with Guided Biopsy in Diagnosis of Cirrhosis--A Prospective Randomized Trial. *Dig Dis Sci* 1983, 28:39.

15. Nord HJ: Biopsy Diagnosis of Cirrhosis: Blind Percutaneous Versus Guided Direct Vision Techniques–A Review. *Gastrointest Endosc* 1982, 28:102.

16. Boyce HW: Diagnostic Laparoscopy in Liver and Biliary Disease. *Endoscopy* 1992, 24:676.

17. Tameda Y, Toshizawa N, Takasa K: Prognostic Value of Peritoneoscope Findings in Cirrhosis of Liver. *Gastrointest Endosc* 1990, 36:34.

18. Kameda Y, Shinji Y: Early Detection of Hepatocellular Carcinoma by Laparoscopy: Yellow Nodules as Diagnostic Indicators. *Gastrointest Endosc* 1992, 38(5):554.

19. Manohar A, Simjee AE, Haffejee AA: Symptoms and Investigative Findings in 145 Patients with Tuberculous Peritonitis Diagnosed by Peritoneoscopy and Biopsy over a Five-Year Period. *Gut* 1990, 31:1130.

20. Sheldon GF, Croom RD, Meyer AA: The Spleen. In *Textbook of Surgery*, 14th ed. Edited by Sabiston DC Jr. Philadelphia: WB Saunders; 1991:1108–1133.

21.•• Berci G, Sackier JM, Pax-Partlow M: Emergency Laparoscopy. *Am J Surg* 1991, 161:332.
A classic report on the use of laparoscopy in the evaluation of trauma performed as a bedside diagnostic modality under intravenous sedation and local anesthesia.

22.• Smith RS, Tsoi EDM, Fry WR, *et al.*: Laparoscopic Evaluation of Abdominal Trauma: A Preliminary Report. *Contemp Surg* 1993, 42(1):13.
A particularly contemporary review of these authors' application of laparoscopy in the evaluation of trauma.

23. Ivatury RR, Simon RJ, Weksler B, *et al.*: Laparoscopy in the Evaluation of the Intrathoracic Abdomen After Penetrating Injury. *J Trauma* 1992, 33(1):101.

24. Nord HJ, Boyd WP: Diagnostic Laparoscopy. *Endoscopy* 1992, 24:133.

25. Gordon SC, Watts JC, Veneri RJ: Focal Hepatic Candidiasis with Perihepatic Adhesions: Laparoscopic and Immunohistologic Diagnosis. *Gastroenterology* 1990, 98:214.

26. Phillips EH, Carroll BJ, Chandra M, *et al.*: Laparoscopic-Guided Biopsy for Diagnosis of Hepatic Candidiasis. *J Laparoendosc Surg* 1992, 2(1):33.

27. Katkhouda N, Fabiani P, Benizri, Mouiel J: Laser Resection of a Liver Hydatid Cyst under Videolaparoscopy. *Br J Surg* 1992, 79:560.

28. Dagnini G, Cladironi MW, Marin G, Patella M: Laparoscopic Splenic Biopsy. *Endoscopy* 1984, 16(2):55.

29.•• Carroll BJ, Phillips EH, Semel CJ, *et al.*: Laparoscopic Splenectomy. *Surg Endosc* 1992, 6:183.
A preliminary report on this group's experience with laparoscopic splenectomy with an excellent description of the operative technique.

30. Hashizume M, Sugimachi K, Ueno K: Laparoscopic Splenectomy With an Ultrasonic Dissector [letter]. *N Engl J Med* 1992, 327(6):438.

Chapter 14

Laparoscopic Colon and Small-Bowel Surgery

Morris E. Franklin, Jr

With the advent of laparoscopic cholecystectomy and its obvious ramifications, the surgical and medical approaches to most intestinal and gastrointestinal tract diseases have changed rapidly. That this new surgical approach would extend to other uses became obvious, and despite some resistance to this type of surgery, laparoscopic techniques are the future for a multitude of patients with colonic, intestinal, and biliary tract disease [1]. The outstanding results obtained in most series for laparoscopic cholecystectomy have indicated the wide range of acceptance and safety of this surgical approach to gallbladder disease. Improvements in technical products and the advent of advanced laparoscopic tools specifically designed for colonic surgery have led to numerous laparoscopic approaches to surgery of the large and small bowel.

HISTORY

Although laparoscopic diagnostic tests have long been used in the evaluation of colonic disease, only after the first report of repair of a colonic injury encountered during a laparoscopic procedure for endometriosis by Dr. Harry Rich was it realized that colonic procedures be approached laparoscopically. Undoubtedly, appendectomies have been performed in Germany for a long time with outstanding results. In the course of performing these procedures, mobilization of the right colon was occasionally necessary; this idea later came to the United States, where a laparoscopically assisted right colectomy was performed by Jacobs in mid-1990 [2]. This procedure was the first truly planned colonic procedure that embodied laparoscopic techniques. Jacobs used the available equipment to mobilize the right colon, perform a minilaparotomy, and complete the procedure by excising the colon, controlling the bleeding with hemostasis, performing an anastomosis outside the abdominal cavity, and returning the completed anastomosis inside. In late 1990, Dennis Fowler performed the first known laparoscopically assisted left-colon resection [3•]. The first totally intracorporeal laparoscopic colon procedure was performed by Franklin and associates also in late 1990 [4,5]. The patients in these early attempts uniformly did quite well and stimulated interest in additional procedures.

EQUIPMENT AND TECHNIQUE

EQUIPMENT

The equipment required for laparoscopic colon surgery is basically the same as that required for laparoscopic cholecystectomy and other laparoscopic procedures, with some notable exceptions. One exception is that the monitors must be placed in accordance with the portion of the colon on which the operation is planned. Operations on the left, sigmoid, low-anterior, or abdominal-perineal sections of the colon require monitors placed at the foot of the operating table. Operations on the left-upper colon, splenic flexure, transverse colon, or hepatic-flexure portion of the colon require monitors placed more toward the head of the table, or at least at the level of the patient's shoulders. Operations on the cecum require monitors placed at the foot of the table. Thus, if a right hemicolectomy or a left hemicolectomy is proposed, the monitors must be movable, or multiple monitors must be used. Monitors must be available for the surgeon and the assistant surgeon because many of these procedures are prolonged and require intense viewing; the presence of a solitary monitor is grossly inadequate.

The operating table used for laparoscopic colon resections also differs somewhat from that used for laparoscopic cholecystectomy. Only infrequently is there a need for roentgenographic evaluation during the procedure; thus, a translucent table is not mandatory. The table must, however, allow for steep Trendelenburg positioning and for left and right lateral tilting. Additionally, the table must allow ready anal access, as this access is an integral part of laparoscopic colon resections, particularly on lesions that require segmental resection, colotomy, or other surgical procedures requiring precise localization using the colonoscope.

Additional equipment required includes a colonoscope with its monitor, an optional laser, a sequential compression device for the legs, and equipment for adequate warming of intravenous fluids, irrigation fluids, and inspired gases.

Trocar placement varies, depending on the segment of the colon involved. In most cases, at least one trocar should be placed at the umbilicus and the laparoscope inserted through this port. If the patient has had prior surgery, auxiliary ports must be used initially to clearly differentiate the presence of adhesions in the subumbilical area. At least two trocars should be placed for use by the surgeon and usually two trocars for the assistant surgeon, as most laparoscopic colon procedures are performed two-handed by both surgeons (Fig. 1). Experience has demonstrated that 10-mm trocars are more useful than isolated 5-mm or 7.5-mm trocars; thus primarily 10- to 11-mm trocars are recommended for use at all port sites for these advanced procedures. Trocar placement sites are depicted for low-anterior and abdominal-peritoneal resections in Figure 2; placement for splenic-flexure and left-colon resection is depicted in Figure 3; placement for right-colon resection is shown in Figure 4. Availability of an instrument set for open laparotomy is also strongly advised, as the need for conversion to an open procedure may become apparent immediately upon inserting the laparoscope or at any point during the procedure, should an untoward event occur.

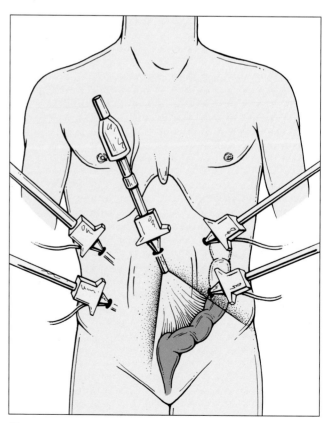

Figure 1. Placement of trocars for sigmoid colon resection.

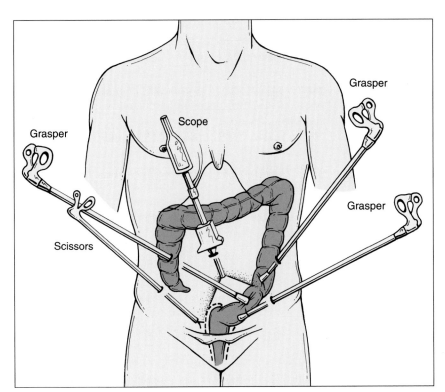

Figure 2. Placement of trocars for low-anterior and abdominal-peritoneal resection.

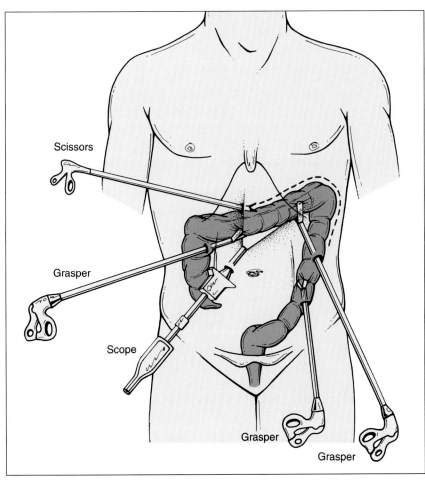

Figure 3. Placement of trocars for splenic-flexure and left-colon resection.

OPERATIVE TECHNIQUE

The operative technique employed for laparoscopic colon resection depends on the area of the colon to be resected, disease process involved, presence or absence of prior surgery, and, most of all, experience of the operating surgeon. The simplest procedure for most laparoscopic colon resections is that of the laparoscopically assisted colon resection popularized by Jacob and Geiss. In this procedure, the involved colon portion is mobilized freely and, in nonmalignant disease, is brought out of the abdominal cavity through a minilaparotomy incision. This step is followed by devascularization, resection, and anastomosis according to the operating surgeon's preferred technique, all done extracorporeally. The colon portion is then reinserted into the abdomen, the abdominal incision is closed, the abdomen is reinsufflated to check for bleeding, and any mesenteric defect is closed. In malignancy, a similar procedure is carried out with the exception that the hemostasis is controlled intracorporeally by identifying, devascularizing and ligating the vessels using clips, ties, or stapling devices [7]. The involved segment is then brought extracorporeally, resected, and the anastomosis constructed. In laparoscopically assisted, intracorporeal low-anterior resections, the anvil is introduced into the proximal segment of the bowel outside the abdominal cavity, sutured into place, and reinserted into the abdominal cavity [8–10]. The head of the stapling device is brought through the previously stapled distal end of the colon, and the anastomosis is completed. These extracorporeally performed procedures obviously are considerably easier to perform than completely intracorporeal procedures and should be the initial procedures attempted by the novice. They do not, however, avoid the greatest problem associated with open procedure—the wound [2,3•].

The totally intracorporeal technique of resection is much more difficult and involves considerably more dexterity and planning. In this technique, the entire procedure save removal of the specimen is performed intracorporeally. The involved segment of colon is isolated, the vasculature is controlled, and the colon is divided. In low-anterior, sigmoid, or left-colon resections, the anvil is placed into the proximal segment of the colon and secured from a transanal approach with intracorporeal suturing technique or endoloops. A similar procedure is carried out on the distal part of the colon. The anvil and the head of the stapling device are then brought together after excess tissue is trimmed (Fig. 5). The resected specimen is placed in a bag and removed transanally if the specimen is small enough (Fig. 6) or is stored in an out-of-the-way place in the abdominal cavity until the anastomosis is completed. The surgeon checks for bleeding, examines the anastomosis for leaks, and then removes the specimen through an extended infraumbilical incision or a right- or left-lower quadrant incision.

The advantage of this intracorporeal procedure, even though it is much more difficult to perform, is that in colon cancer the specimen is totally isolated during the entire procedure and there is little chance of tumor spillage or seeding into the abdominal wall. Spillage and seeding have been reported in laparoscopic thoracotomy and in laparoscopic abdominal procedures. In all cases, the surgeons must have a thorough understanding of, and must constantly review, the anatomy and particularly the relationship of the ureters to any point of the resection. Although multiple methods for identifying the ureters have been expounded, none appears totally adequate for the inexperienced laparoscopic surgeon.

OPERATIVE TECHNIQUE FOR SMALL-BOWEL SURGERY

Small-bowel surgery is in its infancy, and, except for trauma, very few indications exist for it. Certain indications for small-bowel surgery, however, can be accomplished easily laparoscopically. Among these indications are intestinal obstruction, foreign-body removal, perforation, and obstruction (even, as we have noted, in the case of gallstone ileus [11; Franklin *et al.*, Unpublished]. There has been very little experience in resection of the small bowel for carcinoma or Crohn's disease, although these disease entities seem to be good candidates for laparoscopy.

We have approached virtually 100% of intestinal obstructions laparoscopically over the past two years

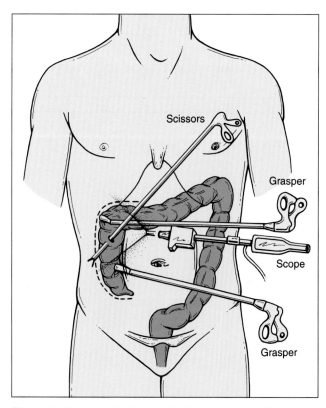

Figure 4. Placement of trocars for right-colon resection.

and found few problems with insufflation or identification of the obstruction. In approximately 90% of the cases, resolution of the small-bowel obstruction was accomplished laparoscopically. Causes of these obstructions include adhesions, internal hernias, volvulus, and foreign bodies such as gallstones in gallstone ileus. In most cases, the small bowel must be examined, and retrograde examination from the cecum is the easiest method. We use primarily 5-mm Glassman-type laparoscopic clamps (Solos, Atlanta, GA) and handle the bowel atraumatically. We strongly urge the avoidance of using routine graspers to hold the small bowel, as this use injures the tissue, much like a hemostat injures the bowel. Using laparoscopy, we could ascertain the location of the obstruction in virtually 100% of the cases of intestinal obstruction and alleviated the problems in 95%. Obviously, this approach is unwise in patients who have had multiple prior operations. If a foreign body such as a gallstone or toothpick is in the small bowel, it can be removed easily by performing an enterotomy. The enterotomy can be closed using either laparoscopic suturing techniques or a stapling device such as an Endo GIA (US Surgical, Norwalk, CT). Resection of the small bowel can also be accomplished laparoscopically with either a hand-sewn anastomosis or a functional end-to-end, side-to-side, triple-stapled anastomosis.

CLINICAL CASES

Case One involves an 85-year-old woman with intestinal obstruction. Roentgenograms of the abdomen reveal an ileus pattern, and air is noted in the biliary tract. Further examination reveals cholelithiasis but no jaundice. The patient is placed on nasogastric suction, and laparoscopy is performed in which the small bowel is examined; a large gallstone is found approximately 20 cm from the ileocecal valve. The small bowel is opened, and a large, irregular staghorn-type gallstone is removed. The proximally dilated bowel is noted as is the nondistended distal bowel. The enterotomy is closed with an Endo GIA 50 stapling device, leaving a good lumen. Testing under pressure revealed no leakage. The liver and the gallbladder fossa are then visualized, and the patient is noted to have a loop of bowel (duodenum) stuck to the wall of the gallbladder. This loop is taken down, and the source of the fistula is found between the gallbladder and the second portion of the duodenum. This fistula is repaired with two layers of absorbable sutures followed by a running laparoscopic suture to obtain a good closure. The gallbladder is then removed. Cholangiography is performed and reveals no evidence of stones in the common bile duct. The patient has an uneventful postoperative course, tolerates liquids in 3 days, and is discharged from the hospital in 4.5 days.

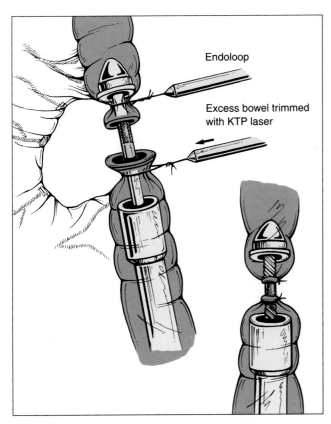

Figure 5. Anastomosis: anvil and head of stapling device are brought together after excess tissue is trimmed.

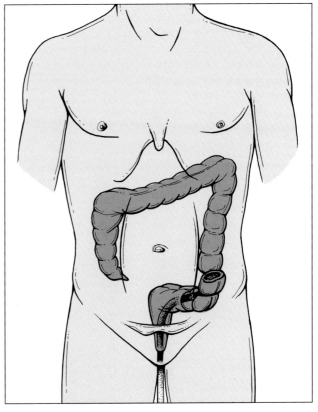

Figure 6. Resected specimen removed through transanal route.

Case Two involves a 68-year-old, steroid-dependent sarcoid patient who has had three episodes of sepsis. Examination reveals a retroperitoneal abscess that extends to the psoas muscle. Further evaluation reveals the patient has severe diverticulitis and a fistula from the colon to the large, above-mentioned abscess. The abscess is drained percutaneously, and the patient is given large doses of antibiotics. Approximately 1 month later, the patient undergoes a laparoscopic sigmoid-colon resection with end-on colostomy. The fistula's tract is identified clearly, and a drain is left in this area. Postoperatively, the patient has virtually no ileus, tolerates liquids within 18 hours, and is ready for discharge within 36 hours of her initial surgery. The patient has an uneventful recovery and at her request has not had the colostomy closed to this date.

Case Three involves a 67-year-old man with acute diverticulitis and signs and symptoms of acute abdominal pain with peritoneal irritation. Roentgenographic study reveals free air under the diaphragm [12•]. The patient is believed to have diverticulitis; he is somewhat septic, as evidenced by a temperature of 38.3°C and a white cell count of 18,000 with a significant left shift. He undergoes laparoscopy, during which a small perforation in the sigmoid colon is found. This perforation is repaired laparoscopically with a patch, using the appendices epiploicae over the injury. The abdominal cavity is irrigated thoroughly, and a drain is put in place. The patient is kept on no parenteral intake until normal bowel activity returns, and he has an uneventful recovery. Approximately 2 months later, after being carefully evaluated to determine the extent of his diverticular disease, he undergoes a laparoscopic sigmoid-colon resection with a primary anastomosis, all performed intra-corporeally. He has an uneventful recovery, tolerates liquids within 24 hours, has a bowel movement within 36 hours, and is discharged approximately 60 hours postoperatively.

CLINICAL APPLICATION

This author believes treatment of the vast majority of small- and large-bowel disease processes can be approached laparoscopically, depending on the skill, expertise, and imagination of the operating surgeon. We currently approach 100% of our colonic problems laparoscopically; we have had extremely good results performing total intracorporeal anastomoses in patients for whom anastomosis was indicated. Tables 1, 2, 3, and 4 indicate our experience with multiple laparoscopic procedures.

CONCLUSION

Laparoscopic colectomy adds a new, exciting dimension to the treatment of colonic disease and multiple small-bowel disease processes. It appears to be as safe as open procedures, and whereas the open and laparoscopic approaches both serve to perform the same procedure, the laparoscopic approach avoids the high risk of complication associated with large abdominal incisions, particularly in elderly, frail patients and patients with expected poor healing from various causes [13]. We expect that between 80% and 90% of future colonic and small-bowel procedures will be performed laparoscopically and, as more surgeons gain experience with this type of surgery, new techniques and instrumentation will be developed.

Table 1. Laparoscopic colotomy with polypectomy

Location	Patients, n
Right colon	7
Left colon	2
Sigmoid colon	2
Rectum	2
Total	13

Table 2. Laparoscopically monitored polypectomy*

Location	Patients, n
Right colon	2
Transverse and left colon	3
Sigmoid colon	2
Rectum	2
Total	9

*Polypectomy performed with colonoscope while colonic is monitored laparoscopically.

Table 3. Laparoscopic colon resections

Location	Patients, n
Right colon	11
Transverse colon	2
Left colon	11
Sigmoid colon	42
Left-anterior colon	24
Abdominal-perineal colon	17
Total	107

Table 4. Complications encountered in 129 colonic laparoscopic procedures

Complication	Patients, n
Pneumonia	1
Death	1*
Anastomotic leak (suspected)	1
Thrombophlebitis	0
Blood transfusion	1
Wound infection	1†
Reoperation	2‡
Cerebrovascular accident	1

*Patient with pneumonia (death 21 days postoperatively).
†Umbilical infection in patient with specimen removed transanally.
‡One bleeding ulcer, one loop ileostomy for anastomotic leak.

REFERENCES

Papers of particular interest, published within the period of review, have been highlighted as:
• Of special interest
•• Of outstanding interest

1. Braasch JW: Laparoscopic Cholecystectomy and Other Procedures. *Arch Surg* 1992, 127:887.

2. Jacobs M, Vergeja GD, Goldstein DS: Minimally Invasive Colon Resection. *Surg Laparosc Endosc* 1992, i:144–150.

3.• Fowler DL, White SA: Laparoscopy-Assisted Sigmoid Resection. *Surg Laparosc Endosc* 1991, 1:183–188.
Early experience with laparoscopy-assisted colon resection.

4. Phillips EH, Franklin ME, Carroll BJ *et al*.: Laparoscopic Colectomy. *Ann Surg* 1992, 216:703–707.

5. Franklin ME, Ramos R, Rosenthal D, Schuessler W: Laparoscopic Colonic Procedures. *World J Surg* 1993, 17:51–56.

6. Franklin ME, Rosenthal D, Ramos D: Laparoscopic Colectomy: Utopia or Reality? *Gastrointest Endosc Clin North Am* 1992, 3:353–365.

7. Blond KI, Copeland EM: Malignant Diseases of the Colon and Rectum. In *Surgical Treatment of Digestive Disease*. Edited by Moody FG. Chicago: Year Book; 1986.

8. Debos JT, Thomson FB: A Critical Review of Colectomy with Anastomosis. *Surg Gynecol Obstet* 1972, 135:747–752.

9. Kyzer S, Gordon PH: Experience with the Use of the Circular Stapler in Rectal Surgery. *Dis Colon Rectum* 1992, 35:696–706.

10. Gillen P, Peel AL: Comparision of Mortality, Morbidity and Incidence of Local Recurrence in Patients with Rectal Cancer Treated by Either Stapled Anterior Resection or Abdominal-Perineal Resection. *Br J Surg* 1986, 73:339–341.

11. Franklin ME, Dorman JP, Pharand D: Laparoscopyic Surgery in Acute Small Bowel Obstruction. *Surg Lap Endosc* 1993, in press.

12.• Hedberg S, Welch CE: Complications in Surgery of the Colon and Rectum. In *Complications in Surgery and Their Management*. Edited by Hardy W. Philadelphia: Saunders, 1985:630–664.
Standard by which everything must be compared.

13. Kenady DE: Management of Abdominal Wounds. *Surg Clin North Am* 1984, 64:803–807.

Chapter 15

Laparoscopic Appendectomy

Keith N. Apelgren

Traditional appendectomy through a right-lower-quadrant incision has become the standard of care for patients with suspected appendicitis. Since the advent of laparoscopic cholecystectomy in the late 1980s, many general surgeons have turned to the laparoscopic approach in treating appendicitis. The advantages of the laparoscopic approach over the open approach for appendectomy are still being debated [1]. The purpose of this chapter is to discuss the technique and the advantages and disadvantages of laparoscopic appendectomy.

INDICATIONS AND CONTRAINDICATIONS

The indications for appendectomy remain the same, whether done open or laparoscopically. In a patient for whom the diagnosis of appendicitis is in doubt, I believe that the laparoscopic approach is better because it allows a more thorough exploration of the entire abdomen and pelvis if the appendix appears normal. This situation is especially true for young women of childbearing age. Another advantage of the laparoscopic approach is in obese patients in whom large incisions will be necessary to gain access to the peritoneal cavity in the right lower quadrant. A final, obvious advantage is the cosmetic appearance of the three or four small scars over one larger, although still small, scar in the right lower quadrant.

Potential advantages of the laparoscopic approach, such as shorter hospital stay, less postoperative pain, earlier return to normal activity, and decreased overall cost, are claimed by enthusiasts for the laparoscopic approach but have not been proven in the retrospective studies! Two prospective, randomized studies have documented some of the above advantages [2,3•]. The advantage of a decreased wound infection rate with the laparoscopic approach seems real, although the rate with the open technique is low.

Relative contraindications to the laparoscopic approach include previous operations that would preclude safe or effective port placement. Other contraindications include coagulopathy and pregnancy. This last, relative contraindication is the least compelling; there are reports of successful laparoscopic appendectomies in pregnant patients [4,5••].

TECHNIQUE

The technique used for laparoscopic appendectomy depends on the experience of the surgeon, the equipment available, and the expertise of the first assistant. There have been several descriptions of the technique of port placement [1,6–8•]. Figure 1 depicts three different diagrams for port placement using the three-port technique. The surgeon generally stands on the patient's left side with the television monitor positioned directly across from or by the patient's feet. In women, the lithotomy position is helpful to use, along with placement of a device on the cervix to manipulate the uterus. I favor port placement as shown in Figure 1*B*, with a 12-mm port being placed initially at the umbilicus. A 5-mm port is placed in the right upper quadrant and a 10-mm port in the left lower quadrant under direct vision. The tele-

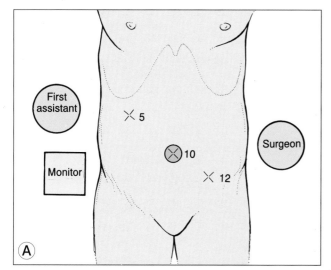

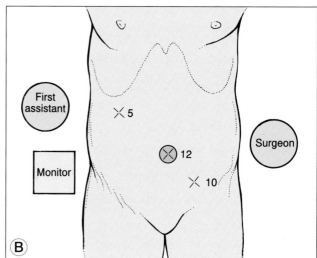

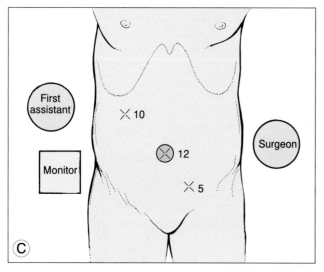

Figure 1. **A**, **B**, **C**, Port placement (three sites) for laparoscopic appendectomy. Ⓧ site of telescope; x = site of other ports (5, 10, 12 = size of port in mm).

scope is then transferred from the umbilicus to the left lower quadrant so that instruments can be seen on the television monitor as coming from the same quadrant. The 12-mm port is used to allow placement of an endostapling device across the appendix or mesoappendix. Other authors favor port placement as in Figure 1A, where the camera stays at the umbilicus and instruments come in from the right and left of the screen on the television monitor [7,8•]. These authors say that this placement avoids the phenomenon of "sword fighting," in which the instruments clash with each other. Figure 1C placement is favored by some experienced laparoscopic surgeons [6] because it allows the procedure to be done entirely by the surgeon while the scrub nurse holds the camera in the right upper quadrant. This technique allows the surgeon to operate with both hands, the right hand operating through the 12-mm port at the umbilicus and left hand through the 5-mm port in the left lower quadrant. As expertise is gained by each laparoscopic surgeon, this two-handed technique becomes easier and preferred. In a training situation, the surgeon in training should initially use only one hand, as done with laparoscopic cholecystectomy.

If the endostapling device is not preferred or not available, the 12-mm port size is not necessary. Two 10-mm ports are necessary, however, because the telescope must be used in one and the appendix extracted through the other. This requirement does not hold if a 5-mm telescope is available.

Figure 2 depicts two different arrangements for port placement using four ports. Occasionally, the fourth port is necessary to stabilize the appendix or the mesoappendix for dissection. This placement is accomplished by adding a 5-mm port in the right lower quadrant as depicted in Figure 2A. In patients with a small abdomen, placement in the right lower quadrant may be too close to the appendix to allow manipulation of the instrument, and this fourth 5-mm port may be placed on the left side above the left-lower-quadrant port. This positioning may result in some difficulty with the instruments' "sword fighting" but can be used by experienced laparoscopic surgeons.

Figure 2. **A**, **B**, Port placement (four sites) for laparoscopic appendectomy. Ⓧ = site of telescope; x = site of other ports (5, 10, 12 = size of port in mm).

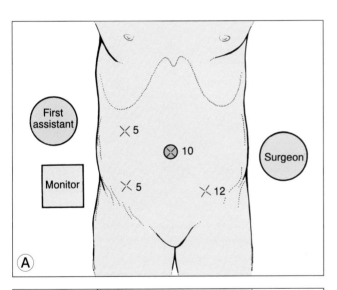

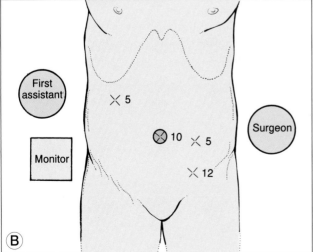

The base of the appendix may be secured using pretied endoscopic sutures; two loops are placed proximal and one distal to the divided appendix. It has also been secured with metallic clips [6] (see Fig. 3), a technique of which I do not approve. It may also be divided using an endostapling instrument, as shown in Figure 3B.

The mesoappendix can be divided using a number of techniques (see Fig. 4). In general, monopolar cautery dissection with clipping of the appendiceal artery has been used successfully. Clips alone may be used, as shown in Figure 4A. Alternatively, a laser may be used to divide the mesoappendix, again with control of the appendiceal artery either by clip or pretied endoscopic

suture. Another method is by using an endostapling instrument, as shown in Figure 4B. The amount of mesoappendix left on the appendix should be minimal (Fig. 5A) to make later extraction easier. If the technique of Figure 5B is used, later extraction techniques may have to be more complex.

The appendix is then removed, generally using the 12-mm port by drawing the appendix into the port and then removing the port with the appendix inside so that the inflamed, infected organ does not touch the fascia or subcutaneous tissue. If the appendix is too large to be drawn into the 12-mm port, it can be placed into a sterile plastic container to aid extraction and prevent conta-

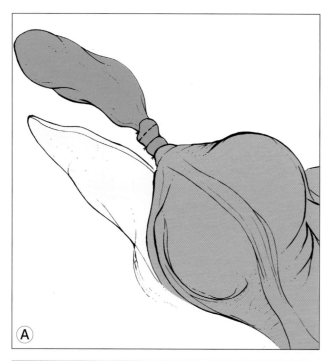

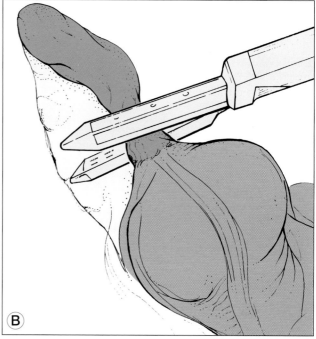

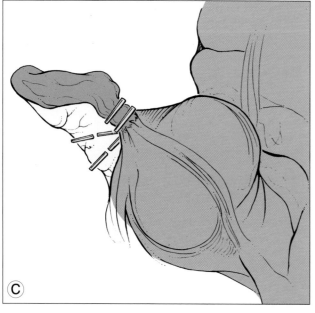

Figure 3. Methods of controlling the appendiceal base. **A,** Pretied sutures (two at base). **B,** Endostapling device. **C,** Large clip (from France).

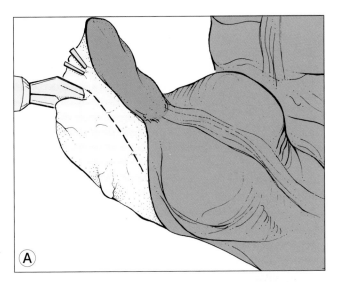

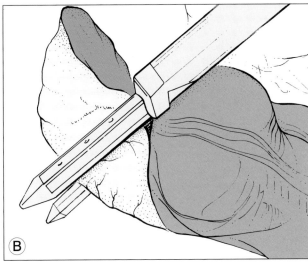

Figure 4. Methods of controlling the mesoappendix. **A**, Metallic clips. **B**, Endostapling device. **C**, Electrocautery.

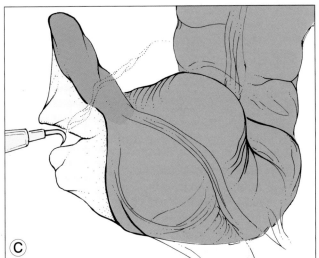

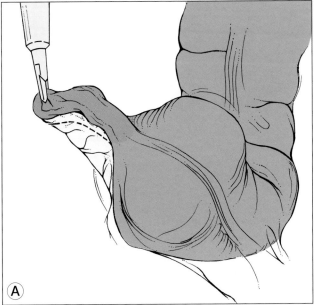

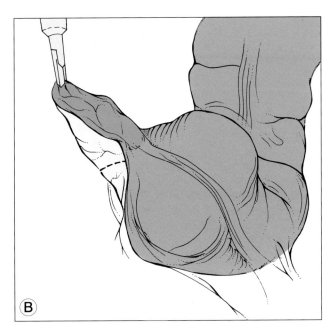

Figure 5. Control of mesoappendix. **A**, Correct, close to the appendix. **B**, Incorrect, excessive tissue.

mination of the abdomen or the subcutaneous space (see Fig. 6). This may be accomplished by a sterile condom (Fig. 6*A*) or by a commercial plastic bag (Fig. 6*B*). This procedure may require enlarging the incision from which the appendix is extracted, a technique now well established for extracting difficult gallbladders.

In extremely difficult situations involving an enlarged, inflamed appendix, the laparoscopic approach may be converted to an open procedure, using a small, right-lower-quadrant incision through which the appendix, attached to the cecum, is withdrawn. The appendectomy is then done extracorporeally [9–11]. The cecum is replaced into the abdominal cavity, and the operative site is inspected laparoscopically to ensure hemostasis. Other, minor refinements in the technique will certainly be described in the future.

DISCUSSION

Patients who undergo laparoscopic appendectomy are generally discharged the following day. Patients who do not fit this general rule include those with ruptured or gangrenous appendices. Such patients can be treated laparoscopically. Patients with ruptured appendices and pus in the right lower quadrant and the pelvis can be treated laparoscopically; proponents of this technique claim that a more thorough suctioning of the entire abdominal cavity can be accomplished laparoscopically than can be done through open procedures. This advantage remains to be demonstrated, although it is possible. Hospital stay, then, is dictated more by the stage of the disease and the temperament of the patient, than by the technique chosen to remove the inflamed appendix. In

fact, in my experience, hospital stay was identical at 2.9 days whether open or laparoscopic techniques were used. Other authors have demonstrated a shorter hospital stay with the laparoscopic approach [2,3•,12].

The issue of whether using an endostapling device is faster and more secure than using endosutures is also hotly debated. Many experienced laparoscopic surgeons claim that they can place sutures and remove the appendix as quickly as other surgeons can use the endostapling device. If this claim is true, it would result in significant cost savings, since the endostapling device is a single-use instrument that costs $200 to $300, with reloads costing $100 to $150 each. My experience and opinion are that the endostapling device does make the operation easier and faster, although I have not objective data to prove this opinion.

The issue of postoperative pain is a difficult one to evaluate. Many authors [2,3•,9] claim that pain is less after the laparoscopic approach but do not supply data. The few studies available [2,3•] suggest that less pain medication is required with the laparoscopic approach.

The issue of hospital cost is significant in this day and age. Clearly, the cost of the operation itself is higher for the laparoscopic approach than for the open approach. If the patient stays in the hospital a shorter time, this cost may be recouped in the overall hospital costs. Some authors claim this experience, although my experience is that the overall cost of the operation and hospitalization is higher for the laparoscopic approach.

The issue of whether to remove a normal appendix during laparoscopy for right-lower-quadrant pain has also been raised. Some surgeons suggest that it should not be removed if normal. Other surgeons argue, how-

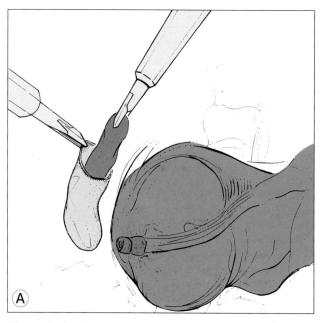

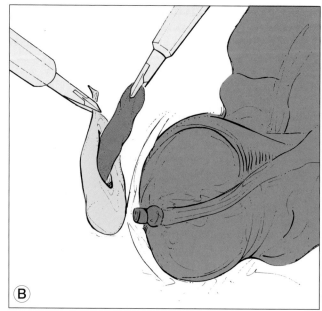

Figure 6. Ancillary methods to remove a bulky, inflamed appendix. **A**, Sterile plastic bag. **B**, Cut-off end of finger of large sterile glove.

ever, that the procedure is done for possible appendicitis, and because the appendix would be removed if the open technique were used it should be removed laparoscopically as well. I agree with the latter argument. One caveat is that the operation must be performed with the same low morbidity and mortality as the open procedure.

The question of when to expect the patient can return to work or normal activity after the laparoscopic approach versus after the open approach has also been raised. The data on laparoscopic cholecystectomy clearly show that patients return to normal activity in a shorter period of time. This advantage may not hold for laparoscopic appendectomy because the incision used for open appendectomy is much smaller than that used for cholecystectomy. Once again, some proponents of laparoscopic appendectomy claim that return to activity is sooner. In examining data, however, I find the issue remains controversial; some studies show an earlier return to activity and others do not. Once again, the motivation and attitude of the patient plays a critical role in this statistic and is a factor that is not constant across all patient groups.

The issue of improved cosmetic result can be important. This point is especially true in an obese patient in whom a large skin incision is necessary to reach the peritoneal cavity. In a young, thin patient, this issue is less compelling, although it is still valid. The umbilical and lower abdominal trocar sites can be hidden in the umbilicus and the hairline suprapubicly. The right-upper-quadrant trocar site is generally a 5-mm one and usually very inconspicuous.

In using the laparoscopic approach, the surgeon must be willing to convert to the open approach for any difficulties encountered. One must be aware of the possible complications of laparoscopy, including injury to intra-abdominal organs caused by placement of the insufflation needle or trocars. Abdominal wall vessel injury is also possible. The following case report serves to illustrate the point.

CASE REPORT

R.M. is a 13-year-old girl who presented with typical appendicitis, including fever, leukocytosis, and right-lower-quadrant pain. She is 1.60 m tall and weighs 103.5 kg. The laparoscopic approach was chosen because of her obesity. Pneumoperitoneum was initially difficult because of preperitoneal insufflation but was established, and acute appendicitis was confirmed. A 5-mm port was placed in the right upper quadrant easily. A 10-mm port placed through the left rectus muscle resulted in brisk arterial bleeding for 15 minutes, obscuring the operative site. The case was converted to an open procedure using a 20-cm incision from the right lower quadrant across the midline to the site of the left 10-mm trocar puncture. The inferior epigastric artery was controlled by suture ligation and an appendectomy was performed without difficulty through a 10-cm fascial-peritoneal incision. Blood loss was 600 mL. Operation duration was 112 minutes, and hospital stay was 6 days. Preoperative and postoperative hemoglobin concentrations were 14.3 and 11.0 g/dL, respectively. The girl returned to school and normal activity three weeks postoperatively.

This case and others heard anecdotally have convinced me that the technical risks of laparoscopy, although small, are significant.

SUMMARY

Laparoscopic appendectomy has become an established procedure. In my experience, it is clearly superior to the open technique for the obese patient or the patient for whom the diagnosis is in question. It is also preferred when cosmetics are a major concern. For the thin patient with obvious appendicitis, however, the open technique remains equally efficacious. As new instruments and techniques are described and competition decreases the costs of instrumentation, laparoscopic appendectomy may overtake open appendectomy as the treatment of choice for appendicitis.

REFERENCES

Papers of particular interest, published within the period of review, have been highlighted as:
• Of special interest
•• Of outstanding interest

1. Apelgren KN, Molnar RG, Kisala JM:Laparoscopic Better Than Open Appendectomy? *Surg Endosc* 1992, 6:298–301.

2. McAnena OJ, Austin O, O'Connell PR, *et al.*: Laparoscopic Versus Open Appendicectomy: A Prospective Evaluation. *Br J Surg* 1992, 79:808–820.

3. • Attword SEA, Hill ADK, Murphy PG, *et al.*: A Prospective Randomized Trial of Laparoscopic Versus Open Appendectomy. *Surgery* 1992, 112:497–501.
   The most recent randomized controlled study of laparoscopic appendectomy.

4. Schreiber JG: Endokopische Chirurgic in Einer Gynakologischen Tagesklinik. *Geburtshilfe Fauenheilkd* 1992, 52:42– 46.

5. •• Perissot J, Collet D, Edge M. Therapeutic Laparoscopy. *Endoscopy* 1992, 24:138–143.
An excellent review of all aspects of laparoscopic general surgery.

6. Grandjean JP, Silverio JM: Appendicectomie Percoe-lioscapique Utilisant L'Endo Clip®. *Lyon Chir* 1991, 87:449– 451.

7. Daniell JF, Gurley LD, Kurtz BR, Chambers JF: The Use of an Automatic Stapling Device for Laparoscopic Appendectomy. *Obstet Gynecol* 1991, 78:721–723.

8. • Scott-Connor CEH, Hall TJ, Anglin BL, Maukkassa FF: Laparoscopic Appendectomy—Initial Experience in a Teaching Program. *Ann Surg* 1992, 215:660–668.
A good description of the technique and review of laparoscopic principles.

9. Valla JS, Limonne B, Valla V, *et al.*: Laparoscopic Appen-dectomy in Children: Report of 465 Cases. *Surg Laparosc Endosc* 1991, 1:166–172.

10. Byme DS, Bell G, Morrice JJ, Orr G: Technique for Laparoscopic Appendicectomy. *Br J Surg* 1992, 79:574–575.

11. Goh P, Tekant Y, Kum CK, *et al.*: Technical Modification to Laparoscopic Appendectomy. *Dis Colon Rectum* 1992, 35:999–1000.

12. Gilchrist BF, Lobe TE, Schropp KP, *et al.*: Is There a Role for Laparoscopic Appendectomy in Pediatric Surgery? *J Ped Surg* 1992, 27:209–214.

Chapter 16

Laparoscopy in the Management of Chronic Abdominal Pain

Stephen Wise Unger

Laparoscopy has undergone a tremendous rise in popularity since Mouret's first laparoscopic cholecystectomy in 1987 and the huge subsequent interest in the surgical community to educate practicing physicians in this new technique. While the use of laparoscopy had been dormant in the general surgical community and instrumentation had been directed toward gynecologic applications, new interest stimulated by the delivery of this technique into the hands of general surgeons has recently directed applications of laparoscopy to more difficult gallbladders, acute cholecystitis, hernia repair, colon resection, peptic ulcer disease, appendicitis, and the acute abdomen. Little has been written, however, about the application of laparoscopy to the management of chronic abdominal pain.

TECHNIQUE

The technique of laparoscopy for the management of chronic abdominal pain is essentially the same as that used for diagnostic laparoscopy for the past 50 years. General anesthesia is used most often, primarily because of surgeons' familiarity with using the laparoscope in operational laparoscopy with patients under general anesthesia. The abdomen is entered using a Veress needle with the patient in slight Trendelenburg position. This position elevates the intestinal viscera and, with the needle directed toward the feet at about 45°, lowers the risk of an impalement injury between the umbilicus and sacral prominence. For patients with prior surgery, the abdomen may be entered by an open technique [1•] or by an alternate puncture technique, closed but away from the site of prior operation [2]. The open technique may also be chosen for patients with abdominal distention or chronic small bowel obstruction.

Once the abdomen is insufflated and the initial trocar is inserted, all other trocars are placed under direct vision. Many surgeons prefer disposable trocars for the initial puncture, since no reusable trocar currently available includes a safety mechanism to retract or cover the sharp portion of the trocar. Once the trocar is inserted, a 10-mm laparoscope is placed with video attachment. Video is probably the most important technical feature of the new era of laparoscopy, for it frees the surgeon's hands to operate and allows viewing of either video or still images.

The surgeon must have a systematic plan for exploring the abdomen. Our method is to first examine the pelvis with the patient in steep Trendelenburg position. This position causes the viscera to move away from the pelvic floor and exposes the rectum, uterus, adnexa, and bladder. In addition, the pelvic floor can be visualized at this point, which is important in hernia repairs. The patient may be rotated side to side or a second trocar inserted under direct vision so that the organs can be separated and examined by moving them with an instrument. Again, side-to-side table rotation may allow visualization of both lateral gutters and may enhance the view of structures within the field. Use of defogging agents also improves the image. With an angled laparoscope and manipulation with a second instrument, greater than an estimated 70% of the liver surface can be seen. Side-to-side rotation allows visualization of the spleen and splenic flexure of the colon. If the surgeon decides to inspect the small bowel, then careful manipulation, using the bowel graspers to "walk" forward or backward from the ligament of Trietz to the ileocecal valve, allows complete inspection of the small intestine (Fig. 1). If necessary, the posterior wall of the stomach or even the pancreas may be inspected by taking down the gastrocolic ligament between clips or with a linear stapling device. This technique, however, is very sophisticated, potentially time consuming, and for the advanced laparoscopic surgeon only. Adequate visualization of the diaphragmatic hiatus is easily accomplished by lifting the left lobe of the liver and pulling down on the stomach (Fig. 2).

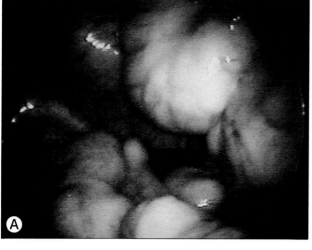

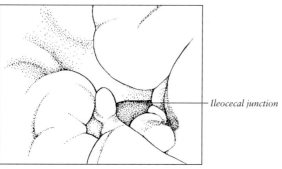

Ileocecal junction

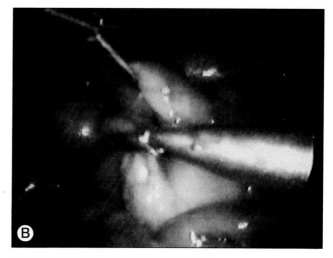

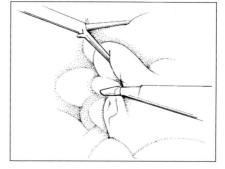

Figure 1. **A,** This picture shows the ileum and cecum, demonstrating the ileocecal juncture and the beginning of the step-by-step inspection of the entire small bowel. **B, C, D,** These three pictures show two bowel graspers being used in a hand-over-hand motion, "walking" down the intestine systematically toward the ligament of Trietz. **E,** This picture demonstrates the jejunum as it turns into the retroperitoneum under the Ligament of Trietz. **F,** This figure demonstrates transsection of an adhesion during the step-by-step inspection of the entire small bowel.

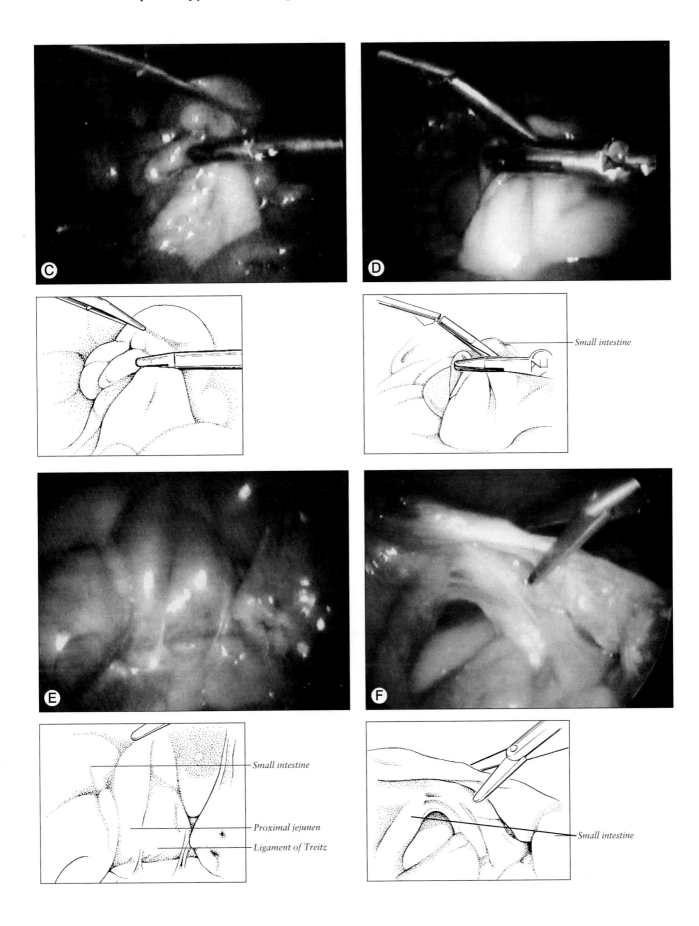

Once general inspection is completed, the area in question may be investigated further and the position changed to maximize exposure of that region. Additional trocars, usually 5 mm, are placed in anatomically favorable areas for manipulation or retraction.

CLINICAL SERIES

Large clinical series analyzing experience with chronic abdominal pain simply do not exist. Recent series, however, consider small, select groups of patients, and through careful review of that information, general guidelines and expectations can be extracted. Many of the series referenced pertain to gynecologic topics or precede the recent era of operative general surgery. Cohen [3] reported eight patients who underwent laparoscopy for chronic abdominal pain; he found two with no demonstrable disease, three with solitary band adhesions, one with inflammatory pancreatic mass, one with chronic cholecystitis, and one with multiple adhesions. In Ferguson's study of 51 cases [4], distinguishing chronic from acute pain is difficult, but the conclusion was that patients with chronic, recurring abdominal pain would benefit from a laparoscopic diagnosis. Lundberg and coworkers [5] similarly evaluated 95 laparoscopic patients with pelvic pain independent of the preoperative physical and pelvic exam diagnosis. Thirty-seven of these patients were normal, 22 had adhesions or masses, and the remainder had gynecologic pathology. Levinson [6] documented 59 patients who underwent laparoscopy for abdominal pain. He diagnosed 19 with irritable bowel syndrome, 12 with "psychiatric pain," 13 with adhesions

(seven of whom were pain free after enterolysis), seven with pelvic inflammatory disease, five with endometriosis, and three with chronic appendicitis. Klimanskaya and coworkers [7] presented an interesting series of pediatric patients who underwent laparoscopy for "chronic and relapsing pain." They found 12 cysts, 12 with no pathology, 10 adhesions, 5 with Meckel's diverticula, and 2 with tumors. Easter and coworkers [8•] used laparoscopy on 70 patients for chronic abdominal pain. Fifty-three percent had positive diagnoses, and 39 of these had subsequent positive outcomes. These 53% included diagnoses that required no further intervention, such as Crohn's disease, adhesions, diverticulosis, and cirrhosis. Interestingly enough, when referrals came from surgical rather than medical colleagues, the yield and outcome were significantly better. Salky and Bauer [9] presented 144 patients with chronic abdominal pain; a definite diagnosis was made in 67%, with laparoscopic intervention possible in almost half of these.

SPECIFIC INDICATIONS

ADHESIONS

The laparoscopic treatment of adhesions as a natural extension of minimally invasive technology is controversial. A recent editorial [10] suggested that there is no indication for laparoscopic adhesiolysis. Amongst many other workers, Daniell [11] and Sutton and Mac Donald [12] believe there is a benefit, however. Peters and coworkers [13] in the Netherlands randomized 48 women with pelvic adhesions to adhesiolysis or control

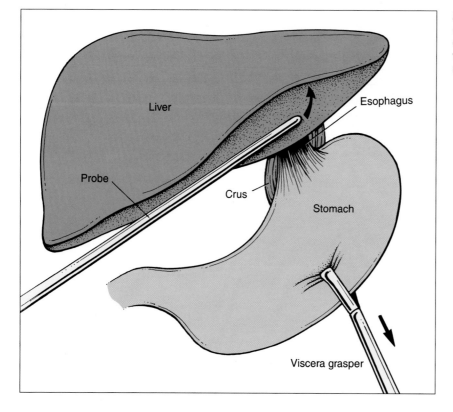

Figure 2. This figure shows that with elevation of the left lobe of the liver and downward traction of the stomach, good visualization of the esophageal hiatal region can be obtained.

after laparoscopic diagnosis. They found that the subgroup of patients with well-vascularized adhesions involving bowel to abdominal wall were likely to benefit from adhesiolysis. Steege and Stout [14] identified a psychological profile, "chronic pain syndrome," that doomed enterolysis to failure but believed that adhesiolysis in the absence of this syndrome was worthwhile. Reiter and Gambone [15] emphasized the psychiatric component of this pain syndrome. Anecdotal reports document hepatic adhesiolysis with pain relief in Fitz-Hugh and Curtis syndrome [16]. The other side of the coin is presented by Baker and Symonds [17], who found 58 of 60 patients unchanged or better six months after diagnostic laparoscopy only, raising the question of the placebo effect of the procedure alone.

UNUSUAL CONDITIONS

RETRACTILE MESENTERITIS

Weiser and coworkers [18] described two cases of retractile mesenteritis or mesenteric peniculitis diagnosed laparoscopically. Clearly nontherapeutic laparotomy is avoided by this approach.

TORSION

Omental torsion with resection is an unusual pain syndrome but could easily be confused clinically with acute or chronic appendicitis. Laparoscopic treatment has recently been reported by Chung and coworkers [19]. Shalev and coworkers [20] reported a case of laparoscopic detorsion of the adnexa in a child.

TUBERCULOSIS

Whereas fever, ascites, and weight loss are the more common symptoms in tuberculosis, abdominal pain may also be a symptom of the disease. Several workers

[21,22] report laparoscopy to be useful and diagnostic in 85% of patients, by using a combination of culture and sensitivity and peritoneal biopsy.

HUMAN IMMUNODEFICIENCY VIRUS

More abdominal pain syndromes, particularly right-lower-quadrant pain, are becoming associated with acquired immune deficiency syndrome. Although there are significant risks and precautions associated with human immunodeficiency virus transmission during laparoscopy, the technique may offer a far less invasive diagnostic approach than laparotomy in these fragile patients [23].

CONCLUSION

Because the worldwide application of laparoscopy in general surgery is just now being realized, the application of laparoscopy to the management of chronic abdominal pain has not reached a steady state or standard of care at this point. As discussed above, there are many examples in which chronic abdominal pain can be diagnosed and even treated laparoscopically, and the clinical surgeon should keep laparoscopy and operative laparoscopic intervention as options in the management of chronic abdominal pain. Each case must be considered individually, and the informed consent on potential laparoscopic interventions must be discussed with the patient and other consultants ahead of time. This informed-consent discussion must include the possibility of an open procedure, both in the event of untoward events occurring during laparoscopy and in the event that the findings yield a diagnosis better treated by laparotomy. Large clinical series investigating laparoscopic management of chronic abdominal pain are eagerly awaited so that a more clear cut and standardized approach may be developed.

REFERENCES

Papers of particular interest, published within the period of review, have been highlighted as:
• Of special interest
•• Of outstanding interest

1. • Fitzgibbons RJ, Salerno GM, Filipi CJ: Open Laparoscopy. In *Surgical Laparoscopy*. Edited by Zucker KA, Baily RW, Reddick EJ. St. Louis, MO: Quality Medical Publishing; 1991:87–97.
To safely laparoscope patients with multiple prior procedures, this technique must be mastered.

2. Reddick EJ, Olsen D, Spaw A, *et al.*: Safe Performance of Difficult Cholecystectomies. *Am J Surg* 1991, 161:377–381.

3. Cohen MM: Peritoneoscopy in General Surgery. *Can J Surg* 1981, 24:490–493.

4. Ferguson IL: Laparoscopy for the Diagnosis of Non-Specific Lower Abdominal Pain. *Br J Clin Pract* 1974, 26:163–165.

5. Lundberg WI, Wall JE, Mathers JE: Laparoscopy in Evaluation of Pelvic Pain. *Obstet Gynecol* 1973, 42:872–876.

6. Levinson JM: The Role of Laparoscopy in Intraabdominal Diagnosis. *Del Med J* 1978, 50:259–270.

7. Klimanskaya EV, Graniko OD, Mirin Y: Operative Endoscopy from the Point of View of the Pediatrician. *Endoscopy* 1983, 15:233–234.

8. • Easter DW, Cuschieri A, Nathanson LK, Lavelle-Jones M: The Utility of Diagnostic Laparoscopy for Abdominal Disorders. *Arch Surg* 1992, 127:379–393.

This report is one of the only series in the literature, since the era of interventional laparoscopy that deals with chronic pain.

9. Salky B, Bauer J: The Use of Laparascopy in the Evaluation of Abdominal Pain [abstract]. *Surg Endosc* 1992, 6:85.

10. Ikard RW: There is no Current Indication for Laparoscopic Adhesiolysis to Treat Abdominal Pain. *South Med J* 1992, 85:939–940.

11. Daniell JF: Laparoscopic Adhesiolysis for Chronic Abdominal Pain. *J Gynecol Surg* 1989, 5:61–66.

12. Sutton C, Mac Donald D: Laser Laparoscopic Adhesiolysis. *J Gynecol Surg* 1990, 6:155–159.

13. Peters AAW, Trimbos-Kemper GCM, Admiral C, Trimbos JB: A Randomized Clinical Trial on the Benefit of Adhesiolysis in Patients with Intraperitoneal Adhesions and Chronic Pelvic Pain. *Br J Obstet Gynecol* 1992, 99:59–62.

14. Steege JF, Stour AL: Resolution of Chronic Abdominal Pain after Laparoscopic Lysis of Adhesions. *Am J Obstet Gynecol* 1991, 165:278–283.

15. Reiter RC, Gambone JC: Nongynecologic Somatic Pathology in Women with Chronic Pelvic Pain and Negative Laparoscopy. *J Reprod Med* 1991, 36:253–259.

16. Owens S, Yeko TR, Bloy R, Maroulis GB: Laparoscopic Treatment of Painful Perihepatic Adhesions in Fitz-Hugh-Curtis Syndrome. *Obstet Gynecol* 1991, 78:542–543.

17. Baker PN, Symonds EM: The Resolution of Chronic Pelvic Pain after Normal Laparoscopy Findings. *Am J Obstet Gynecol* 1992, 166:835–836.

18. Weiser J, Salky B, Slepian A, Dikman S: Laparoscopic Diagnosis of Retractile Mesenteritis. *Gastroint Endosc* 1992, 38:615–617.

19. Chung SCS, Ng KW, Li AKC: Laparoscopic Resection for Primary Omental Torsion. *Aust NZ J Surg* 1992, 62:400–401.

20. Shalev E, Mann S, Romano S, Rehav D: Laparoscopic Detorsion of Adnexa in Childhood: A Case Report. *J Pediatr Surg* 1991, 26:1193–1194.

21. Hossain J, Al-Aska AK, Mofleh IA: Laparoscopy in Tuberculous Peritonitis. *J R Soc Med* 1992, 85:89–91.

22. Mimica M: Usefulness and Limitations of Laparoscopy in the Diagnosis of Tuberculous Peritonitis. *Endoscopy* 1992, 24:588–591.

23. Eubanks S, Newman L, Lucas G: Reduction of HIV Transmission During Laparoscopic Procedures. *Surg Laparosc Endosc* 1993, 3:2–5.

Chapter 17

Laparoscopy in the Intensive Care Unit Patient

Jonathan M. Sackier

Richard Bright (1789–1858) is perhaps the person we should thank for the concept of an intensive care unit (ICU). He was the innovator who proposed gathering patients together in one special ward to study and treat a given group of diseases [1]. The ICU, therefore, is a place where the most ill patients may be assembled and where staff and equipment are concentrated to enable intensive observation and therapy to be undertaken. The purpose of this chapter is to highlight conditions that may be approached laparoscopically, either for diagnosis or therapy, in patients already being cared for in the ICU. Where relevant, specific differences between healthier patients and patients in the ICU are contrasted. Primarily, the subject matter is timing. Critically ill patients have a narrow window of opportunity during which treatment may be instituted. Therefore, the same time latitude in selecting tests that is such a luxury in the elective setting is not available. Probably the most important point in treating ICU patients is to avoid being too dogmatic in designing an algorithm for a diagnosis or therapy; any algorithm must be adaptable to given patients, diseases, and other variables such as local expertise. No investigation is perfect, and one must rely on the expertise of the person performing or interpreting each test. Therefore, making a diagnosis in a catastrophically ill patient places the physician under an unusual amount of stress. This situation has led many physicians to select diagnostic exploratory laparotomy in such patients [2,3]; however, even this bold move, which may not be well tolerated by such ill patients, has high false positive rates [4,5].

LAPAROSCOPY

Laparoscopy was developed at the turn of the century by Ott [6] in Petrograd and Kelling [7] in Dresden. The Swede Jacobaeus [8] was the first to accumulate and publish broad experience with the technique. Few general surgeons showed an interest in laparoscopy [9–11], however, and gynecologists were primarily those who used this approach, especially to examine female genitalia and attempt tubal ligation, patency studies, and other more difficult maneuvers [12••].

Not until the advent of laparoscopic cholecystectomy did general surgeons embrace this technique. The first gallbladder to be removed under laparoscopic control was probably by Mühe [13] of Germany, although most authors acknowledge Philippe Mouret from southern France, whose work was never published. Many others in Europe [14–16] and the United States [17–19] performed the operation, which rapidly gained in popularity. At this stage, the long-ignored technique of laparoscopy was venerated as providing easy access to the peritoneal cavity in a more rapid and less traumatic fashion than diagnostic laparotomy [20].

As mentioned, all investigations rely on the skill, interest, and motivation of the person performing the test; this caveat is certainly true of laparoscopy. For a surgeon with no laparoscopic experience under stressful circumstances to evaluate a severely ill patient by this method is as inappropriate as doing one's first laparotomy in the middle of the night on a severely ill patient with multisystem organ failure. Hospital credentialling committees, therefore, should have a clearly defined set of guidelines as to who should perform the procedure, what their training should be, and what peer review mechanisms should be in place.

Of course, the burning issue is, is laparoscopy potentially better than laparotomy? Several advantages are conveyed, and the most important ones are to the patient. The amount of time taken to perform a laparoscopy is less than for laparotomy, as no large incisions need to be opened and closed. This difference results in less pain for the patient, which in turn results in less catabolic insult as detected by the level of acute phase proteins [21••]. Such reduced pain may also result in less diaphragmatic splinting, thereby leading to better oxygen exchange and a lower incidence of postoperative pneumonia. The patient's mobility is improved, and if the laparoscopy uncovers no pathology, the effect on the patient is far milder than if a laparotomy had been undertaken.

Several factors probably contribute to these advantages. In most operations, trauma to the integument is greater than internal trauma, the abdominal wall is retracted both by mechanical and human means, and the bowel is handled and packed, which leads to serosal drying and mechanical trauma. These factors are not true for laparoscopy. There are, in addition, advantages to the laparoscopic surgeon in that the investigation may be initiated sooner, allowing for earlier diagnosis and treatment. There may also be benefits for the hospital and the third-party payor, as the cost of laparoscopy

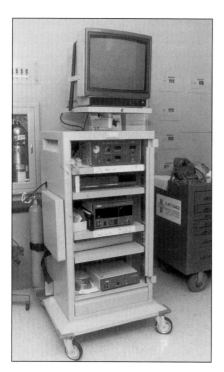

Figure 1. A cart that contains all the equipment necessary for performing laparoscopy.

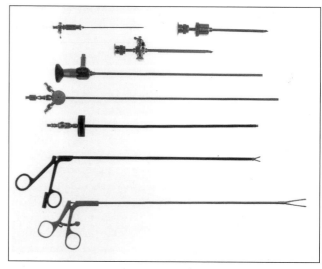

Figure 2. The ideal set for emergency laparoscopy: Veress needle, laparoscope, trocars, suction probe, coagulation probe, coarse grasper, bowel grasper.

should be less than the open equivalent, especially if carried out in the ICU, thereby avoiding incurring the additional costs of using the operating room.

LOGISTICS

The majority of laparoscopic examinations in ICU patients take place in the operating room, but they may be performed in the ICU at the bedside for those in whom transfer is inadvisable. Regardless of setting, proper consent must be obtained, and the assistants present must include a well-trained nurse. In addition, the surgeon should be totally familiar with all the apparatus required to complete the laparoscopy. Such familiarity will ensure the rapid, smooth, and elegant completion of the procedure and allow for troubleshooting when things go wrong.

EQUIPMENT

The standard laparoscopy equipment should be kept on a cart that can be moved from one part of the hospital to another. The equipment should be bolted into place so that it is not damaged in transit. The cart should include a television monitor, light source (preferably 300-W xenon light source), insufflator, two tanks of carbon dioxide gas, camera control unit, and video recorder, and possibly a still-image capture unit (Fig. 1). The choice of whether to use reusable or disposable instruments is largely personal, but issues to consider include sterility, cost, ecologic effect of disposable instruments, and the subjective, but important "feel" of a well-crafted metal instrument. A set of instruments should be sterile wrapped, and several sets should be available for diagnostic procedures to avoid delays waiting for equipment.

The ideal set should consist of the Veress needle, trocar-cannulae assemblies, telescope, light cable, blunt probe, suction-coagulation-irrigation probe, grasping forceps, and bowel forceps (Fig. 2). In addition, devices such as Trucut (Baxter Healthcare, Deerfield, IL) needles or forceps may be needed for obtaining biopsies.

The choice of telescope is a critical decision. The 4.2-mm telescope that passes through the 5-mm cannula is sufficient for most diagnostic purposes but does not transmit as much light as the larger 10-mm scope. The smaller cannula is obviously easier to insert with its accompanying trocar. The 10-mm telescope allows more light but does require a larger cannula. The 0° forward optic telescope has limitations, and the surgeon will want to become familiar with the use of the 30° forward oblique telescope because it provides five perspectives on given structure: straight-on and from above, below, right, and left.

ANESTHESIA

Many ICU patients are already intubated and, if not anesthetized, are sedated enough to allow the laparoscopy to take place. As long as the procedure is explained carefully to the patient, laparoscopy can be performed with merely mild sedation. If the patient is not intubated, then lower insufflation pressures must be used (no greater than 10 mm Hg), and the patient should be told to expect some abdominal and shoulder discomfort. The use of epidural anesthesia in laparoscopy has been discussed [21••], but I have no personal experience with it. Regardless of the anesthesia chosen or the setting, adequate monitoring should include blood pressure, pulse, electrocardiogram, and pulse oximetry. Obviously, in such sick patients, having an anesthesiologist present is preferable.

The choice of gas to induce the pneumoperitoneum is extremely interesting. Carbon dioxide is readily available, inexpensive, and familiar to most surgeons. It does, however, lower the pH, raise the carbon dioxide partial pressure, lower the oxygen partial pressure, and cause vasodilation, which may lead to vascular collapse [22]. Nitrous oxide reportedly causes far less discomfort, but objective evidence for this supposition is lacking [23]. Another concern has been that nitrous oxide supports combustion, whereas carbon dioxide does not. Other problems relating to carbon dioxide stem from inadvertent insertion of the needle into a great vessel, causing gas embolism [24], although this complication may be avoided by careful positioning of the needle during blind puncture. The surgeon has the responsibility to be aware of all the physiologic effects of pneumoperitoneum [25].

TECHNIQUES

In all patients, the bladder and the stomach should be decompressed. Obviously, many ICU patients already have urine output measured with a Foley catheter, thereby obviating the inclusion of this step. Passage of a nasogastric tube is extremely valuable. Awareness of the position of intra-abdominal adhesions may be useful in such patients, and the technique of ultrasound mapping described by Siegel and coworkers [26••] is of value. After the abdomen is shaved, the elected site of needle entry, usually the umbilicus, is anesthetized with lidocaine if the patient is awake. The needle is introduced, and testing is performed twice with saline to ensure that no blood or intestinal content is retrieved and that saline flows freely. The hanging drop test is then carried out, and saline should easily drip into the peritoneal cavity from the needle.

On commencing insufflation, never use a rapid flow rate, as this may lead to cardiac dysrhythmias or diaphragmatic rupture. Once the pneumoperitoneum has been completed to 15 mm Hg pressure in the anesthetized patient, or no greater than 10 mm Hg for the alert, sedated patient, a trocar-cannula is introduced. Several devices are available, some of which include a "safety shield"; however, a certain amount of time is required for these shields to retract, and great care should be taken to avoid pointing the trocar at important structures such as the aorta [27].

Alternatively, the "Hasson" technique of open laparoscopy may be used [28]. All subsequent trocars must always be introduced under direct vision to prevent injuring any underlying structure.

The position of the trocar must allow the surgeon to reach the area under consideration and not be at too acute an angle with the telescope, as this positioning would cause "swordfighting." Conversely, additional trocars should not be placed at too obtuse an angle, for this arrangement would hinder depth perception.

To gain access to different areas of the abdominal cavity, relying on the movements allowed by modern electric hospital beds is extremely useful. By tilting the patient into the Trendelenburg position, the surgeon can view the pelvic organs and fixed portions of the ascending and descending colon. By using reverse Trendelenburg position, the surgeon can see the hiatus and domes of the liver. Rolling the patient to either right or left will allow the opposite side to be visualized. The small bowel may be packed away to the opposite side of the abdomen by gentle "hand-over-hand" maneuvers with bowel graspers.

TRAUMA

Patients admitted to the hospital with penetrating trauma to the abdomen that renders them unstable obviously require immediate exploration. In such patients, laparoscopy is not ideal, but in patients with penetrating trauma to the abdomen who are stable, laparoscopy may be valuable to ascertain whether the peritoneal cavity has been breached or organs have been injured [29,30].

Often, in the multiply injured patient who has suffered blunt trauma (motor vehicle accident, falls, etc.), head injuries, associated orthopedic injuries, and chest trauma may together necessitate intensive care resuscitation and evaluation before an operative algorithm is decided upon. In such patients, the laparoscope may be used at the most appropriate time to ascertain whether an abdominal catastrophe has occurred that would dictate changing the order of priorities, a decision often difficult in these patients. This procedure may take place in the emergency room, operating room, or most appropriately in the ICU. The minilaparoscope set designed by Berci [31••] is excellent for this purpose. The purpose of the laparoscopy is to determine the presence and grade of any injury found. If intestinal content is seen, then the surgeon should search for the injury briefly to guide placement of the laparotomy wound. If a pancreatic injury is suspected and serosanguinous fluid is seen, the fluid should be sent for determination of amylase content. If a hemoperitoneum is noted, it should be graded as follows:

- *Minimal.* Small flecks of blood cover the serosa of the bowel, liver, or paracolic gutters. These flecks may be washed away with irrigation and will either not reaccumulate or the bleeding source will be seen and attended to laparoscopically (Fig. 3).
- *Moderate.* Pools of blood are seen in the paracolic gutters; they may be washed away and a bleeding source sought.
- *Severe.* On introduction of the Veress needle, frank blood is aspirated or on entering the abdomen, the intestines are seen to float on a pool of blood. No

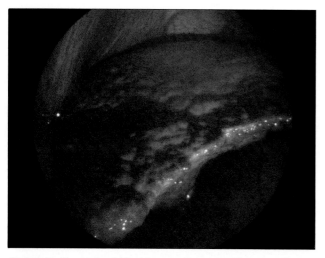

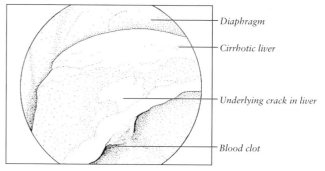
Diaphragm
Cirrhotic liver
Underlying crack in liver
Blood clot

Figure 3. Example of blunt trauma that caused a minor liver fracture that was sufficient to cause a positive peritoneal lavage but was capable of being arrested under laparoscopic control after irrigation and minimal electrosurgery.

time should be wasted in such patients in going straight to laparotomy [32,33]. Obviously, a small injury may be treated laparoscopically using either cautery or surgical suturing (Fig. 4). Alternatively, a laparoscopically assisted procedure may be performed. For instance, if the patient has overwhelming neurosurgical, orthopedic, or chest injuries and a small bowel laceration is seen, this laceration may be exteriorized. Another less conventional approach is to create a controlled fistula [33].

SEPSIS

Locating the source of sepsis in an extremely ill ICU patient is often extremely challenging, and occasionally one has a patient in septic shock who requires resuscitation and then evaluation of the cause. In this setting,

laparoscopy is a valuable tool, and examples are given below.

A patient with abdominal pain, sepsis, and a confusing clinical picture along with normal roentgenograms may have a sealed, perforated duodenal ulcer with intra-abdominal loculation. Under laparoscopic control this ulcer may be lavaged copiously and drains placed (Fig. 5). In patients with noncommunicating diverticular disease [34] when the diagnosis is suspected, laparoscopy may be used to confirm the situation and to place a drain into the large pericolic abscess cavity [35]. Similarly, patients with postoperative sepsis after major surgery may have laparoscopic evaluation (bearing in mind that open cannula placement will probably be necessary) as an alternative to percutaneous computed-tomography-scan-guided drainage; the advantage is that larger drains can be positioned.

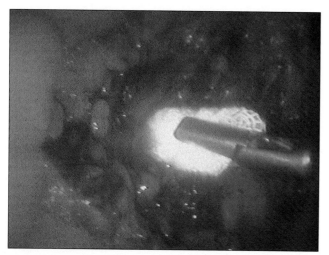

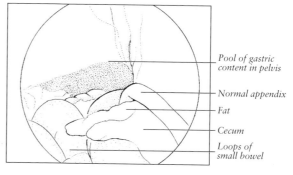

Figure 4. Blunt trauma may cause mesenteric injury as shown here. Hemostasis may be achieved with topical agents after ensuring the bowel is viable.

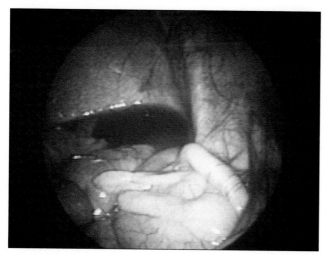

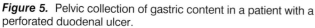

Figure 5. Pelvic collection of gastric content in a patient with a perforated duodenal ulcer.

In patients with fever of unexplained origin, laparoscopy is indicated only after all other appropriate tests have not been diagnostic or in the presence of abdominal signs and symptoms [36]. Obviously, in a carefully selected group of patients who are likely to have unusual infections, laparoscopy may be valuable. This group includes those with tuberculosis [37] (Fig. 6) or coccidiomycosis.

In other circumstances, the patient may have a confusing clinical picture and a fever. One such case was that of a 15-year-old girl with a history of Ewing's sarcoma of the hip that was purportedly treated successfully with chemotherapy and radiation. Her platelet count was reduced to 7000, and computed tomography scan demonstrated multiple lesions in the liver and spleen. Percutaneous aspiration had yielded necrotic tissue, and because of the swinging nature of the fever, the cause was thought to be metastatic abscesses. Laparoscopy was performed, and under careful control, samples were obtained that clearly demonstrated metastatic Ewing's

sarcoma [38]. This information allowed the patient to be discontinued from painful, distressing, and unhelpful intensive treatment. To control hemorrhage that would otherwise occur in this circumstance, through-and-through sutures were used to close the portal entry sites. The sutures were then tied over bolsters until hemostasis was achieved and then tied snugly to the skin. A recent report [39] demonstrated laparoscopy to be valuable in seven ICU patients with sepsis.

LIVER DISEASE

For patients awaiting liver transplantation, the shortage of donor livers means that especially those in stage IV failure, *ie*, confined to the ICU, will most likely be the ones chosen to receive a transplant. Often, these patients have cirrhosis, and ensuring whether or not hepatoma is superimposed upon the macronodular picture of cirrhosis is extremely valuable (Fig. 7). Laparoscopy may be performed before the transplantation.

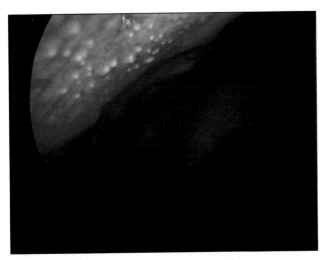

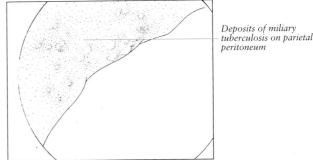

Deposits of miliary
tuberculosis on parietal
peritoneum

Figure 6. Miliary tuberculosis on the parietal peritoneum.

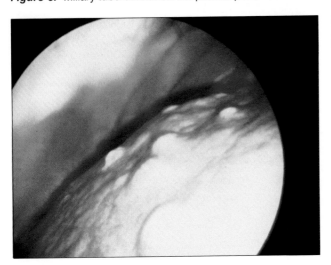

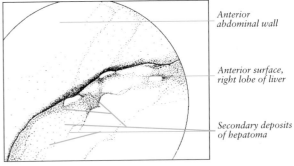

Anterior
abdominal wall

Anterior surface,
right lobe of liver

Secondary deposits
of hepatoma

Figure 7. Multifocal hepatoma in a cirrhotic liver.

Often, patients with cholecystitis suffer from severe cardiopulmonary disease, for arteriosclerosis is associated with gallstone disease [40–42]. Several treatment options for these patients include percutaneous cholecystostomy, open cholecystectomy (which, in this circumstance, has a high morbidity and mortality), or laparoscopic cholecystectomy or cholecystostomy. Laparoscopic cholecystectomy has been performed in a patient who was so severely ill with myocardial infarction that he was a heart transplant candidate [43]. Obviously, careful, continuous assessment is required with a Swan-Ganz catheter and an arterial line in addition to the usual monitoring. This approach is reasonable because of the significant mortality from septic complications in patients with acute cholecystitis [44].

Another group of patients in whom cholecystitis is challenging are the morbidly obese. These patients present a special challenge, and laparoscopic cholecystotomy should be considered. Although laparoscopic cholecystectomy is feasible [45–47], the time taken to perform the operation and the amount of gas necessary to maintain the pneumoperitoneum works against a safe outcome. Additionally, such obese patients, if extremely ill and in the ICU, need considerable assistance from medical and support personnel to be moved to the operating room; a quick, simple cholecystotomy performed laparoscopically is ideal.

The laparoscope is placed through the umbilicus, and a grasping forceps is inserted through a cannula below the xiphisternum. The gallbladder's mobility is ascertained, and a trocar is introduced below the right costal margin such that the tip of the trocar can be brought directly into the gallbladder. Through the cannula, a Malecot catheter is inserted; the cannula is then with-

drawn over this tube. If the surgeon has any concern about leakage from the insertion site, a simple suture may be placed using the subxiphisternal cannula, and an additional cannula may be introduced in the midclavicular line below the right costal margin. Alternatively, a suture may be passed from outside into the gallbladder, and later, when the patient's condition has improved, the stones may either be dissolved through this tube or a laparoscopic cholecystectomy performed.

Patients in crisis with sickle cell anemia may have acute cholecystitis because of gallstones superimposed on the clinical picture. Laparoscopic cholecystectomy is a valid option in this circumstance [48]. As this scenario is often in children, the subxiphisternal trocar should be placed below the left costal margin, the 4.2-mm instead of 10-mm telescope should be used, and the two lateral graspers should be moved further from the right costal margin to give space to manipulate instruments.

HYPOTENSION

If an elderly patient with hypotension and an irregular heartbeat also has metabolic acidosis, distended abdomen, and blood per rectum, the diagnosis of mesenteric ischemia is seldom in doubt. These patients are, however, extremely delicate, and do not tolerate intervention well. Bedside laparoscopy is beneficial to confirm the diagnosis of ischemia. If totally necrotic or gangrenous bowel is seen, then the situation can be treated conservatively. Similarly, if patchy ischemia is seen, especially if it affects the colon (Fig. 8), a policy of watch and wait while maximizing cardiac output may be appropriate. In the event of an early localized ischemia, however, the window of opportunity for sur-

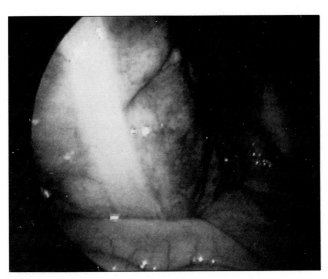

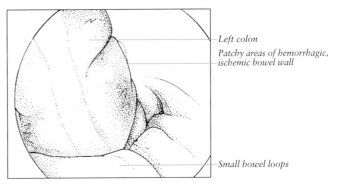

Left colon

Patchy areas of hemorrhagic, ischemic bowel wall

Small bowel loops

Figure 8. Ischemic colitis viewed laparoscopically.

gical intervention has been identified (Fig. 9). Although laparoscopic small or large bowel resection is feasible, an emergency situation in the ICU is hardly the setting in which to attempt it. In such patients, leaving a cannula in place after the laparoscopy or positioning one after the subsequent laparotomy is valuable. This placement will allow for second-look diagnostic laparoscopy at the bedside 24 hours later. A purse-string suture holds the cannula in the fascia and is tied to the device to prevent it from falling out. It is beyond the scope of the chapter to discuss this situation further. Similar scenarios occur in patients who have undergone cardiopulmonary bypass; bowel ischemia may occur and laparoscopy may be used as described for classical mesenteric ischemia.

PANCREATIC CARCINOMA

Up to 30% of patients with pancreatic carcinoma have metastases undetected by conventional imaging [49]. Often, these patients present with obstructive jaundice, and if they are elderly, this obstruction may be sufficient to create problems with urinary output and may confine the patient to the ICU. Before considering resection, a laparoscopy to confirm the diagnosis may be worthwhile. If, indeed, cure is impossible, an internal bypass can be fashioned with a cholecystoenterostomy or cholecystojejunostomy using sutures or staples [50]. No doubt, such patients are better served by having their bile diverted internally rather than externally.

BOWEL

In patients with intestinal obstruction and who must remain in the ICU because of other organ dysfunction, laparoscopy may be used as a quick, simple method to decompress the patient by bringing out a proximal loop of bowel. The laparoscope should be placed at the umbilicus and a mobile section of bowel above the obstruction selected. Two grasping forceps should be used, one in each iliac fossa or in the subcostal area. By carefully examining the bowel, an appropriate region may be selected. When a site for the stoma has been chosen, a larger trocar (20 mm) is inserted after a disk of skin is cut away. Grasping forceps are placed through this cannula, pneumoperitoneum is released, and the bowel is brought up to the skin. The instruments are removed, the wounds are closed, and the stoma is matured in the usual fashion [35,51].

In patients in whom an obstruction is caused by a volvulus, sigmoid decompression usually suffices. In the presence of a cecal volvulus [52] or sigmoid volvulus [53] that cannot be decompressed from the outside, however, the laparoscopic route may be ideal.

FEEDING ACCESS

Often, ICU patients require supplemental nutrition, and using the gastrointestinal tract is always preferable to the parenteral route. Percutaneous endoscopic gastrostomy and jejunostomy are well-known, effective techniques,

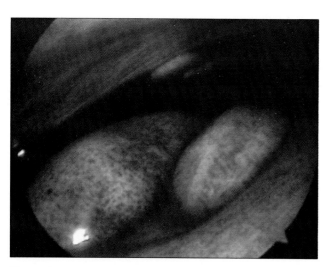

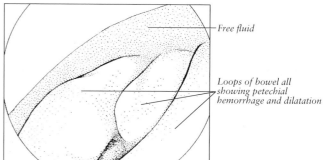

Figure 9. A laparoscopic view of ischemic small bowel. This approach allows the surgeon to evaluate the abdominal contents earlier in the disease process.

but in some patients (*eg*, those with obstructing esophageal lesions, burns, or stricture), they are just not possible. In this setting, either ultrasound-guided or laparoscopic gastrostomy may be used. The latter has the advantage of allowing evaluation of other intra-abdominal organs that may be involved. Additionally, the goal is to choose the least invasive method with the least chance of complications, for this technique is selected so as to *avoid* laparotomy—having to take a patient to the operating room for a complication of a minimally invasive approach would be extremely depressing!

One may insert the laparoscope through the umbilicus, then use T-bar fasteners to lift the stomach or jejunum to the anterior abdominal wall, and introduce the tube through the appropriate stoma site into the bowel. The T-bar fasteners ensure the bowel adheres to the abdominal wall [54,55]. In patients in whom the thickness of the abdominal pannus makes another technique preferable, the laparoscopic linear stapler can be used to create a gastric tube by repeatedly firing across the anterior wall of the stomach. This gastric tube may then be brought up to the abdominal wall and sutured in place as a gastrostomy [56].

RENAL TRANSPLANTATION

Patients undergoing cadaveric renal transplantation often have a stormy postoperative course that includes rejection, infection, and other complications. The laparoscope provides a means of accessing the transplanted organ to perform biopsies and draining lymphoceles that sometimes accumulate after such surgery [57].

THORACOSCOPY

As the range of uses for the laparoscope broadens, the diaphragm ceases to present a barrier. The laparoscope may be used to reveal emphysematous blebs that have led to recurrent pneumothorax. Occasionally, patients have rapidly worsening dyspnea as a result of pericardial tamponade. When the cause is a malignant effusion, obviously as little intervention as possible is the desire. In this setting, laparoscopy is ideal. After creating the pneumoperitoneum, the surgeon places additional trocars to the left side of the abdomen for the passage of instruments. An incision may be made into the region of the central tendon of the diaphragm, where the pericardium is attached. This incision should result in a gush of fluid, which may be aspirated. Simultaneous inspection can be made inside the pericardium to check for secondary deposits of the primary malignancy [58].

CONCLUSION

Laparoscopy or thoracoscopy does not represent a new specialty but a means of access to the body cavities. They enable surgeons to perform techniques that are extremely familiar. Those who use these methods must be well trained, must understand all the limitations, and must be prepared to convert to the open variant if needed. Recent reports demonstrate the value of this modality in severely ill patients [59••].

The surgeon should also be aware of all physiologic effects of laparoscopy, for in the course of an elective procedure, such a patient may be converted from a straightforward case to an ICU patient simply as a result of physician ignorance (*eg*, from the effects of retained carbon dioxide in subcutaneous emphysema after a lengthy procedure). For this reason, a thorough preoperative history is required, for it may reveal contraindications to the laparoscopy. Similarly, a careful preoperative examination should always include a search for signs of previous surgery, liver disease (portal hypertension and therefore increased tendency to bleed), or lumbar lordosis, which may increase the risk of aortic injury. The patient should be monitored carefully throughout surgery, and because of the raised intra-abdominal pressure and reverse Trendelenburg position often involved in laparoscopic cholecystectomy, deep venous thrombosis prophylaxis should be instituted to prevent disastrous postoperative pulmonary embolism. Lengthy laparoscopic operations may be better performed using gasses other than carbon dioxide or performed gasless by using an abdominal lift [60•], although this method may well be found to cause more pain and discomfort for the patient and therefore serve as no real advance.

As in all medical treatment, the doctor should always ask, "Is this investigation or therapy going to make a substantial difference to the patient's life?" If the answer is no, then laparoscopy is as inappropriate as any other investigation. Merely because it can be done does not mean it should be done.

ACKNOWLEDGMENT

I thank my colleagues, especially, Stephen Shoop, MD and David Easter, MD, for allowing me to discuss their cases.

REFERENCES

Papers of particular interest, published within the period of review, have been highlighted as:
• Of special interest
•• Of outstanding interest

1. Lyons AS, Petrucelli RJ: *Medicine: An Illustrated History.* New York: Abrams; 1987.

2. Ferraris VA: Exploratory Laparotomy for Potential Abdominal Sepsis in Patients with Multiple Organ Failure. *Arch Surg* 1993, 118:1130–1133.

3. Hinsdale JG, Jaffe BM: Reoperation for Intra-Abdominal Sepsis: Indications and Results in Modern Critical Care Setting. *Ann Surg* 1984, 199:31–36.

4. Bunt TJ: Non-Directed Laparotomy for Intra-abdominal Sepsis: A Futile Procedure. *Am Surg* 1986, 452:294–298.

5. Nell CJC, Pretorius DJ, DeVall JB: Reoperation for Suspected Intra-Abdominal Sepsis in the Critically Ill Patient. *S Afr J Surg* 1986, 24:60–62.

6. Ott D: Die Direkte Beleuchtung der Bauchhole, der Haranblase, des Dichdarams und des Uterus zu Diagnostichen Zwecken. *Rev Med Tcheque* 1909, 2:27–30.

7. Kelling G: Zur Coelioskopie. *Arch Klin Chir* 1923, 126:226–229.

8. Jacobaeus HC: Kurze Ubersicht uber meine Erfahrungen Mit der Laparoskopie. *Munch Med Wschr* 1923, 58:2017–2019.

9. Ruddock JC: Peritoneoscopy. *Surg Clin North Am* 1957, 37:1249–1253.

10. Cuschieri A: Laparoscopy in General Surgery and Gastroenterology. *Br J Hosp Med* 1980, 24:252– 258.

11. Berci G, Cuschieri A: Practical Laparoscopy. London: Baillierre Tindall; 1986.

12.•• Semm K: Operationsehre fur Endoskipische Abdominal Chirurgie: Operatiave Pelviskopie, Operative Laparoskopie. Stuttgart, Germany: Shattanuer Verlag Gmbh; 1984.

The most compelling text of laparoscopic surgery, of great interest due to its early publication.

13. Mühe E: The First Cholecystectomy Through the Laparoscope. *Langenbecks Arch Chir* 1986, 39:804.

14. DuBois F, Bertholet G, Lavard H: Cholecystectomy et par Celioscopie. *Presse Med* 1989, 18:980–984.

15. Perissat J, Collet DR, Belliard R: Gallstones: Laparoscopic Treatment, Intracorporeal Lithotripsy Followed by Cholecystostomy or Cholecystectomy: A Personal Technique. *Endoscopy* 1989, 21:373–374.

16. Nathanson LK, Shimi S, Cuschieri A: Laparoscopic Cholecystectomy: The Dundee Technique. *Br J Surg* 1991, 78:155–159.

17. Reddick EJ, Olson DO: Laparoscopic Laser Cholecystectomy. *Surg Endosc* 1989, 3:131–133.

18. Berci G, Sackier JM, Paz-Partlow M: Laparoscopic Cholecystectomy: Mini-Access Surgery—Reality or Utopia? *Postgrad Gen Surg* 1990, 2:50–54.

19. Bailey RW, Imbembo AL, Zucker KA: Establishment of a Laparoscopic Cholecystectomy Training Program. *Am Surg* 1991, 57:231–236.

20. Boyce HW, Henning H: Diagnostic Laparoscopy 1992: Time For a New Look. *Endoscopy* 1992, 24:671–673.

21.•• Mealy K, Gallagher H, Barry M, *et al.*: Physiological and Metabolic Responses to Open and to Laparoscopic Cholecystectomy. *Br J Surg* 1992, 79:1061–1064.

The first report to document objective differences.

22. Muller HO, Gundel E, Kollmeier H: Laparoskopie mit Kohlensauregas. Mogliche, Fehldeutung and Eines E. Endoskopichen Gefasse Befunds. *Endoskopie* 1970, 2:58–60.

23. Nakatsuka I, Okada M, Konishi M, Noguchi J: Blood Gas Changes After Laparoscopy. *Masui* 1991, 40:1616–1619.

24. Yacoub OF, Cardona I, Coveler LA, Dodson MG: Carbon Dioxide Embolism During Laparoscopy. *Anaestheliology* 1982, 57:533–535.

25. Rademaker BM, Ringers J, O'Doom JA, *et al.*: Pulmonary Function of Stress Response After Laparoscopic Cholecystectomy: Comparison With Subcostal Incision and Influence of Thoracic Epidural Anesthesia. *Reg. Anesth Analg* 1992, 75:381–385.

26.•• Siegel B, Golub RM, Loiacano L, *et al.*: Techniques of Ultrasonic Defection and Mapping of Abdominal Wall Adhesions. *Surg Endosc* 1991, 5:161–163.

A valuable and simple technique that I have found to be reproducible.

27. Dunn DC, Watson CJE: Disposable Guarded Trocar and Cannula in Laparoscopic Surgery: A Caveat. *Br J Surg* 1992, 79:927.

28. Hasson HN: A Modified Instrument and a Method for Laparoscopy. *Am J Obstet Gynecol* 1971, 110:886–887.

29. Sackier JM: Emergent Laparoscopy. In *Endoscopic Surgery*. Edited by Greene FL, Ponsky JG. Philadelphia: Saunders; 1993, in press.

30. Ivatury RR, Simon RJ, Weksler B, *et al.*: Laparoscopy in the Evaluation of the Intrathoracic Abdomen After Penetrating Injury. *J Trauma* 1992, 33:101– 109.

31.•• Wood D, Berci G, Morgenstern L, Paz-Partlow M: Mini-Laparoscopy in Blunt Abdominal Trauma. *Surg Endosc* 1988, 2:184–189.

The landmark article on this subject by the first proponent of trauma laparoscopy.

32. Berci G, Sackier JM, Paz-Partlow M: Emergency Laparoscopy. *Am J Surg* 1991, 161:355–360.

33. Birns MT: Inadvertent Instrumental Perforation of the Colon During Laparoscopy: Nonsurgical Repair. *Gastrointest Endosc* 1989, 35:54–56.

34. Hinchey EJ, Schaal PGH, Richards GK: Treatment of Perforated Diverticular Disease of the Colon. *Adv Surg* 1978, 12:85–109.

35. Sackier JM: Laparoscopic Colon and Rectal Surgery. In *Minimally Invasive Surgery.* Edited by Hunter JG, Sackier JM. New York: McGraw-Hill; 1993.

36. Henning H: The Value of Laparoscopy in Evaluating Fever of Unexplained Origin. *Endoscopy* 1992, 24:687–688.

37. Bhargava DK, Shriniwas, Chopra P, *et al.*: Peritoneal Tuberculosis: Laparoscopic Patterns and its Diagnostic Accuracy. *Am J Gastroenterol* 1992, 87:109–112.

38. McKenzie DJ, James B, Geller SA, Sackier JM: Laparoscopic Diagnosis of Ewing's Sarcoma Metastatic to the Liver. Case Report and Review of the Literature. *J Pediatr Surg* 1992, 27:93–95.

39. Bender JS, Talamini MA: Diagnostic Laparoscopy in Critically Ill Intensive Care Patients. *Surg Endosc* 1992, 6:302–304.

40. Kaye MD, Kern F: Clinical Relationship of Gallstones. *Lancet* 1977, 1:1028–1030.

41. Bortinchak EA, Freeman DH, Ostfeld AM, *et al.*: The Association in Cholelithiasis and Coronary Heart Disease in Farmingham, Massachusetts. *Am J Epidemiol* 1985, 121:19–30.

42. Paul O, Lepper MJ, Phelan WH, *et al.*: A Longitudinal Study of Coronary Heart Disease. *Circulation* 1963, 28:20–31.

43. Carroll BJ, Chandra M, Phillips EH, Harold JG: Laparoscopic Cholecystectomy in the Heart Transplant Lung Candidate With Acute Cholecystitis. *J Heart Lung Transplant* 1992, 11:831–833.

44. Boline GB, Gifort RRM, Yang HC, *et al.*: Cholecystectomy in the Potential Heart Transplant Patient. *J Heart Lung Transplant* 1991, 10:269–274.

45. Collet D, Eddye M, Mangne E, Perrisat J: Laparoscopic Cholecystectomy in the Obese Patient. *Surg Endosc* 1992, 6:186–188.

46. Miles RH, Carballo RE, Prinz RA, *et al.*: Laparoscopy: The Preferred Method of Cholecystectomy in the Morbidly Obese. *Surgery* 1992, 112:818–823.

47. Sackier JM: The Complicated Laparoscopic Cholecystectomy. *Gastrointest Endosc Clin North Am* 1993; 3:283–295.

48. Ware RE, Kinney TR, Casey JR, *et al.*: Laparoscopic Cholecystectomy in Young Patients With Sickle Hemoglobinopathies. *J Pediatr* 1992, 120:58–61.

49. Spinelli P, Di Felice G: Laparoscopy in Abdominal Malignancies. *Prob Gen Surg* 1991, 8:329–347.

50. Fletcher DR, Jones RM: Laparoscopic Cholecystojejunostomy as Palliation for Obstructive Jaundice in Inoperable Carcinoma of Pancreas. *Surg Endosc* 1992, 6:147–149.

51. Lange V, Meyer G, Schardey HM, *et al.*: Laparoscopic Creation of a Loop Colostomy. *J Laparosc Endosc Surg* 1991, 1:307–312.

52. Shoop S, Sackier JM: Laparoscopic Cecopexy, Laparoscopic Treatment of Cecal Volvulus. *Surg Endosc, in press.*

53. Miller R, Roe AM, Eltringham WK, Espiner HJ: Laparoscopic Fixation of Sigmoid Volvulus. *Br J Surg* 1992, 79:435.

54. Reiner DS, Leitman IM, Ward RJ: Laparoscopic Stamm Gastrostomy with Gastropexy. *Laparosc Endosc Surg* 1991, 1:189–192.

55. Morris JB, Mullen JL, Yu JC, Rosato EF: Laparoscopic Guided Jejunostomy. *Surgery* 1991, 112:96–99.

56. Haggie JA: Laparoscopic Tube Gastrostomy. *Ann R Coll Surg Engl* 1992, 74:258–359.

57. Slavis SA, Gardener LD, Swift C, Gross ML: Laparoscopic Drainage of Lymphocele After Renal Transplantation. *J Urol* 1992, 148:96–97.

58. Ready A, Black J, Lewis R, Roscoe B: Laparoscopic Pericardial Fenestration for Malignant Pericardial Effusion [Letter]. *Lancet* 1992, 339:1609.

59.•• Forde KA, Treat BR: The Role of Peritoneoscopy (Laparoscopy) in the Evaluation of the Acute Abdomen in Critically Ill Patients. *Surg Endosc* 1992, 6:219–221.

A concise review of the topic and a good clinical experience.

60.• Araki K, Yamumoto H, Doiguchi M, *et al.*: Abdominal Wall Retraction During Laparoscopic Cholecystectomy. *World J Surg* 1993, 17:105–108.

An interesting approach that may owe more to ingenuity than real need.

Chapter 18

Laparoscopic Herniorrhaphy

Elizabeth J. Redmond
Giovanni M. Salerno
Riccardo Annabali
Robert J. Fitzgibbons, Jr

Inguinal hernias remain a common problem. At least 500,000 hernia repairs are performed in the United States each year [1]. Most options available for primary hernia repair have their roots in Bassini's repair, which he described in 1884 [2]. Bassini recognized that the cause of the problem was a weakness in the floor of the inguinal canal and that to prevent recurrence, high ligation of the sac was required. His method relies on approximating the inguinal ligament to the conjoint tendon, which reinforces the floor of the canal.

The technique has been modified by many surgeons over the years to reduce its associated complications and improve its efficacy. For example, the Shouldice repair involves the identification and repair of four separate layers of fascial tissues. In expert hands, the recurrence rate using this technique is as low as 0.6% [3]. In routine hospital practice, however, a recurrence rate of 10% is not uncommon [4]. For recurrent hernias, the prospect of a further recurrence is as high as 35% [5]. Other problems associated with routine hernia repair relate to the incision and dissection required to expose the area. The incision is painful and causes patients to miss a minimum of 2 weeks of work. This absence is further prolonged for patients whose occupations involve physical exertion. In patients who develop complications, as occurs in approximately 5% of cases, the total amount of time they are incapacitated may be considerable [6]. Infection of the material used for the hernia repair may ensue; exploration and removal of the foreign material are usually required. This complication results in a high recurrence rate. The dissection of the cord may damage the structures contained therein; such complications include inadvertent vasectomy and vessel damage, which lead to hematomas or testicular atrophy and pain. Groin dissection affects the lymphatic drainage and may result in excessive swelling.

The most troublesome long-term complications of hernia repair include hypoesthesia and painful neuromas. These neuromas are caused by inadvertent nerve division or trapping of the nerve in scar tissue and may affect the ilioinguinal, iliohypogastric, or genitofemoral nerves. A proportion of patients with these complications require further surgical exploration to repair the neuroma.

To summarize, conventional hernia repair is not without risk. Nevertheless, it is generally safe and effective. It may be performed readily using local anesthesia, thus minimizing risks to the frail patient. It allows an accurate diagnosis of the problem, and complications such as irreducibility and sliding contents can be appreciated and managed readily.

THE ROLE OF LAPAROSCOPY IN THE MANAGEMENT OF HERNIA

Laparoscopic cholecystectomy has become the approach of choice more rapidly than almost any other surgical innovation [7]. This rapid acceptance is because of the procedure's decreased postoperative pain and lack of scarring, which make the technique so acceptable to patients, and the decreased hospital stay and excellent visualization, which make the procedure so attractive to surgeons. Therapeutic laparoscopy was, therefore, bound to be extended to other surgical fields. It now has an established role in antireflux surgery and colorectal surgery and is being evaluated for use in upper gastrointestinal resections and for expansion of its traditional role in gynecologic surgery and diagnosis. The hernia repair is the latest and perhaps the most unlikely indication to be evaluated [8].

THE INTRA-ABDOMINAL APPROACH TO HERNIORRHAPHY

Surgeons have for many years repaired hernias found incidentally during laparotomy for other indications, when repair was appropriate. This use was recognized and described by Andrews [9] in 1924. A formal intra-abdominal approach was first described by Marcy [10] in 1887, and later modified in 1932 by LaRoque [11], who performed and reported 1700 such repairs. LaRoque pointed to the advantage of easy dissection of the sac, which allowed the essential high ligation without risk to the cord structures. LaRoque also believed the procedure was particularly appropriate for the safe

management of the irreducible hernia, as it allows for inspection of the hernia contents and, if required, safe resection. A series of hernia repairs performed during laparotomy was reported by Ger and coworkers [12] in 1990. The basis of this procedure was simple closure of the hernia defect intra-abdominally using Michel clips. The final patient in the series had a hernia discovered during a diagnostic laparoscopy. Ger applied Michel clips under laparoscopic guidance. This procedure is the first recorded laparoscopic hernia repair and was actually performed in 1979, before the use of the laparoscope for cholecystectomy.

The intra-abdominal approach has empirical appeal, as the hernia can be approached at its origin. Most surgeons, however, consider this method too invasive for a primary herniorrhaphy. The introduction of therapeutic laparoscopy in general surgery as an alternative method to gain access to the peritoneal cavity has enabled surgeons to reconsider this approach.

THE PROBLEM OF RECURRENCE

Most of the many described modifications to the Bassini repair have been developed to reduce the incidence of recurrence. The importance of excess tension as a cause of recurrence was recognized, and the relaxing incision was added. Lichtenstein and coworkers [13] stress the importance of tension and poor tissue quality in recurrence. To negate this problem, they advocated the routine use of prosthetic materials to produce strong, tension-free repairs with minimal chances of recurrence. They also believed that the lack of tension relieves discomfort and allows the patient a quicker return to normal function. The question of infection in these repairs has not been fully addressed but has been negligible in their experience.

CONVENTIONAL PREPERITONEAL HERNIORRHAPHY

The preperitoneal approach to femoral hernias was first described by Cheatle [14] in 1920 but popularized by Henry in 1936 [cited in 15]. Henry discovered this approach independently while operating to treat urologic complications of Bilharzia in Egypt [15].

The French surgeons Stoppa and Rives also considered the preperitoneal space ideal for the placement of a prosthetic patch to reinforce the fascia. This placement provides a mechanical advantage by using the intra-abdominal pressure to maintain the position of the prosthesis rather than allowing such pressure to be a factor in recurrence, as occurs in prostheses placed in more superficial positions. The patch is covered by the peritoneum, which eliminates the potential problems of contact between the prosthesis and the intra-abdominal organs.

Rives [16] uses an inguinal incision as in conventional hernia repair. The cord is mobilized and a high ligation of the sac performed. The transversalis fascia is then incised parallel to the inguinal canal to enter the preperitoneal space. The peritoneum is separated by blunt dissection, and Cooper's ligament, the iliac vessels, and the femoral ring are exposed in the process. A piece of Dacron mesh is then introduced and sutured along the symphysis pubis and Cooper's ligament. It is tailored around the cord, anchored to either side of the cord, and sutured at its upper border.

Stoppa and coworkers [17] use a more extensive prosthesis in a manner termed the "great prosthesis reinforcement of the visceral sac." Through a lower midline incision, the recti are split, and the extraperitoneal space is developed by gauze dissection. The hernia defect is thus exposed and the hernia sac reduced. The cord is mobilized and moved laterally, as Stoppa believes in the importance of "parietalizing" the cord structures. A bilateral dissection is performed routinely. A piece of Dacron, 24 cm by 16 cm, is introduced into this space to cover all potential hernia defects. The important landmarks are the symphysis pubis, Cooper's ligament, the inferior epigastric vessels, the internal inguinal ring, and the anterior superior iliac spines. The patch is sutured only at the symphysis pubis and the umbilicus and is maintained in position by intra-abdominal pressure. These techniques are important, as they have provided the logical basis for the laparoscopic methods.

JUSTIFICATION OF LAPAROSCOPIC HERNIA REPAIR

The three key factors that led to the development of laparoscopic hernia repair are the acceptance of prosthetic materials for herniorrhaphy, the apparent efficacy of the preperitoneal approach, and the development and widespread use of therapeutic laparoscopy in general surgery. To justify replacing a safe and effective technique such as the classical hernia repair with laparoscopic herniorrhaphy, four aims must be met:
1. Reduced postoperative pain and a shortened period of time away from work
2. Reduced rate of recurrence
3. Decreased incidence of postoperative neuralgias
4. Reasonable cost

In achieving these aims, laparoscopic repair must be at least as safe as the conventional approach. The routine use of prosthetic materials must not cause an excessive increase in the rate of infection, and traversing the peritoneal cavity must not cause later problems secondary to adhesions.

In considering these problems, issues of safety must be of prime importance. A small but definite incidence of cardiac dysrhythmia is associated with the induction of pneumoperitoneum [18]. This complication may be minimized by using careful technique and avoiding rapid insufflation and high pressures within the peritoneal cavity. These techniques must always be carried out with full facilities for resuscitation. Laparoscopy usually requires general anesthesia and complete muscle relaxation with their attendant risks. Epidural or spinal anesthesia are theoretically possible but have not been used extensively with therapeutic laparoscopy [19].

The work of Stoppa and coworkers [17] implies little excess risk of infection using prosthetic materials. Monofilament meshes are theoretically less likely to allow late postoperative infection to develop. Evidence from the use of prosthetic arthroplasties suggests that the organisms that cause infection are usually implanted at the time of surgery. Therefore, adopting a "no-touch" technique appears logical, and the use of prophylactic perioperative antibiotics should be obligatory [20].

The possibility of bowel damage during entry to the peritoneal cavity can be minimized by using careful technique and adopting an open laparoscopic technique when possible. This technique was developed to counter the dangers of "blind" access to the peritoneal cavity normally encountered when using a Veress needle to insufflate the abdomen. A small incision is made immediately beneath the umbilicus and deepened through the subcutaneous fat until the midline raphe is identified as it leads up to the umbilicus. Even in the obese patient, this raphe is usually found close to the skin. The raphe should be grasped with two Kocher's clamps and divided with heavy scissors. The peritoneum closely adheres to the fascia and may be divided in the same action [21•]. The possibility that adhesions form subsequent to the insertion of foreign materials into the peritoneal cavity has been investigated in the laparoscopic laboratory in our department and will be considered later.

THE CHOICE OF PROSTHETIC MATERIAL

Numerous materials have been used for the reinforcement of herniorrhaphy. These materials range from natural substances such as fascia lata to specially developed polymers. The most effective prostheses are believed to be those of a mesh configuration, as these allow incorporation of fibroblasts into the patch, thereby reinforcing the repair. Two commonly available materials are polypropylene mesh (Prolene [Ethicon, Somerville, NJ], Marlex [C & R Bard, MA]) and polyester (Dacron, Mersilene [Ethicon, Somerville, NJ]). Both materials are nonabsorbable and incite a tissue reaction that encourages scarring and therefore strength. Polypropylene has the advantage that it is a monofilament structure and thus theoretically has a lower risk of infection. Absorbable materials are attractive, as they pose an even lower risk of infection once implanted. Materials with an absorption time longer than 90 days are available; in theory, the time allows adequate strength to be acquired by the scar. There is little published experience using these meshes in herniorrhaphy. Expanded polytetrafluoroethylene has been advocated for use in hernia repairs. It is of low reactivity, which makes it attractive for use intraperitoneally, but this same property reduces scarring so the repair is solely dependent on the intrinsic strength of the patch [22].

PERTINENT ANATOMY

Within the abdominal cavity several important structures need to be identified to perform a repair safely. In the midline lies the median umbilical ligament, which passes from the dome of the bladder to the umbilicus.

This structure is the remains of the urachus and may occasionally be patent. Lateral to this ligament lies the medial umbilical ligament, which is formed by a fold of peritoneum over the remains of the umbilical artery. The inferior epigastric arteries originate from the external iliac artery and run rostrally into the rectus sheath to supply the rectus muscle. These vessels may be viewed from the peritoneal aspect as the lateral umbilical ligaments; they mark the medial border of the internal inguinal ring. Indirect hernias occur laterally to this border, and direct hernias occur medially through Hesselbach's triangle. The spermatic vessels course over the psoas muscle to reach the internal inguinal ring. Laparoscopically, these vessels can be identified through the peritoneum and protected during the dissection. The vas

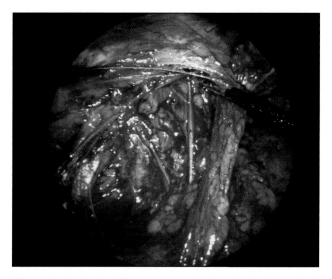

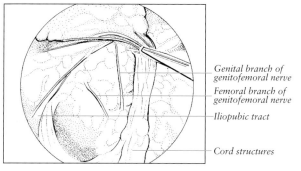

Genital branch of genitofemoral nerve

Femoral branch of genitofemoral nerve

Iliopubic tract

Cord structures

Figure 1. Anatomy of importance to the herniorrhaphist. Cord structures have been retracted by forceps. The femoral branch of the genitofemoral nerve and the lateral cutaneous nerve of the thigh are displayed passing beneath the iliopubic tract.

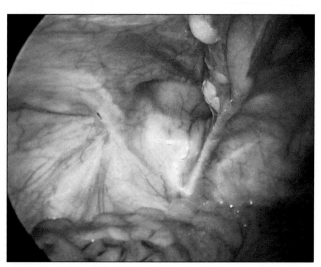

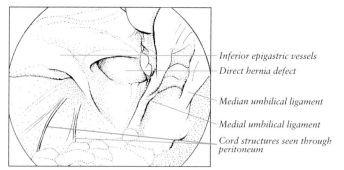

Inferior epigastric vessels

Direct hernia defect

Median umbilical ligament

Medial umbilical ligament

Cord structures seen through peritoneum

Figure 2. Interior view demonstrating direct hernia and the anatomic landmarks.

deferens emerge from behind the base of the bladder and pass medially to cross the external iliac vessels and join the spermatic vessels as they enter the inguinal canal. Throughout their course, they are covered only by peritoneum. The genitofemoral nerve appears at the medial border of the psoas muscle at about the level of L-3 and crosses behind the ureter beneath the psoas fascia. It divides a variable distance above the iliopubic tract into the genital branch and femoral branch. The genital branch joins the cord structures and passes through the inguinal canal to innervate the cremaster muscle and supply sensation to the scrotum and adjacent thigh. The femoral branch, the lateral cutaneous nerve of the thigh, and the femoral nerve are at risk as they pass beneath the iliopubic tract.

The iliopubic tract is an important structure to the laparoscopic surgeon. It is a condensation of the endoabdominal fascia over the psoas muscle and originates from the inner lip of the iliac crest, the anterior superior iliac spine, and the iliopectineal arch. It passes parallel to the inguinal ligament, on the surface of the iliacus and psoas muscles, crosses the femoral vessels anteriorly, and forms the inferior border of the deep inguinal ring and the anterior border of the femoral canal. It inserts at the pubic tubercle and medial portion of Cooper's ligament [23]. The iliopubic tract serves as a landmark. Staples inserted inferior to this structure and lateral to the femoral vessels may impinge upon either the femoral branch of the genitofemoral nerve or the lateral cutaneous nerve of the thigh and produce troublesome neuralgias. The laparoscopic herniorrhaphist must take great care to avoid applying staples inferior to the iliopubic tract and lateral to the spermatic vessels (Fig. 1). The ilioinguinal nerve passes through the inguinal canal along with the genital branch of the genitofemoral nerve but enters the canal by piercing the transversalis and internal oblique muscles near the anterior superior iliac spine. The external iliac vessels run on the psoas muscle and pass over Cooper's ligament and beneath the inguinal ligament into the femoral triangle. Cooper's ligament is a fascial condensation that extends from the pubic tubercle along the pectineal line of the superior pubic ramus and is formed by the periosteum and the insertion of the iliopubic tract and transversalis fascia. Cooper's ligament is exposed when the peritoneum is reflected downward during hernia repair, and this is the structure to which the inferomedial border of the prosthetic patch is applied.

SPECIFIC LAPAROSCOPIC HERNIORRHAPHIES

TRANSABDOMINAL PREPERITONEAL HERNIORRHAPHY

Transabdominal herniorrhaphy is particularly attractive to the laparoscopic surgeon because it is so similar to conventional preperitoneal hernia repair. The only difference is that the preperitoneal space is entered through an incision in the peritoneum instead of through a conventional skin and abdominal-wall incision. To minimize the risks associated with blind entry to the abdomen, the open laparoscopy technique using a Hasson cannula is recommended. The inguinal regions are inspected to confirm the pathology and check the contralateral side (Fig. 2). Two further cannulae are then inserted under direct vision. A large, 11- or 12-mm operating port is introduced contralaterally, just lateral to the rectus muscle, and a 5- or 11-mm cannula is introduced in an equivalent position ipsilaterally (Fig. 3). The medial umbilical ligament is identified and

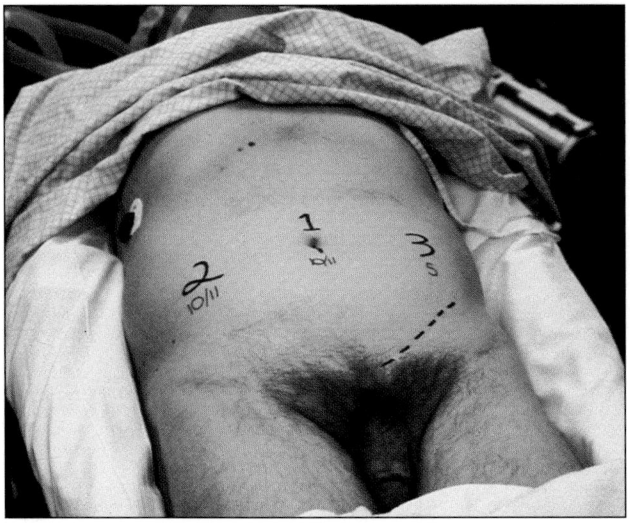

Figure 3. Correct port positions for the transabdominal preperitoneal herniorrhaphy or intraperitoneal onlay mesh technique.

divided if it appears to compromise exposure (Fig. 4). Bleeding from small vessels is secured by using electrocautery. A peritoneal flap is then created by incising the peritoneum from the medial umbilical ligament to the anterior superior iliac spine 2 cm above the myopectineal defect (Fig. 5). The flap is then mobilized downward using sharp and blunt dissection. The inferior epigastric vessels and cord structures are thus exposed (Fig. 6). For direct hernias, the sac is reduced from the hernial orifice by using gentle traction (Fig. 7). The preperitoneal fat and pseudosac are left behind; they are separated by sharp dissection if necessary. As the dissection continues inferiorly, Cooper's ligament and the iliopubic tract are exposed (Fig. 8). The dissection is completed by mobilizing the cord structures away from the peritoneal flap.

Indirect hernias are clearly more difficult to manage (Fig. 9). If the sac is small, it can be mobilized from the cord structures and reduced back into the abdomen. If the hernia extends into the scrotum, complete mobilization would lead to an unacceptably high risk of spermatic cord and testicular complications. In this situation, the best approach is to divide the neck of the sac at a convenient point distal to the internal ring and to mobilize only the proximal portion off the cord. After completely dissecting the preperitoneal space and identifying the critical anatomic structures, the surgeon commences the repair. First, a decision must be made whether the cord structures are to be encircled with mesh or merely covered. If a direct hernia is large and extends to the internal ring or if an indirect hernia has destroyed the ring (Nyhus Type III, Table 1), we prefer

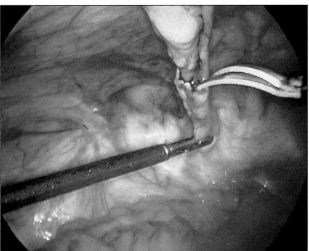

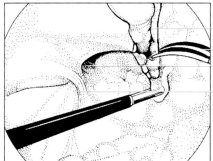

Medial umbilical ligament

Scissors

Direct hernia defect

Internal ring with cord structures

Figure 4. Peritoneal incision is commenced by dividing the medial umbilical ligament.

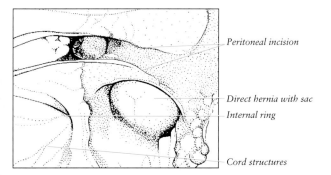

Peritoneal incision

Direct hernia with sac

Internal ring

Cord structures

Figure 5. Complete peritoneal incision.

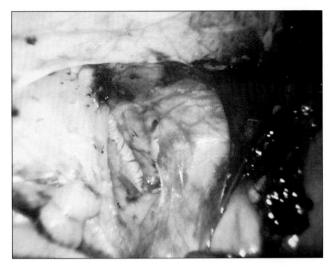

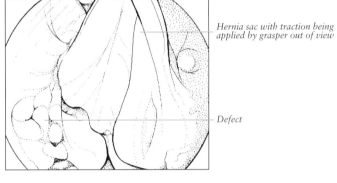

Upper edge peritoneum

Hernia in defect

Inferior epigastric vessels

Lower edge of peritoneal flap mobilized downward

Figure 6. Peritoneal flap is mobilized downward to display epigastric vessel and cord structures. The hernia sac remains in the defect.

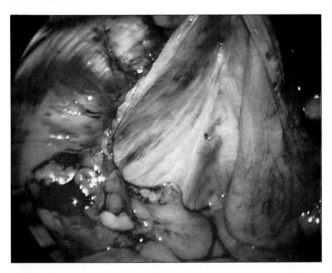

Hernia sac with traction being applied by grasper out of view

Defect

Figure 7. Hernia sac is reduced.

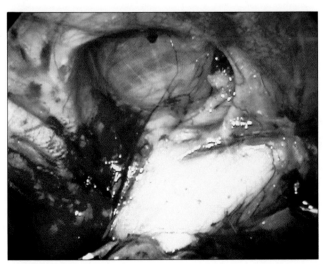

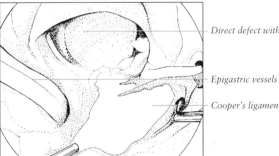

Direct defect with pseudosac

Epigastric vessels

Cooper's ligament

Figure 8. Cooper's ligament and the iliopubic tract with the pseudosac seen in the defect.

to place a slit to accommodate the cord structures. This procedure requires additional mobilization of the cord posteriorly to accommodate the mesh. In other circumstances, the mesh is simply laid over the cord structures, and this dissection is avoided.

We prefer polypropylene mesh, but different materials are used by other surgeons. The size of the mesh is important, and we generally use an 11- by 6-cm patch. This size is sufficiently large to cover the defect and provide an extensive overlap. It allows the intra-abdominal pressure to act on strong, healthy tissue, which tends to keep the patch in position rather than encourage it to herniate through the defect. The mesh is folded in half along its longitudinal axis and loosely sutured together. This procedure facilitates manipulation of the patch intra-abdominally. The folded patch is introduced into the abdominal cavity and placed over the myopectineal defect behind the cord. The loose sutures are divided and the patch unfolded and positioned around the cord. The upper border of the patch is stapled to the transversalis fascia approximately 1 or 2 cm above the internal ring. If a slit has been made in the patch, it is repaired around the cord. The inferior edge is stapled to the symphysis pubis and Cooper's ligament medially and to the iliopubic tract laterally. Staples must not be placed below the level of the iliopubic tract lateral to the external iliac vessels, or the patient will have an inordinately high risk of neuralgia that involves the lateral cutaneous nerve of the thigh or the femoral branch of the genitofemoral nerve. The lateral edge is stapled at a point just medial to the anterior superior iliac spines. The patch is then trimmed to fit the preperitoneal space before the peritoneum is repaired.

The final step is to close the peritoneum with staples, thus isolating the patch from the abdominal contents. This step is facilitated by reducing the pneumoperitoneum. A long-acting local anesthetic may be left in the preperitoneal space to reduce postoperative discomfort. Bilateral hernias can be repaired using one long transverse peritoneal incision and a large piece of mesh fashioned similarly to that described by Stoppa [17] for conventional preperitoneal repair. Two separate pieces of prosthetic material are preferable, however, because the smaller pieces are easier to manipulate and the possibility of incising a patent urachus is avoided. Some surgeons prefer to suture the patch in position, but the recently developed stapling devices greatly facilitate stabilization of the prosthesis and are therefore preferable.

This approach to herniorrhaphy has, at least with short-term follow-up, an acceptably low recurrence rate and good patient acceptance [24••]. Considerable dissection is required, but with experience the surgeon will have an operating time similar to that for conventional herniorrhaphy. The preperitoneal dissection causes some pain, but the tension-free nature of the repair means pain is not prolonged, and most patients return to normal activities within a week. Although diagnostic laparoscopy is possible using local anesthetic, the considerable preperitoneal dissection involved in this procedure precludes its use.

INTRAPERITONEAL ONLAY MESH TECHNIQUE

The reason for the preperitoneal dissection described in the above technique is threefold: to allow for ligation or reduction of the sac as classically required for herniorrhaphy, to allow for fixation of the prosthesis directly to the transversalis fascia, and to provide a covering for the mesh to minimize the theoretical risk of adhesions between the prosthetic patch and the bowel. To establish whether a scientific basis existed for these rationales, an animal model for the insertion of prosthetic material into the abdominal cavity was developed in our department. We posed the question, if an inguinal hernia could be repaired so successfully with a prosthesis placed in the preperitoneal space, could the same

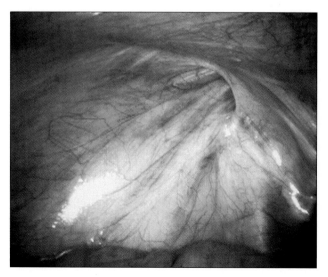

Figure 9. Indirect hernia viewed laparoscopically.

Table 1. Nyhus groin hernia classification[*]

Type	Description
Type I	Indirect inguinal hernia with normal internal ring (*ie*, pediatric hernia)
Type II	Indirect inguinal hernia with dilated internal ring, anatomically intact
Type III	A) Direct inguinal hernia
	B) Indirect inguinal hernia with anatomic destruction of the ring
	C) Femoral hernia
Type IV	Recurrent hernia

*Modified from Nyhus [29].

results be obtained with a prosthesis placed one "layer" deeper, on the peritoneal surface itself? This idea assumes that the prosthesis could be fixed to the same landmarks described earlier for the transabdominal preperitoneal procedure.

Yorkshire crossfeeder pigs, with either unilateral or bilateral indirect inguinal hernias, underwent intraperitoneal hernia repairs. The control group of pigs underwent laparotomy and had their hernias repaired by using a polypropylene (Prolene) patch sutured over the defect and overlapping the defect significantly. The treatment group underwent an identical procedure, except that the prosthesis was placed laparoscopically and was stapled rather than sutured. All hernia repairs in both groups were successful. Examination of these patches at postmortem 6 weeks after operation showed that they had been covered by a tissue layer; histologic examination demonstrated this layer to be peritoneum [25]. The staples had become flush with the new surface (Fig. 10). Interestingly, the percentage of the patch covered by adhesions and the tenacity of the adhesions were significantly less in the laparoscopy group than in the controls [26].

Encouraged by these results, we obtained permission to begin performing intraperitoneal operations in patients. Only patients with indirect hernias were routinely offered the procedure, because only data on indirect inguinal hernias in pigs were presented to our university's Institutional Review Board. Operating ports are placed as for the transabdominal preperitoneal procedure. The site of the hernia is inspected to ensure its suitability for this type of repair. The anatomic landmarks are identified and the patch is placed into position and stapled at 1-cm intervals. Landmarks used for staple placement are essentially the same as those used in the transabdominal preperitoneal procedure. Again, great care is taken not to place staples below the iliopubic tract lateral to the internal spermatic vessels.

Because the iliopubic tract can be hard to identify with the peritoneum still in place, a rule of thumb is that the staples should be placed only once the surgeon can feel the head of the stapler with the opposite hand.

To date, more than 50 intraperitoneal onlay mesh procedures have been performed in patients at Creighton University [27•]. The authors have had the opportunity to inspect the patch in four patients: one patient developed a painful neuralgia involving the lateral cutaneous nerve of the thigh before it became apparent that great care should be taken to place staples above the iliopubic tract. This patient underwent a second laparoscopy to remove the offending staple. Another patient developed symptomatic biliary tract disease and required laparoscopic cholecystectomy. A third patient suffered a gunshot wound to the abdomen. The fourth patient developed an infection of the prosthesis. Adhesions between the prosthesis and the bowel were observed in the first two patients, though no clinical sequelae had occurred. The gunshot-wound patient had no adhesions, and the mesh appeared completely covered by a "neoperitoneum." Approximately 18 months after his procedure, the final patient, developed fever and a fluctuant mass in his groin. The mass was drained using general anesthesia and found to contain purulent material. The patient underwent laparoscopy and was found to have an inflammatory mass that involved the cecum in the right iliac fossa, where the patch had been placed. The appendix could not be identified. The inflammatory mass was entered and the mesh removed. Because of the infective process, the mesh was quite loose and easily removed along with its staples. The findings in this patient caused us, in consultation with the university's Human Research Committee, to suspend the use of the intraperitoneal operation using polypropylene mesh in patients, pending further observation of the rest of the group.

In summary, the intraperitoneal operation is an effec-

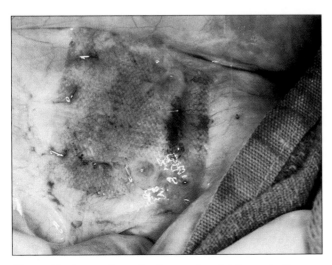

Figure 10. Intraperitoneal onlay mesh patch from pig 6 weeks postinsertion. Note the smooth "neoperitoneal" covering.

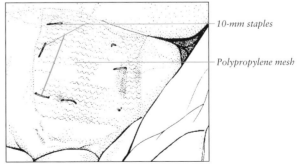

tive technique for correction of an indirect inguinal hernia in patients. Other investigators have used the technique in direct hernias with success, although it is almost certainly not suitable for large direct hernias, as obtaining adequate fixation of the prosthesis would be difficult. A biological material with less reactivity than polypropylene will probably be required to prevent adhesions that involve abdominal organs and the risk of subsequent erosion into these structures.

EXTRAPERITONEAL LAPAROSCOPIC HERNIORRHAPHY

To avoid the possible complications of entering the peritoneal cavity and in an attempt to adopt a similar approach to the preperitoneal dissection described by Stoppa and Rives [16,17], McKernon [28] developed an extraperitoneal approach. This procedure employs the principles of minimal-access surgery and is performed using laparoscopic instrumentation.

To use this technique, the surgeon adopts a modified open laparoscopy approach. When the midline raphe is divided, however, the surgeon does not divide the peritoneum but enters the preperitoneal space. Once this space has been identified, it should be enlarged, initially with hemostats and subsequently by the use of a hydrodissector introduced through an operating laparoscope. Two further ports are introduced to facilitate the dissection as the space becomes large enough to accommodate them. When the hernia orifice is identified, a patch of polypropylene mesh is inserted and secured with staples. This method avoids the dangers associated with entering the peritoneal cavity and of placing the prosthetic material within the abdominal cavity. It has the intrinsic advantages of a tension-free repair and the mechanical advantage of a preperitoneal repair. This seemingly ideal approach is limited, however. The extensive dissection required is painful, and technical problems have been encountered. An indirect sac must be opened to ensure it has no contents before it can be ligated. The operating space is small and inadvertent breach of the peritoneum is not infrequent; this complication further limits operating space by allowing a pneumoperitoneum to develop. Although this approach is based on a well-known open technique, the perspective is difficult to interpret through the laparoscope, and approach requires considerable experience to become completely familiar with the resulting visualization.

RECURRENT HERNIAS

Even the most skeptical surgeons would agree that laparoscopic herniorrhaphy may be the procedure of choice for the management of recurrent hernias, especially bilateral ones. Recurrent hernias are usually direct, and a previous repair under tension may have further weakened the transversalis fascia. Scarring from the previous repair may make the extraperitoneal approach difficult, and the transabdominal preperitoneal procedure is the logical choice. This approach is ideal because of its use of a prosthetic patch to avoid further tension and the avoidance of a potentially very difficult dissection around the cord. If this operation is reserved only for this indication, however, surgeons will not gain the experience necessary to use it for this more difficult application.

CONCLUSIONS

Laparoscopic hernia repair has advanced rapidly. Questions about its long-term efficacy and safety remain, and surgeons electing to use these new techniques must remain vigilant and open minded with regard to the limitations of these procedures. Patients are well informed as to the existence of laparoscopy and may request it when presenting their problem for attention. Patients need to be made aware that laparoscopic hernia repair is still under evaluation and is considered investigational. Ideally, these repairs should be performed as part of a controlled trial with careful follow-up to allow the eventual recommendations and limitations to be defined.

REFERENCES

Papers of particular interest, published within the annual period of review, have been highlighted as:
• Of special interest
•• Of outstanding interest

1. *Socio-economic Factbook for Surgery.* American College of Surgeons; 1980.

2. Bassini E: Sulla Cura Radicale dell' Ernia Ingiunale. *Arch Soc Ital Chir* 1887, 4:380.

3. Glassow F: Short Stay Surgery (Shouldice Technique) for Repair of Inguinal Hernia. *Ann R Coll Surg Engl* 1976, 58:133–139.

4. *Conceptualization and Measurements of Physiological Health for Adults.* Santa Monica, CA: Rand; 1983 (3):3–120.

5. Berliner S, Burson L, Katz P, *et al.*: An Anterior Transversalis Fascia Repair for Adult Inguinal Hernias. *Am J Surg* 1978, 135:633–636.

6. Iles JDH: Specialization in Elective Herniorrhaphy. *Lancet* 1965, i:751–755.

7. Soper NJ, Stockman PT, Dunnegan DL, Ashley SW: Laparoscopic Cholecystectomy: The New "Gold Standard"? *Arch Surg* 1992, 127:917–923.

8. Macintyre IMC: Laparoscopic Herniorrhaphy. *Br J Surg* 1992, 79:1123–1124.

9. Andrews E: A Method of Herniotomy Utilizing Only White Fascia. *Ann Surg* 1924, 80:250–238.

10. Marcy HO: The Cure of Hernia. *JAMA* 1887, 8:589–592.

11. LaRoque GP: The Intra-abdominal Method of Removing Inguinal and Femoral Hernia. *Arch Surg* 1932, 24:189–203.

12. Ger R, Monroe K, Duvivier R, *et al.*: Management of Indirect Inguinal Hernias by Laparoscopic Closure of the Neck of the Sac. *Am J Surg* 1990, 159:371–XX.

13. Lichtenstein IL, Shulman AG, Anid PK, Motller MM: The Tension-free Hernioplasty. *Am J Surg* 1989, 157:188–193.

14. Cheatle GL: An Operation for the Radical Cure of Inguinal and Femoral Hernia. *Br Med J* 1920, 2:68.

15. Henry AK: Special Comment: The Preperitoneal Approach and Ilio-pubic Tract Repair of Femoral Hernias. In *Hernia*, 3rd ed. Edited by Nyhus LM, Condon RE. Philadelphia: Lippincott; 1989:195–198.

16. Rives J: Surgical Treatment of the Inguinal Hernia with Dacron Patch. *Int Surg* 1967, 47:360–361.

17. Stoppa R, Petit J, Henry X, *et al.*: Plastrie de l'Aine par Vote Mediane Sous-Peritoneale. *Acta Chir*, AFC Paris Masson Editeur 1972.

18. Harris MNE, Plantevin OM, Crowther A: Cardiac Arrhythmias During Anaesthesia for Laparoscopy. *Br J Anaesth* 1984, 56:1213–1216.

19. Hanley ES: Anesthesia for Laparoscopic Surgery. *Surg Clin North Am* 1992, 72, 1013–1019.

20. Salvati EA, Chekofse KM, Brause BD, *et al.*: Infections Associated with Orthopedic Devices. In *Infections Associated with Prosthetic Devices. Edited by Sugarman B, Young EJ. Boca Roaton: CRC Press; 1983:181–218.*

21. • Hart RO, Fitzgibbons RJ Jr, Filipi CJ, Salerno GM: Open Laporoscopy for Laparoscopic Herniorrhaphy. In *Surgical Laparoscopy*. Edited by Zucker K, Reddick EJ, Bailey BW. St. Louis: Quality Medical; 1991:87–97.
Describes the open laparoscopic approach to hernia repair. An important modification to improve the safety of this technique.

22. Toy FK, Smoot RT Jr.: Toy-Smoot Laparoscopic Hernioplasty. *Del Med J* 1992, 64:23–28.

23. Condon RE: The Anatomy of the Inguinal Region and its Relation to Groin Hernia. In *Hernia*. 3rd ed. Edited by Nyhus LM, Condon RE. Philadelphia: Lippincott; 1989:18–64.

24.•• MacFayden B: Complications of Laparoscopic Herniorrhaphy [abstract]. *SAGES Symposium* 1992, 5:9–10.
A pertinent reminder of the problems and the need for vigilance in the development of this technique.

25. Salerno GM, Fitzgibbons RJ Jr, Filipi CJ: Laparoscopic Herniorrhaphy. In *Surgical Laparoscopy Update*. Edited by Zucker K, Reddick EJ, Bailey BW. St. Louis: Quality Medical; 1993:87–97.

26. Filipi CJ, Fitzgibbons RJ Jr, Salerno GM, Hart RO: Laparoscopic Herniorrhaphy. *Surg Clin North Am* 1992, 72:1109–1124.

27. • Fitzgibbons RJ Jr, Salerno GM, Filipi CJ, Hart RO: Intraperitoneal Onlay Mesh Technique for the Repair of Inguinal Hernia. *Ann Surg*, submitted.
An animal model to establish the safety of the onlay procedure and the materials used.

28. McKernan JB, Laws HL: Laparoscopic Repair of Inguinal Hernias Using a Totally Extraperitoneal Prosthetic Approach. *Surg Endosc* 1993, 7:26–28.

29. Nyhus LM: Inguinal Hernia. *Curr Prob Surg* 1991, 28:407–450.

Chapter 19

Laparoscopy for Urologic Conditions

Kevin R. Loughlin

When considered within the context of all urologic surgery, laparoscopy plays a relatively minor role in the armamentarium of the urologic surgeon. For laparoscopy to achieve a larger role in urologic surgery, continued advances in instrumentation are required. In this chapter, we review the current status of laparoscopic varicocelectomy, pelvic lymphadenectomy, and nephrectomy. We also examine the current applications of laparoscopy in pediatric urology. Finally, we review the rather early, preliminary experience of laparoscopic retroperitoneal lymph node dissection, lymphocele drainage, ureterolysis, ureteral reimplant, diverticulectomy, cystectomy, ileal conduit, and bladder neck suspension.

LAPAROSCOPIC VARICOCELECTOMY

Laparoscopic varicocele ligation has been performed by many urologists, and reports from several medical centers have been published. The data suggest that laparoscopic varicocele ligation is therapeutically equivalent to open surgical (inguinal and retroperitoneal) and radiographic (embolization) techniques. Laparoscopic varicocelectomy appears to reduce postoperative morbidity [1,2••,3•]. Experimental work in a canine model by Klee and coworkers [4] verified that successful ligation of the gonadal veins can be achieved laparoscopically.

Whether it is necessary to identify and preserve the testicular artery during laparoscopic varicocelectomy remains controversial. Loughlin and Brooks [5••] reported on the use of a laparoscopic Doppler probe (Fig. 1) that they believe facilitates the identification and preservation of the testicular artery (Fig. 2). Matsuda and coworkers [6] claim the testicular artery does not have to be preserved; they clip the testicular artery and veins en bloc. Further multicenter experience is needed to resolve whether the testicular artery should be preserved during laparoscopic varicocele ligation. Because the testicular artery is preserved during open surgical repair or radiographic embolization procedures, however, intuition would suggest that the laparoscopic surgeon do the same.

TECHNIQUE

The technique of laparoscopic varicocele ligation is straightforward. The procedure is usually performed using general anesthesia, although Matsuda and coworkers [6] have recently reported using local anesthesia alone for laparoscopic varicocelectomy. A urethral catheter is placed to empty the bladder, and a Veress needle is placed at the umbilicus to inflate the peritoneal cavity with approximately 5 L of carbon dioxide. Alternatively, a minilaparotomy can be performed at the inferior margin of the umbilicus, and the trocar can be placed into the peritoneum under direct vision. Three laparoscopic trocars are placed for unilateral varicoceles. Four laparoscopic trocars are placed for bilateral varicocele repair. Ten-millimeter trocars are positioned at the umbilicus and at two-finger breadths above the symphysis pubis. A 5-mm trocar is placed lateral to McBurney's point on the side of the varicocele. A laparoscopic videoendoscope is placed through the umbilical trocar port, and the procedure is performed using a video monitor.

The next step is to identify the pertinent anatomy. The intra-abdominal vas deferens can be seen joining the spermatic cord above the internal inguinal ring (Fig. 3). The gonadal vessels are visualized easily in the retroperitoneum. The posterior peritoneum is excised with cautery, laser, or endoscopic scissors (Fig. 4). The gonadal vessels are then mobilized; however, reliably identifying the spermatic artery and its branches is sometimes difficult through the laparoscope. Therefore, we prefer to use the laparoscopic Doppler mentioned previously to facilitate identification of the spermatic artery during laparoscopic varicocele ligation. The Doppler is 28.58 cm long and fits through a 5-mm laparoscopic trocar port. It is connected to a speaker that can be placed on or off the surgical field at the discretion of the surgeon. After identifying the gonadal artery, the surgeon isolates the gonadal vein or veins using blunt dissection with atraumatic graspers. A disposable endoscopic clip applier is used to ligate the gonadal vein or veins while sparing the artery. The pneumoperitoneum is vented and the trocars are removed. Subcuticular stitches are used to close the puncture sites on the abdominal wall.

LAPAROSCOPIC PELVIC LYMPHADENECTOMY

Laparoscopic pelvic lymphadenectomy has the potential to have the widest application of laparoscopy in urology. This potential stems from the importance of the status of the pelvic lymph nodes in the treatment of prostate cancer, the most common male malignancy. Most urologists embrace the philosophy that if the

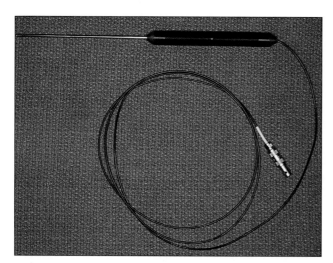

Figure 1. Endoscopic Doppler probe that can be placed through a 10-mm port. (*From* Loughlin and Brooks [5]; with permission.)

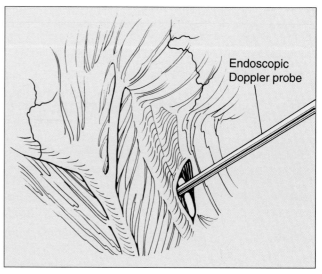

Figure 2. Endoscopic Doppler probe is used to identify spermatic artery. (*From* Loughlin and Brooks [5]; with permission.)

pelvic lymph nodes are involved in prostate cancer, cure cannot be achieved with radical prostatectomy or radiation therapy, and hormonal therapy is indicated in these patients for palliation.

Two crucial questions need to be answered before laparoscopic pelvic lymphadenectomy can be accepted. First, can a laparoscopic node dissection be performed safely? Second, can a laparoscopic node dissection be performed as completely as an open node dissection? Kavoussi and coworkers [7••] reported a retrospective multicenter review of 372 patients who underwent laparoscopic pelvic lymph node dissections. The complication rate was 15%. A total of 55 complications occurred, 14 intraoperatively and 41 postoperatively. Complications included vascular injury (11 patients), viscus injury (8), genitourinary problems (10), functional or mechanical bowel obstruction (7), lower extremity deep venous thrombosis (5), infection or wound problems (5), lymphedema (5), anesthetic complications (2), and obturator nerve palsy (2).

Vascular injuries occurred during both trocar placement and dissection. Trocar injuries were most commonly associated with the epigastric vessels. Green and coworkers [8•] describe a useful method to manage trocar injuries.

Bowel injury occurred in three patients. It was recognized intraoperatively in one, and postoperatively in two. Ureteral injuries were noted in two patients; one was recognized intraoperatively, and an open repair was performed in the other patient in conjunction with

a radical retropubic prostatectomy. The second case was not recognized until 3 days postoperatively, when the patient became febrile and computed tomography scan revealed a fluid collection in the pelvis consistent with a urinoma. The patient underwent an open repair of the ureter.

Many of the complications occurred early in the experience of the respective institutions. Urologists performing laparoscopic pelvic node dissections, however, must be aware that significant complications occurred throughout the collective experience of the eight institutions. Adherence to good laparoscopic technique and familiarity with the anatomy are the most reliable ways to avoid complications.

The second question—whether laparoscopic pelvic node dissection is as complete as open pelvic lymph node dissection—also needs to be addressed. Parra and coworkers [9•] compared 12 open and 12 laparoscopic pelvic node dissections and found no statistical difference in the number of nodes removed by either technique. Experience in our institution also showed that laparoscopic and open node dissections were comparable in efficacy [10••].

TECHNIQUE

The pneumoperitoneum is established in the standard manner. Trocar placement is then performed. The size and location of trocar sites for the procedure vary with the surgeon's preference. Most use the diamond configuration (Fig. 5, *left*). An alternative used by some surgeons

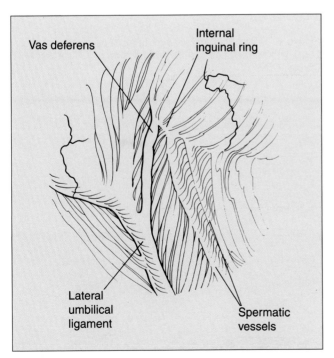

Figure 3. Anatomy of spermatic cord above the internal inguinal ring. (*From* Loughlin and Brooks [5]; with permission.)

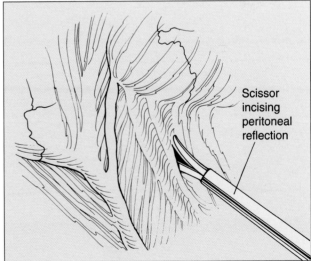

Figure 4. The posterior peritoneum is incised parallel to the spermatic cord. (*From* Loughlin and Brooks [5]; with permission.)

is the so-called fan configuration for trocar placement (Fig. 5, *right*). This configuration allows the surgeon and the surgical assistant to manipulate instruments with both hands during the dissection. It is also helpful in obese patients or in those with a prominent urachus. The size of the trocars used at each site may vary. A 10-mm trocar is usually placed in the umbilicus for the videoendoscope. An additional 10- or 11-mm trocar is placed in at least one other site for tissue removal. Another 10- or 11-mm port is used for the endoscopic clip applier. Usually, 5-mm trocars are used for the remaining trocar sites.

After completion of trocar placement, the laparoscopic landmarks for pelvic node dissection are identified. These landmarks include the medial umbilical ligament (remnant of the obliterated umbilical artery), urachus, bladder, vas deferens, iliac vessels, spermatic vessels, and internal ring (Fig. 6). The next maneuver is to incise the posterior peritoneum parallel and lateral to the medial umbilical ligament (Fig. 7). Early identification of the ureter is important to avoid ureteral injury. The vas deferens is then divided to facilitate operative access to the obturator space. Using primarily blunt dissection, the

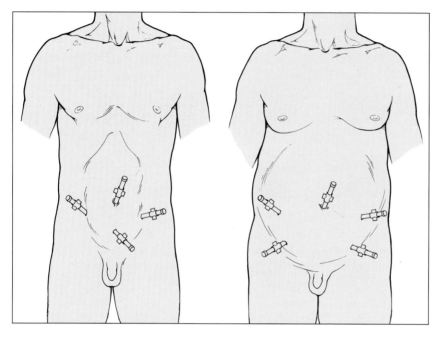

Figure 5. Two alternatives for trocar placement for pelvic lymphadenectomy. The diamond configuration is shown on the left, and the fan configuration on the right. (*From* Loughlin and Kavoussi [10]; by permission of J. Foerster, Fort Collins, CO.)

Figure 6. Pelvic anatomy viewed laparoscopically. (*From* Loughlin and Kavoussi [10]; by permission of J. Foerster, Fort Collins, CO.)

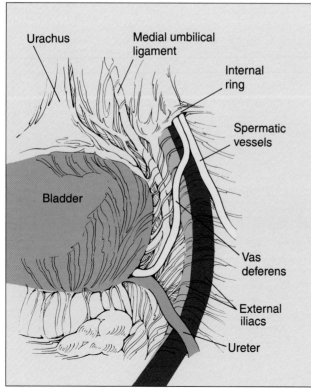

iliac vein and artery are identified (Fig. 8). The nodal tissue overlying the external iliac vein is then teased medially to expose the internal obturator muscle. A laparoscopic vein retractor can be used to retract the external iliac vein laterally and permit easier, more complete dissection of the nodal tissue beneath the vein. The dissection proceeds with removing tissue off the vein distally until Cooper's ligament and the pubic bone are identified.

Blunt dissection is continued and the medial border of the packet is identified by clearing off the pubic bone just lateral to the medial umbilical ligament (Fig. 9). Electrocautery is used to fulgurate small vessels and lymphatics, and the distal extent of the packet is freed from the pubic bone. The packet is pulled proximally and freed from the underside of the pubic bone. At this point, the obturator nerve is identified (Fig. 10).

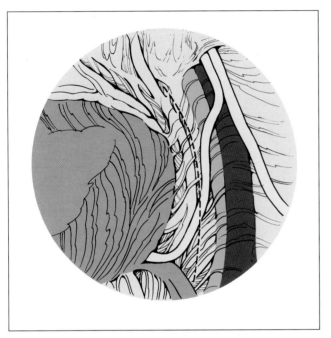

Figure 7. Posterior peritoneum is incised parallel and lateral to medical umbilical ligament to start dissection. (*From* Loughlin and Kavoussi [10]; by permission of J. Foerster, Fort Collins, CO.)

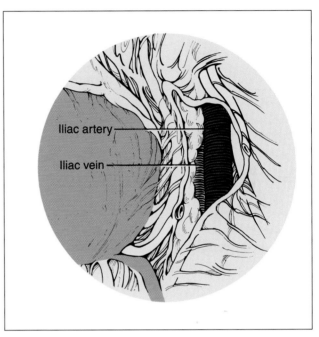

Figure 8. Exposure of iliac vessels. (*From* Loughlin and Kavoussi [10]; by permission of J. Foerster, Fort Collins, CO.)

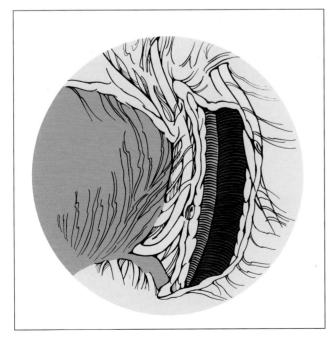

Figure 9. Nodal packet ready to be delivered. (*From* Loughlin and Kavoussi [10]; by permission of J. Foerster, Fort Collins, CO.)

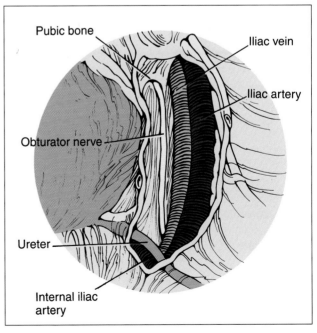

Figure 10. Completion of node dissection. (*From* Loughlin and Kavoussi [10]; by permission of J. Foerster, Fort Collins, CO.)

Because nodal tissue can be quite bulky and difficult to grasp, adequate forceps, such as the endoscopic Russian forceps, can ensure a more reliable grasp of the specimen. With blunt dissection, the obturator nerve is cleaned off proximally, and endoscopic clips are used to divide the distal portion of the dissection. At the completion of the laparoscopic pelvic lymphadenectomy, the iliac artery, vein, pubic bone, and obturator nerve can be seen clearly. The field is checked for hemostasis, and the dissection is performed in an identical manner on the opposite side. The trocars are removed, and the puncture sites are closed in the usual manner.

LAPAROSCOPIC NEPHRECTOMY

Clayman and coworkers [11••] pioneered the development of laparoscopic nephrectomy. They reported their cumulative experience of 16 cases of laparoscopic nephrectomy. Thirteen patients had benign disease, one had a solid renal mass that ultimately proved to be an oncocytoma, and two patients had transitional cell carcinoma of the upper tract. Several obstacles are preventing this technique from being more widely embraced. The first is the time factor. The average operating time was 5.6 hours, which is considerably longer than for an open nephrectomy. The second is the handling of the renal pedicle. Clayman and coworkers [11••] have used endoscopic clips (Endoclip, United States Surgical, Norwalk, CT) to control the renal artery and vein. Ehrlich and coworkers [12] used an endoscopic stapler to control the pedicle. Despite the fact that Clayman's group did not report any significant intraoperative or postoperative bleeding because of inadequate pedicle control, many urologists feel uneasy with this aspect of the operation. The third and perhaps most serious concern is the applicability of this technique to cases of renal malignancy. Currently, the adrenal gland is not included in the laparoscopic radical nephrectomy; although this exclusion is probably more a theoretical concern in lower pole and midpole tumors, it would be a limiting factor in upper pole tumors.

Tumor spillage during laparoscopy is a practical and not a theoretical concern. Several reports [13–17] have documented tumor implantation during laparoscopy. Clayman and coworkers have tried to answer this problem by developing an entrapment system for the kidney [11••] and the lymph nodes [18]. These systems consist of impermeable bags inserted through the laparoscopic trocar. The surgical specimen is then placed within the bag or pouch; a drawstring around the opening of the bag allows for closure and acts as a handle to remove the pouch from the abdominal cavity through the laparoscopic trocar. In nephrectomy, the renal specimen is fragmented and aspirated using a specially designed electrical tissue morcellator placed through the neck of the kidney sack. The development of this type of technology decreases but does not eliminate the potential for tumor spillage. Undoubtedly, more work is needed to address the concern of tumor implantation, if this technique is to be applied to malignant renal tumors.

TECHNIQUE

The patients early in the series all underwent preoperative renal artery embolization [11••]; however, this procedure is no longer done. After induction of general anesthesia, a 7F occlusion balloon catheter is passed up the ureter of the kidney to be removed. A bladder drainage catheter is also used as well as a nasogastric tube. The patient is placed in a supine position. A Veress needle is placed at the umbilicus, and a carbon dioxide pneumoperitoneum is created in the usual manner. Then two 11-mm laparoscopy ports are placed, one at the umbilicus and one immediately subcostal along the midclavicular line (MCL). A 5-mm port is also placed in the MCL, 2 to 3 cm below the level of the umbilicus. The patient is then placed in the lateral decubitus position and secured to the operating table. Two 5-mm ports are placed in the anterior axillary line (AAL), one on a level with the umbilicus and one off the tip of the 11th or 12th rib.

Dissection commences by incising the line of Toldt and reflecting the colon medially. The ureter is then identified and secured with a 5-mm locking forceps. The lower pole lateral surfaces, upper pole lateral surfaces, and upper pole of the kidney are dissected free. The adrenal gland is left in place.

The kidney is then lifted upward, which places the renal hilum on traction. The renal artery and vein are then dissected. Three endosurgical clips are placed on the distal portion of each vessel, and two clips are placed on the proximal portion of each vessel; an endoscopic scissors is then used to divide the vessels.

The ureter is divided between two metal clips and the kidney is free. An impermeable nylon surgical sack (Cook Urological, Spencer, IN) is introduced through an 11-mm port. Three 5-mm graspers are used to open the mouth of the sack, and the kidney is pushed into the opened sack. The drawstrings on the sack are grasped by a 5-mm forceps and pulled through the 11-mm umbilical port, thereby closing the neck of the sack on the kidney. The mouth of the sack is then brought out through the skin, and the metal shaft of the electrical tissue morcellator (Cook OB/GYN, Spencer, IN; Cook Urological, Spencer, IN) is introduced into the sack. The morcellator is activated, and the renal tissue is fragmented and aspirated. When all the renal tissue is removed, the empty sack is removed from the abdomen. The port sites are closed in the standard fashion.

In the two cases of transitional cell carcinoma [11], the ureter was dissected down to the bladder, and a laparoscopic GIA stapler (Endo-GIA, United States Surgical, Norwalk, CT) was used to include the distal ureter and a cuff of bladder.

Clayman and coworkers [11] and Gaur and coworkers [19] also described a retroperitoneal approach to laparoscopic nephrectomy. A key advance to this approach has been the use of a retroperitoneal balloon dissector that facilitates the development of working space within the retroperitoneal space.

LAPAROSCOPIC PEDIATRIC UROLOGY

In some respects, because of their decreased intra-abdominal and retroperitoneal fat, children may be better suited for laparoscopic procedures than adults. The major application of laparoscopy in pediatric urology thus far, however, has been in the management of undescended testicles [20••–22]. Diamond and Caldamone [20••] demonstrated the value of laparoscopy in three situations. For unilateral impalpable testes with a contralateral normal testes, laparoscopy identified testicular absence in 27%; intra-abdominal testes were found in 16%. For bilateral undescended testes (one or both impalpable), laparoscopy was diagnostic in 75% of cases (17% had blind-ending spermatic vessels above the internal ring, and 58% had intra-abdominal testes. Finally, in patients with previous negative inguinal exploration, laparoscopic diagnosis was made in 100% of cases. Laparoscopy also enables the pediatric urologist to plan a surgical approach and incision if an orchiopexy is to be done. In a young child, if an intra-abdominal testis is confirmed, a Fowler-Stephens procedure can be considered, whereas if laparoscopy demonstrates the testis is just above or at the internal inguinal ring, then the traditional transinguinal incision and approach can be used. In the older child or adolescent in whom the surgeon believes orchiectomy is preferable to orchiopexy, the orchiectomy can be accomplished laparoscopically [22].

LAPAROSCOPIC RETROPERITONEAL NODE DISSECTION

The proper role for laparoscopic retroperitoneal node dissection in the management of testicular cancer is still unclear. Several case reports [23,24] demonstrate the feasibility of the procedure. As with many other laparoscopic procedures, however, increased operating time is a consideration in applying laparoscopic techniques to a procedure. Although Hulbert and Fraley [23] report a laparoscopic retroperitoneal node dissection that took 4 hours, Rukstalis and Chodak [24] report a case that required 8.5 hours to complete. As with pelvic node dissection, the question has also been raised as to the completeness of the laparoscopic retroperitoneal node dissection. Although Rukstalis and Chodak [24] harvested 28 nodes and Hulbert and Fraley [23] report 29 and 17 nodes in their two cases, laparoscopic retroperitoneal node dissection does not now include suprahilar nodes,

and dissecting out the nodal tissue behind the aorta and vena cava is difficult laparoscopically.

Therefore, laparoscopic retroperitoneal node dissection appears, for now, best applied to patients without evidence of bulk disease in the retroperitoneum who would otherwise be candidates for observation rather than surgical exploration. Although the laparoscopic procedure does not currently appear to be as thorough a dissection as open node dissection, it offers the opportunity to have some pathologic documentation of nodal status in patients considered for observation. The technique for laparoscopic retroperitoneal node dissection has not been standardized and is still evolving, therefore, the reader is referred to the case reports [23,24] for the authors' individual techniques.

LAPAROSCOPIC MANAGEMENT OF LYMPHOCELES

Lymphoceles are not uncommon after renal transplantation, and an incidence of 0.6% to 18% has been reported [25–27]. Lymphoceles can also occur after pelvic lymphadenectomy, and an incidence of 5.6% has been reported in this circumstance [28]. Most of these patients are asymptomatic and do not require treatment. When the lymphocele becomes symptomatic or is associated with fever and potential infection, however, drainage of the lymphocele is indicated. Several investigators report successful laparoscopic drainage of lymphoceles [29–31••]. Khauli and coworkers [31••] report a cogent analysis of the indications for laparoscopic management of lymphoceles. An adaption of their proposed algorithm for management appears in Figure 11.

TECHNIQUE

After induction of general endotracheal anesthesia, the surgeon places a urethral catheter to drain the bladder, and a nasogastric tube is inserted. A Veress needle is inserted into the peritoneal cavity in the left upper quadrant to avoid the transplant allograft. A pneumoperitoneum is achieved in the usual manner. The Veress needle is removed, and an 11-mm trocar sheath is inserted through the same site into the peritoneal cavity. The videoendoscope is placed through this port, and two additional 5-mm ports are inserted under direct vision in the periumbilical area in the right upper quadrant at the level of the midclavicular line. The abdomen is carefully inspected, and the renal transplant and associated lymphocele are visualized. They appear as two extrinsic bulges in the retroperitoneum. The lymphocele is distinguishable by its superolateral location to the graft and the soft consistency on probing. In addition, the lymphocele transmits light readily when the light source is placed at its wall.

The patient is then placed in Trendelenburg position to allow the small bowel to fall cephalad and to accentuate the visibility of the lymphocele. The lymphocele is then entered using electrocautery. The peritoneum and its attached lymphocele wall are grasped, and the incision is extended circumferentially using endoscopic scissors. An ellipse of lymphocele wall is removed, thereby creating a window that is approximately 7 cm by 3 cm. After careful coagulation of the edges of the window, the lymphocele is inspected, and all internal loculations are lysed and excised to create a single cavity. The cavity is then irrigated and inspected for adequate hemostasis prior to the usual completion of the laparoscopic procedure.

LAPAROSCOPIC URETEROLYSIS

Kavoussi and coworkers [32] published a case report of laparoscopic ureterolysis. This procedure was performed in a 15-year-old girl with right flank pain. Her intravenous pyelogram demonstrated moderate right hydronephrosis and medial deviation of the right midureter, which suggested the diagnosis of retroperitoneal fibrosis. A computed tomography scan confirmed a retroperitoneal mass. The patient underwent laparoscopic ureterolysis via a transperitoneal approach. An external ureteral stent was placed to help identify the ureter as is done with laparoscopic nephrectomy.

The ureter was successfully mobilized laparoscopically, and laparoscopic biopsy forceps were used to obtain multiple biopsies of the periurethral tissue. The pathology revealed chronic inflammation and fibrosis. The procedure was successful, but the patient remained hospitalized for 6 days. Again the total operative time of 5.5 hours was considerably longer than a comparable open procedure would require. Only additional experience will help determine how applicable laparoscopic ureterolysis will become in the future.

LAPAROSCOPIC URETERAL REIMPLANT

Nezhat and coworkers [33] published a case report of a laparoscopic ureteral reimplant for ureteral obstruction secondary to endometriosis. Given the current status of laparoscopic instrumentation, this technique seems extremely arduous and is unlikely to achieve widespread acceptance. Another limitation of the technique they reported is that a nonrefluxing reimplant could not be performed laparoscopically. Clearly in children and young women, a nonrefluxing reimplant is required. Major advances in instrumentation are needed before this procedure can be done routinely laparoscopically.

LAPAROSCOPIC DIVERTICULECTOMY

Parra and coworkers [34] report a case in which a large bladder diverticulum was excised laparoscopically in an 87-year-old man. The indication for removal was chronic infection. An endoscopic stapler was used to divide the diverticulum at the base. The case was suc-

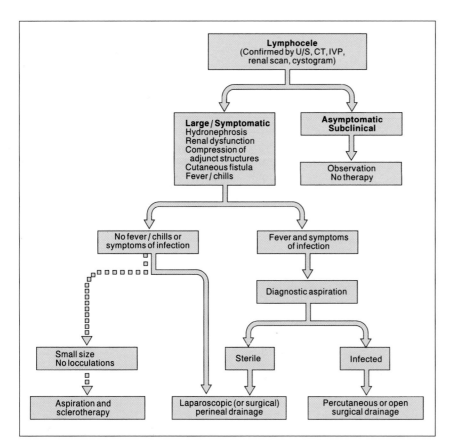

Figure 11. Management algorithm suggested for posttransplant lymphoceles. U/S—ultrasound; CT—computed tomography; IVP— excretory urography. (*Adapted from* Khauli *et al.* [31]).

cessful, but again there was a prolonged operative time of 4.8 hours, which in an 87-year-old seems imprudent. This procedure appears to be another laparoscopic technique with limited applications.

LAPAROSCOPIC CYSTECTOMY

Parra and coworkers [35] also report a case in which a laparoscopic cystectomy was performed in a retained bladder of a 27-year-old paraplegic woman with recurrent pyocystis. Again, although this case was successful, few patients present with pyocystis in a retained bladder. In selected cases, this approach may be a useful alternative to open surgery, but many of these patients can be drained transvaginally with much less potential morbidity than with the laparoscopic procedure.

LAPAROSCOPIC ILEAL CONDUIT

Kozminski and Partamian [36] reported the first laparoscopic ileal loop conduit. The procedure was performed for palliation of obstruction in an 83-year-old man with fibrosarcoma of the prostate. The ileal loop itself was fashioned laparoscopically using endoscopic stapling devices. To perform the ureteral anastomosis, however, the distal ureters and a portion of the conduit had to be brought in through a trocar site, and an extracorporeal, hand-sewn, ureteroileal anastomosis was performed on each side.

The report emphasizes the limitation of laparoscopic instrumentation at this time. Laparoscopic suturing is cumbersome, and the ureteroileal anastomoses could not have been completed easily laparoscopically. Until either tissue-welding techniques or better suturing techniques are available, only limited applications are available for laparoscopic reconstructive surgery such as that outlined in this case report.

LAPAROSCOPIC BLADDER-NECK SUSPENSION

Albala and coworkers [37] report on the use of a laparoscopic bladder neck suspension to treat female urinary stress incontinence. They performed the procedure successfully in 22 patients. Using standard laparoscopic technique, they placed Ethibond 2-0 sutures (Ethicon, Somerville, NJ) between the periurethral tissue and pubic bone and tied the sutures endoscopically. Although they report a successful series with few complications, laparoscopic bladder neck suspension appears to offer no advantage over several widely used transvaginal needle suspension techniques [38–40].

The role of laparoscopy in urologic surgery continues to evolve. Laparoscopic instrumentation remains a major factor in limiting further applications of laparoscopic techniques in urology. Many urologists are committed to laparoscopic surgery, and undoubtedly new techniques will be developed in the near future.

REFERENCES

Papers of particular interest, published within the period of review, have been highlighted as:
• Of special interest
•• Of outstanding interest

1.   Aaberg RA, Vancaillie TG, Schuessler WW: Laparoscopic Varicocele Ligation: A New Technique. *Fertil Steril* 1991, 56:776–777.

2.•• Hagood PG, Mehan DJ, Worischeck JH, *et al.*: Laparoscopic Varicocelectomy: Preliminary Report of a New Technique. *J Urol* 1992, 147:73–76.
Provides a very good description of the base technique of laparoscopic varicocelectomy. Easy-to-follow pictures and illustrations are included in the report.

3.• Donovan JF, Winfield HN: Laparoscopic Varicocele Ligation. *J Urol* 1992, 147:77–81.
A clear presentation of the technique of laparoscopic varicocele ligation.

4.   Klee LW, Brito CG, Bihrle F, *et al.*: Laparoscopic Spermatic Vein Ligation in Dogs. *J Endourol* 1991, 5:341–344.

5.•• Loughlin KR, Brooks DC: The Use of a Doppler Probe to

Facilitate Laparoscopic Varicocele Ligation. *SGO* 1992, 174:326–328.
Introduces the use of a Doppler probe to more reliably identify the spermatic cord structures.

6.   Matsuda T, Horii Y, Higashi S, *et al.*: Laparoscopic Varicocelectomy: A Simple Technique for Clip Ligation of the Spermatic Vessels. *J Urol* 1992, 147:636–638.

7.•• Kavoussi LR, Sosa E, Chandhoke P, *et al.*: Complications of Laparoscopic Pelvic Lymph Node Dissection. *J Urol* 1993, 149:322–325.
This article presents a multicenter review of laparoscopic complications. It is a thorough presentation of the subject.

8.• Green L, Loughlin KR, Kavoussi LR: Management of Epigastric Vessel Injury During Laparoscopy. 1992, 6:99–101.
A concise description of the technique for managing potentially serious laparoscopic complications.

9.• Parra RO, Andrus C, Boullier J: Staging Laparoscopic Pelvic Node Dissection: Comparison of Results With Open Pelvic Lymphadenectomy. *J Urol* 1992, 147:875–878.

A report from a single center comparing the thoroughness of laparoscopic versus open pelvic node dissection.

10.•• Loughlin KR, Kavoussi LR: Laparoscopic Lymphadenectomy in the Staging of Prostate Cancer. *Contemp Urol* 1992, 4:69–82.

This article contains a good overview of the indications for laparoscopic pelvic lymphadenectomy and a clear description as to how the procedure is performed.

11.•• Clayman RV, Kavoussi LR, McDougal EM, *et al.*: Laparoscopic Nephrectomy: A Review of 16 Cases. *Surg Laparosc Endosc* 1992, 2:29–34.

This article is a comprehensive review of the technique of laparoscopic nephrectomy.

12. Ehrlich RM, Gershman A, Mee S, *et al.*: Laparoscopic Nephrectomy in a Child: Expanding Horizons for Laparoscopy in Pediatric Urology. *J Endourol* 1992, 6:463–465.

13. Cava A, Roman J, Gonzalez O, *et al.*: Subcutaneous Metastasis Following Laparoscopy in Gastric Adenocarcinoma. *Eur J Surg Oncol* 1990, 16:63–67.

14. Dubrante Z, Wittmann T, Karascony G: Rapid Development of Malignant Metastases in the Abdominal Wall After Laparoscopy. *Endoscopy* 1978, 10:127–130.

15. Stockdale AD, Pocock TJ: Abdominal Wall Metastases Following Laparoscopy: A Case Report. *Eur J Surg Oncol* 1985, 11:373–375.

16. Pezet D, Fondrinier E, Rotman N, *et al.*: Parietal Seeding of Carcinoma of the Gallbladder After Laparoscopic Cholecystectomy. *Br J Surg* 1992, 79:845.

17. Keate RF, Shaffer R: Seeding of Hepatocellular Carcinoma to the Peritoneoscopy Insertion Site. *Gastroint Endosc* 1992, 38:203.

18. Kavoussi LR, Clayman RV: Organ Entrapment System for Removing Nodal Tissue During Laparoscopic Pelvic Lymphadenectomy. *J Urol* 1992, 147:879–880.

19. Gaur DD, Agarwal DK, Purohit KC: Retroperitoneal Laparoscopic Nephrectomy: Initial Case Report. *J Urol* 1993, 149:103–105.

20.•• Diamond DA, Caldamone AA: The Value of Laparoscopy for 106 Impalpable Testes Relative to Clinical Presentation. *J Urol* 1992, 148:632–634.

The authors present a coherent discussion on the impact of laparoscopy on the management of impalpable testes.

21. Plotzker ED, Rushton HG, Belman AB, *et al.*: Laparoscopy for Nonpalpable Testes in Childhood: Is Inguinal Exploration Also Necessary When Vas and Vessels Exit the Inguinal Ring? *J Urol* 1992, 148:635–638.

22. Thomas MD, Mercer LC, Saltzstein EC: Laparoscopic Orchiectomy for Unilateral Intra-abdominal Testis. *J Urol* 1992, 148:1251–1253.

23. Hulbert JC, Fraley EE: Laparoscopic Retroperitoneal Lymphadenectomy: New Approach to Pathologic Staging of Clinical Stage 1 Germ Cell Tumors of the Testis. *J Endourol* 1992, 6:123–125.

24. Rukstalis DB, Chodak GW: Laparoscopic Retroperitoneal Lymph Dissection in a Patient With Stage 1 Testicular Carcinoma. *J Urol* 1992, 148:1907–1910.

25. Howard RJ, Simmons RL, Najarian JS: Prevention of Lymphoceles Following Renal Transplantation. *Ann Surg* 1976, 18:166–169.

26. Schweizer RT, Cho SI, Koutz SL, *et al.*: Lymphoceles Following Renal Transplantation. *Arch Surg* 1972, 104:42–44.

27. Braun WE, Banowsky LH, Stratton RA, *et al.*: Lymphocytes Associated With Renal Transplantation. Report of 15 Cases and Review of the Literature. *Am J Med* 1974, 57:714–718.

28. McDowell GC, Babaian RJ, Johnson DE: Management of Symptomatic Lymphocele Via Percutaneous Drainage and Sclerotherapy With Tetracycline. *Urology* 1991, 37:237–239.

29. Waples MJ, Wegenke JD, Vega RJ: Laparoscopic Management of Lymphocele After Pelvic Lymphadenectomy and Radical Retropubic Prostatectomy. *Urology* 1992, 39:82–84.

30. Bardot SF, Montie JE, Jackson CL, *et al.*: Laparoscopic Surgical Technique for Internal Drainage of Pelvic Lymphocele. *J Urol* 1992, 147:908–909.

31.•• Khauli RB, Mosenthal AC, Caushaj PF: Treatment of Lymphocele and Lymphatic Fistula Following Renal Transplantation by Laparoscopic Peritoneal Window. *J Urol* 1992, 147:1353–1355.

A thorough, cogent review of the indications for laparoscopic versus percutaneous or open drainage of lymphoceles.

32. Kavoussi LR, Clayman RV, Brunt LM, *et al.*: Laparoscopic Ureterolysis. *J Urol* 1992, 147:426–492.

33. Nezhat C, Nezhat F, Green B: Laparoscopic Treatment of Obstructed Ureter due to Endometriosis by Resection and Ureteroureterostomy: A Case Report. *J Urol* 1992, 148:865–868.

34. Parra PG, Jones JP, Andrus CH, *et al.*: Laparoscopic Diverticulectomy: Preliminary Report of a New Approach for the Treatment of Bladder Diverticulum. *J Urol* 1992, 148:869–871.

35. Parra RO, Andrus CH, Jones JP, *et al.*: Laparoscopic Cystectomy: Initial Report on a New Treatment for the Retained Bladder. *J Urol* 1992, 148:1140–1144.

36. Kozminski M, Partamian KO: Case Report of Laparoscopic Ileal Loop Conduit. *J Endourol* 1992, 6:147–150.

37. Albala DM, Schuessler WW, Vancaillie TG: Laparoscopic Bladder Neck Suspension. *J Endourol* 1992, 6:137–141.

38. Stamey TA: Endoscopic Suspension of the Vesical Neck for Urinary Incontinence. *Surg Gynecol Obstet* 1973, 136:547–559.

39. Raz S: Modified Bladder Neck Suspension for Female Stress Incontinence. *Urology* 1981, 17:82–85.

40. Gittes RF, Loughlin KR: No-Incision Pubovaginal Suspension for Stress Incontinence. *J Urol* 1987, 138:568–570.

Chapter 20

Thoracoscopy and Video-Assisted Thoracic Surgery

Steven J. Mentzer

David J. Sugarbaker

The principles of thoracoscopy were established by Jacobeaus [1] more than 70 years ago: to obtain diagnostic tissue and treat diseases of the thorax with a minimum of operative morbidity. The primary focus of early thoracoscopy was the diagnosis and treatment of cavitory diseases of the thorax [2]. The early thoracoscopy instruments, however, were hampered by a lack of adequate light sources and generally poor optics. Because of these limitations, thoracoscopy was applied only to pleural biopsies, the drainage of pleural effusions, and the cautery of pleural adhesions [1,2].

Improvements in thoracoscopic technology began with improved light sources. Fiberoptic illumination was incorporated into a variety of thoracic operations to improve intraoperative visibility. More recently, advances in video optics and surgical instrumentation have dramatically expanded the applications of thoracoscopy. Video optics have provided improved vision for not only the surgeons but assistants as well. The common perspective of the surgical and anesthetic team is particularly valuable in thoracic operations. Equally important has been the development of thoracoscopic surgical instrumentation with precision comparable to standard thoracic instruments. In particular, reliable vascular and lung stapling devices have facilitated video-assisted anatomic resections of the lung. Together these developments have allowed thoracic operations to be performed through minimally invasive thoracic incisions.

The technologic developments have extended the spectrum of thoracic diseases that can be effectively diagnosed and treated by thoracoscopic technique. These improvements have been integrated into almost all thoracic surgical procedures. They have expanded the focus of thoracoscopy and led to the more general and inclusive term of *video-assisted thoracic surgery* (VATS) [3•]. The purpose of this review is to provide a basic perspective on the integration of video-assisted thoracic techniques into the diagnosis and treatment of thoracic disease.

BASIC OPERATIVE STRATEGY

Video-assisted thoracic surgery requires a fully equipped operating room and a surgical and anesthetic team capable of performing all thoracic surgical procedures. The operating room equipment should include at least one video monitor that is easily visible to the operating surgeons, assistants, and anesthetists. Standard open thoracotomy instruments, in addition to specialized thoracoscopic instruments, should always be available for emergency thoracotomy. The small incision commonly used with VATS operations limits access to the pulmonary hilum, heart, and mediastinal vessels. Any injury to these structures requires the capability of emergently converting the procedure to an open thoracotomy.

Anesthesia for most video-assisted operations requires a familiarity with the principles of selective, or single-lung, ventilation. Because the pleural cavity is a potential space in most patients, thoracoscopic inspection of the pleural cavity depends on deflation of the lung. Selective ventilation of either the left or right lung is commonly achieved with a left-sided double-lumen endotracheal tube. The preference for a left-sided double-lumen endotracheal tube is based on the increased length of the left main-stem bronchus. The extra length facilitates placement of the tube and avoids the inadvertent occlusion of the left upper lobe orifice with the bronchial cuff. Also, the longer left-sided double-lumen endotracheal tube is less likely to be dislodged during surgical manipulation. Selective deflation of a lung or lobe can also be achieved with a single-lumen endotracheal tube and the use of a bronchial blocker. The most common type of bronchial blocker is a 5-mL vascular embolectomy catheter placed in the appropriate airway. After the distal airway is aspirated and deflated, the catheter balloon is inflated to occlude the airway and maintain selective deflation.

For most VATS, the patient is positioned in a full lateral thoracotomy position. The lateral position facilitates access to all the anatomic structures in the ipsilateral hemithorax. In the lateral position, access ports can be placed anteriorly, laterally, and posteriorly. If the patient is appropriately prepared and draped, access ports can be placed in any intercostal space. The posi-

tion of thoracoscopic access ports is important in developing operative strategies because appropriately spaced access ports permit triangulation of the intrathoracic lesion. Triangulation facilitates manipulation of the lesion and safe dissection from several viewpoints. Alternatively, the supine position can be used for the resection of bilateral metastatic lesions in the lung and, less commonly, for mediastinal lesions. We prefer the semiprone position to provide exposure to the esophagus and posterior mediastinum.

Access to the chest cavity is obtained through a combination of blunt and sharp dissection. To prevent injury to adherent lung tissue, we make the initial entry into the chest by direct digital exploration. Once we confirm the absence of pleural adhesions, additional incisions can be made under direct vision using sharp trocars or blunt-tipped access ports. The initial access port is typically located in the seventh or eighth intercostal space in the midaxillary line. This location is low in the chest cavity and provides a panoramic view of the hemithorax contents. In addition, the gravity-dependent location of this port is convenient for chest-tube drainage at the conclusion of the procedure. If extensive adhesions are found at the time of the initial exploration, an alternative site is used. The presence of extensive pleural adhesions, however, typically requires the conversion of the video-assisted procedure to an open thoracotomy.

An advantage of video-assisted surgery in the chest, as opposed to laparoscopic surgery, is the rigidity of the chest wall. When the lung is partially deflated, the thoracoscope provides a view of the entire hemithorax. Deflation of the lung is almost always possible with proper anesthetic airway management. Even in patients with gas trapping in severe bullous lung disease, proper aspiration and occlusion of the airway provides better exposure than carbon dioxide insufflation. Carbon dioxide insufflation is rarely required for VATS. In patients with hypercompliant lung disease, such as bullous emphysema, avoiding increased intrathoracic pressure and the risk of cardiopulmonary compromise is particularly important.

The common operative strategy in most laparoscopic and thoracoscopic procedures is the orientation of surgical instruments and the video camera in the same direction. Similar orientation avoids the video disorientation of mirror-imaging that results when surgical instruments are pointed toward the video camera. Whereas this principle is useful generally, the concavity of the chest often requires that thoracoscopic instruments be inserted from complementary angles. The small distances in the chest and the need to triangulate the lesion result in an unavoidable degree of mirror-imaging. In the early stages of thoracoscopic training, however, frequent changes of the video-camera port can limit the degree of distracting mirror-imaging.

To facilitate the change of instruments and video

ports, we generally use thoracoscopy ports or channels. A variety of ports are currently available and range from bluntly inserted plastic channels to more elaborate fixed and reusable instruments. Many of these instruments are inserted with a sharp trocar. Although thoracoscopy ports are not necessary to maintain insufflation, the channels provide operative flexibility by facilitating the frequent exchange of instruments and video ports. Thoracoscopy ports also improve visibility by keeping the video-camera lens clean. We favor the use of antifogging agents on the video-camera lens to optimize visibility.

BENIGN LUNG DISEASE

FOCAL LUNG DISEASE

A variety of benign lung diseases present as focal parenchymal lesions. In many patients, biopsy of the parenchymal lung lesion can be important in establishing the diagnosis and guiding management decisions. The conventional surgical approach to focal parenchymal lesions has been a limited thoracotomy and wedge resection. This procedure provides an adequate sample of lung tissue but limited access to other areas of the lung.

Thoracoscopy has proven to be an effective approach to the diagnosis of localized disorders of the lung [4–6]. It permits examination of the entire visceral surface of the lung [7,8]. Subpleural nodules can be examined, and representative biopsies can be obtained. We routinely obtain two biopsies to ensure a representative specimen. The biopsies should be taken not only of the abnormal-appearing lung tissue but also of a transition zone between normal and abnormal lung. The transition zone often reflects different stages of the evolving parenchymal process. The application of thoracoscopic biopsy is particularly important in diseases that require sufficient tissue for immunohistologic or genetic studies.

DIFFUSE LUNG DISEASE

Diffuse lung diseases often present with characteristic chest roentgenogram findings, physical findings, and spirometry. Lung tissue is often not required to establish a diagnosis. In patients who do require tissue confirmation, the conventional, minimally invasive approach to obtaining lung tissue has been transbronchial biopsy. In contrast to the situation for focal lung disease, sampling error is not a problem in diffuse lung disease.

Thoracoscopy plays a limited role in diffuse lung disease but may be helpful when extensive testing is required. A large transbronchial biopsy specimen can provide several hundred alveoli; nonetheless, this number may not be adequate for extensive histopathologic processing. We have used thoracoscopic biopsies in patients for whom additional tissue or more detailed histopathologic examination is required.

BULLOUS LUNG DISEASE

Most patients with chronic obstructive lung disease (COPD) have diffuse parenchymal disease. A few patients with COPD, however, develop rapid deterioration in respiratory function associated with a dominant bullous lesion apparent on chest roentgenograms. The bullous disease may expand over weeks to months with the associated compression of surrounding lung tissue.

A surgical approach to the treatment of progressive, unilateral bullous lung disease has been thoracotomy and bullectomy. The disadvantages of this approach are primarily related to the use of general anesthesia and the morbidity of thoracotomy. Most patients with bullous lung disease have significantly compromised lung function. General anesthesia, even without a painful incision, poses a substantial risk of postoperative ventilatory support. This risk is enhanced with the morbidity associated with a standard posterior lateral thoracotomy.

We have used thoracoscopy as an alternative to standard thoracotomy in the treatment of bullous lung disease. Thoracoscopy appears to limit postoperative pain and the compromised respiratory mechanics associated with posterior lateral thoracotomy [9].

The primary limitations to thoracoscopic resection of bullous lung disease include the need for general anesthesia and single-lung ventilation. Patients with end-stage obstructive lung disease may not adequately ventilate or oxygenate with single-lung ventilation. The major problem during single-lung ventilation is the prolonged expiratory phase in patients with severe COPD. The long expiratory phase limits the amount of compensatory hyperventilation that can be used during general anesthesia. The fixed minute ventilation can result in hypercarbia, acidemia, and impaired hemodynamics. An additional problem of the compliant lungs in COPD is gas trapping within the bulla. Because the bullae have little elasticity, they are not readily deflated even after aggressive airway aspiration. The persistent inflation of large bullae can significantly limit visualization.

In patients who have rapidly progressive unilateral bullous disease and can tolerate single-lung ventilation, we prefer a thoracoscopic bullectomy of the dominant bulla. A critical technical consideration is the accurate identification of the base of the bulla. Whereas air trapping within the bulla can hinder the general view of the lung, it often aids in identifying the interface between functioning lung parenchyma and the bulla. The resection is carefully planned to minimize the amount of functioning parenchyma compromised by the procedure. In addition, we minimize traction on the lung to prevent injury to the diseased parenchyma and limit postoperative air leaks. We have found that persistent air leaks have been more troublesome than residual space problems or prolonged postoperative ventilation.

SPONTANEOUS PNEUMOTHORAX

Primary spontaneous pneumothorax is caused by rupture of subpleural blebs in otherwise normal lungs. The blebs are found at the apex of the lung in more than 95% of patients. In approximately 5% of patients, associated subpleural blebs are found at the margin of the lower lobe. This distribution of subpleural blebs underscores the importance of careful inspection of the visceral pleura during any operative procedure.

The preferred treatment of a first episode of uncomplicated pneumothorax is either observation or tube thoracostomy. In healthy young patients with a less than 20% pneumothorax, observation is the treatment of choice. In patients with a larger pneumothorax, tube thoracostomy is required to evacuate the air and re-expand the lung. Most patients with primary spontaneous pneumothorax do not have ongoing air leaks with insertion of the chest tube and re-expansion of the lung.

Although most spontaneous pneumothoraces are uncomplicated, 3% to 20% of patients with pneumothoraces develop complications, such as tension pnemothorax, persistent air leaks, or recurrent pnemothoraces. In patients with complicated or recurrent disease, we favor thoracoscopic resection of subpleural blebs.

Patients with recurrent pneumothorax have an 80% chance of a third recurrence within 2 years. The conventional approach to the treatment of recurrent pneumothoraces has been the removal of subpleural blebs. This procedure, commonly referred to as apical bullectomy, is usually approached through an axillary incision. Axillary incisions provide exposure to the apical blebs and limited views of the lower lobe. An advantage of the axillary incision is that despite the limited exposure, it permits testing of the apex for persistent air leaks. In addition, the small axillary incision is generally well tolerated, and persistent air leaks are unusual.

Thoracoscopy has recently been advocated as an alternative to standard apical bullectomy [10–18]. The thoracoscope can be placed in any port along the midaxillary line for adequate visualization of the apex of the lung. We prefer an additional axillary port to facilitate manipulation of the lung apex. In most cases, we also use a single posterior port for the stapling device. A disadvantage of thoracoscopy is the inability to combine visualization and ventilation of the lung. Insufflation of the lung results in compromised visualization and the potential for a missed residual air leak. Despite this potential disadvantage, the apex of the lung is generally well seen during the procedure and recurrences are unusual.

LUNG NODULES AND CANCERS

SOLITARY PULMONARY NODULES

Solitary pulmonary nodules are spherical tumors of less than 3 cm that are completely surrounded by normal lung tissue. These lesions usually present in the outer half of the lung beyond the reach of the fiberoptic bronchoscope. Almost all lesions eventually prove to be cancer, granuloma, or hamartoma. The solitary pulmonary nodule represents a malignancy in more than 50% of patients over the age of 50 who have a significant smoking history. The risk of cancer increases with the length of smoking history. Further evidence for malignancy is growth of the nodule based on recent chest roentgenograms.

The conventional approach to establishing a histologic diagnosis in patients with solitary pulmonary nodules has involved the use of transbronchial biopsies, percutaneous transthoracic needle aspiration, or both. These procedures have been used to avoid the unnecessary morbidity of thoracotomy in patients with benign lung nodules. A problem with transbronchial and needle-aspiration biopsies has been their relatively high sampling error; moreover, the limited tissue available for testing can complicate attempts to establish a definitive diagnosis.

In contrast to transbronchial or needle-aspiration biopsy, thoracoscopy resects the entire nodule. The histopathologic analysis of the entire nodule eliminates sampling error and provides ample tissue for detailed testing. Using standard thoracoscopic techniques, a solitary lung nodule can be identified and excised during an overnight hospitalization. Thoracoscopic procedures can be performed with minimal postoperative pain and morbidity. For solitary nodules that prove to be granulomas or hamartomas, no further treatment is necessary.

Thoracoscopic resection of a malignant lesion provides the entire lesion for detailed histopathologic analysis. The histopathology may indicate that the nodule is a metastasis and no further resection is indicated. Alternatively, the histopathology may indicate the tumor is a primary lung cancer.

In most cases of primary lung cancer, thoracoscopic resection is inadequate, and a standard anatomic resection is indicated to decrease the incidence of local recurrence. Patients who can tolerate general anesthesia and single-lung ventilation for the thoracoscopic resection are generally able to tolerate an anatomic segmentectomy or lobectomy. Although thoracoscopic resections of primary lung cancers have not been studied in a randomized setting, the available evidence indicates that a parenchymal margin within 2 cm results in a 20% incidence of local recurrence [19]. In addition, a recent lung-cancer study group report demonstrated a 2.5-fold increase in local recurrence rates with limited resections [20].

Another disadvantage to limited parenchymal wedge resections is the lack of staging information obtained by the procedure. A peripheral wedge resection does not provide segmental or lobar nodal staging. In patients with isolated regional metastases, this staging information could provide important information for additional regional therapy.

ANATOMIC LUNG RESECTIONS

The use of the thoracoscope in video-assisted surgical techniques has significantly modified our approach to primary lung cancers. We have incorporated the video thoracoscope and thoracoscopic instrumentation into a variety of anatomic resections of the lung. In the majority of patients with stage I or II lung cancer, we perform an anatomic lobectomy. VATS has allowed us to minimize the length of the incision and the associated postoperative morbidity.

We typically anticipate the size of the resected lung and make one access port sufficiently long to permit removal of the specimen. For anatomic lobectomy, this incision is typically 40 to 45 mm. Most left-lung VATS

lobectomies can be performed through three access ports (Fig. 1). Right-sided lobectomies typically involve the use of four ports (Fig. 2). Although the intercostal spaces used in the procedure vary, the general orientation of the instruments is generally consistent for a particular lobe.

VATS UPPER LOBECTOMY

VATS right-upper lobectomy requires excellent visualization of both the superior vein and upper lobe artery. We have frequently used both an anterior video port and an anterior dissection port. A posterior access port is necessary for dissection of the upper lobe bronchus and the division of the major and minor fissures.

In a standard right-upper lobectomy, our routine is to divide the superior vein and the upper lobe artery before transecting the upper lobe bronchus. This division usually provides excellent exposure of the recurrent artery and both fissures.

A similar approach is used in a VATS left-upper lobectomy. We typically use only one anterior access port for the dissection of the upper lobe vein and bronchus. A posterior incision is used to expose the upper lobe arteries. In a standard VATS left-upper lobectomy, we initially transect the superior vein and upper lobe bronchus. Because of variations in normal arterial anatomy, the upper lobe arteries are exposed after division of the fissure and transected at the conclusion of the procedure.

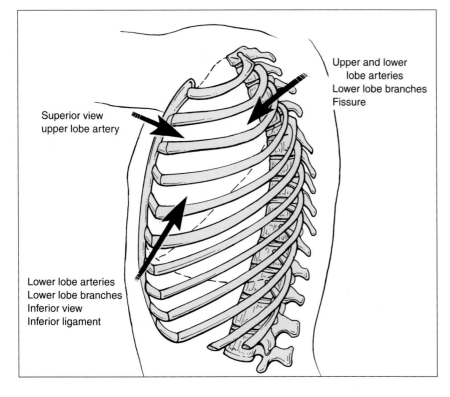

Superior view
upper lobe artery

Upper and lower
lobe arteries
Lower lobe branches
Fissure

Lower lobe arteries
Lower lobe branches
Inferior view
Inferior ligament

Figure 1. Schematic diagram of the access ports used in video-assisted anatomic resections of the left lung.

VATS LOWER LOBECTOMY

The surgical approach to a VATS lower lobectomy is considerably more predictable than in upper lobectomies. We orient our anterior and posterior access ports in the major fissures. This orientation permits visualization of both the artery and the bronchus to the lower lobe. After the division of the major fissure is completed, the inferior pulmonary vein is transected.

The video thoracoscope can also be incorporated into the evaluation of resectability. For example, the thoracoscope can be used to assess mediastinal involvement without a standard thoracotomy (Fig. 3). The parietal pleural surface can be examined for evidence of intrapleural metastatic spread. In several patients with computed tomography evidence of localized parenchymal lymphatic spread, we found metastatic pleural disease without pleural effusion. Thoracoscopy permits biopsy of these lesions as well as nodal sampling and staging.

VATS lobectomies have been successful in decreasing postoperative pain and its associated respiratory compromise. VATS procedures are commonly performed with hospital stays of 2 to 3 days. The primary obstacle to early discharge has been persistent air leaks. We believe that limiting postoperative air leaks with improved approaches to dividing incomplete fissures will further decrease hospital lengths of stay.

PERICARDIAL AND PLEURAL EFFUSIONS

Most patients with malignant pericardial effusions have associated malignant pleural effusions (Fig. 4). Because of the limited life expectancy of patients with malignant pleuropericardial effusions, thoracoscopy offers a minimally invasive approach to simultaneously treating the pericardial and the pleural disease [15,21–23].

The conventional subxiphoid approach to pericardial resection has been associated with a 20% to 30% recurrence rate within 3 months. This failure rate has led to the suggestion that a larger pericardial window would decrease the likelihood of recurrence. Some authors have advocated a phrenic nerve-to-phrenic nerve pericardial resection to limit recurrent effusions. We continue to use a subxiphoid approach to pericardial window in patients who cannot tolerate general anesthesia. Despite some discomfort, a subxiphoid window can be performed under local anesthesia.

Thoracoscopy offers a complementary approach to pericardial resections. Thoracoscopic pericardial windows require general anesthesia and single-lung ventilation in most patients. The thoracoscope can be introduced into either hemithorax and allows the surgeon to visualize the ipsilateral pericardium. A left-sided thoracoscopic approach exposes much of the pericardium

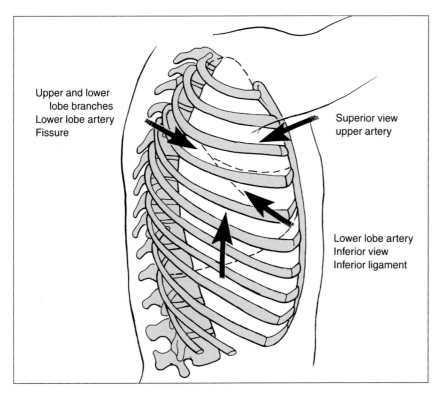

Figure 2. Schematic diagram of the access ports used in video-assisted anatomic resections of the right lung.

Upper and lower lobe branches
Lower lobe artery
Fissure

Superior view upper artery

Lower lobe artery
Inferior view
Inferior ligament

and permits windows to be placed both anterior and posterior to the phrenic nerve. This option is particularly useful in patients with a posterior loculated effusion. A right-sided approach permits access to the anterior pericardium, and an adequate window can be performed for most effusions.

In patients with an associated malignant pleural effusion, we use the thoracoscope to drain the effusion, create the pericardial window, and perform a talc poudrage. This procedure provides maximal benefit from the general anesthesia and minimizes patient discomfort. Although we were initially concerned about epicardial irritation with simultaneous pericardial window and talc poudrage, we have not had any complications from the combined procedure.

MEDIASTINAL DISEASES

ANTERIOR MEDIASTINUM

Radiographically apparent anterior mediastinal masses are typically caused by a goiter, thymoma, teratoma, or lymphoma. The thyroid gland is rarely located in the thorax. The diagnosis is usually made as an incidental finding on routine chest roentgenograms and confirmed by a radionuclide thyroid scan. In contrast, thymomas, lymphomas, and teratomas are anterior mediastinal masses that require histologic diagnosis. Needle-aspiration biopsies are of limited usefulness because of the importance of histologic architecture in establishing a diagnosis. Therefore, surgical biopsy plays a central role in these diseases.

Despite the need for surgery, anterior mediastinal masses are rarely an indication for thoracoscopic surgery [24,25]. The thyroid and thymus glands are

bilateral structures that are not fully visualized with a transpleural thoracoscopic approach. We prefer a trans-cervical or transsternal mediastinoscopy approach to provide exposure to the anterior mediastinum. Both mediastinoscopy approaches ensure adequate visualization of both lobes of the thyroid and thymus glands. In addition, the diagnosis of invasive thymoma is based on an assessment made at the time of surgery. We believe this assessment is difficult with a thoracoscopic approach.

To obtain tissue for diagnosis, we prefer to use a standard mediastinoscope. The mediastinoscope can be inserted through a small anterior mediastinotomy incision. The single working port of the mediastinoscope, used with the appropriate mediastinoscopy biopsy instruments, provides excellent exposure with minimal morbidity. Another advantage of anterior mediastinotomy is that it does not require single-lung ventilation.

MIDDLE MEDIASTINUM

Biopsies of mediastinal lymph nodes play an important role in the staging and treatment of lung cancer patients [26,27]. Patients with lung cancer confined to the lung have 5-year survival rates in excess of 50% to 60%. Involvement of mediastinal lymph nodes, however, decreases the expected 5-year survival rate to less than 10%.

The involvement of mediastinal lymph nodes is important not only to clarify the prognosis but to identify patients who might benefit from adjuvant therapy. Several multi-institutional studies are currently evaluating multimodality therapy in patients with early metastatic disease. The preliminary results of these investigations have been encouraging and underscore the importance of nodal staging. In most current multi-

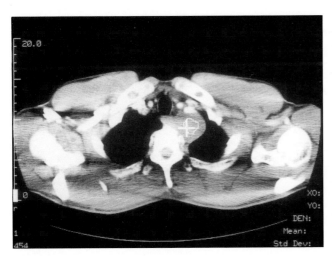

Figure 3. Chest computed tomography scan showing a left-upper lobe mass staged with the thoracoscope and resected using a video-assisted technique.

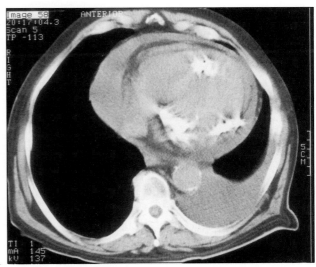

Figure 4. Chest computed tomography scan showing a malignant pericardial effusion and left pleural effusion. The pericardial window was performed through a left-sided thoracoscopy port. A pleurodesis was also performed.

modality protocols, not only are mediastinal lymph node biopsies mandatory, but mediastinal mapping is also required (Fig. 5) [28]. The distinction between ipsilateral (stage IIIA) and contralateral (stage IIIB) lymphnode involvement is particularly important in defining the role of surgical therapy.

The conventional approach for staging right-sided lung cancer is through a cervical mediastinoscopy incision. The patient is positioned supine, and the incision is made in the suprasternal notch. The mediastinoscope is introduced into the pretracheal fascia and advanced to the level of the subcarinal space. This approach provides access to the upper (level 2R) and lower (level 4R) paratracheal and subcarinal (level 7) lymph nodes. In most of our patients, the lymph node samples are examined by frozen section at the time of the operation. Negative frozen sections are an indication for resection of the primary tumor. Cervical mediastinoscopy is especially useful in providing access to both the anterior and posterior compartments of the subcarinal (level 7) nodal station.

Despite the development of thoracoscopic instrumentation, we still prefer cervical mediastinoscopy in all patients with enlarged paratracheal lymph nodes apparent on chest computed tomography scans. Cervical mediastinoscopy provides access to the right paratracheal and subcarinal lymph nodes as well as access to the contralateral paratracheal lymph nodes. Biopsies of the contralateral lymph nodes are important in distinguishing stage IIIA and IIIB lung cancer.

Cervical mediastinoscopy is also performed on all patients with right lower lobe tumors. Lower lobe lung cancers preferentially metastasize to the subcarinal space. The subcarinal nodal station is more readily explored through a cervical approach than a transpleural thoracoscopic approach. An additional reason to perform routine cervical mediastinoscopy in lower lobe tumors is that the subcarinal space is difficult to image, and subcarinal lymph node enlargement is difficult to assess by computed tomography.

In patients with right upper lobe cancers and no apparent metastatic disease, we have frequently used thoracoscopy to stage the right paratracheal lymph nodes. To perform a right paratracheal lymph node biopsy, the patient is turned to a lateral thoracotomy position and prepared for resectional surgery. Using access ports commonly used during a video-assisted procedure, the mediastinal pleura is incised cephalad to the azygos vein. The right lower (level 4R) and upper (level 2R) paratracheal lymph nodes are readily identified as a nodal cluster, and biopsies can be obtained. This approach has the additional benefit of permitting visual assessment of the tumor and preliminary dissec-

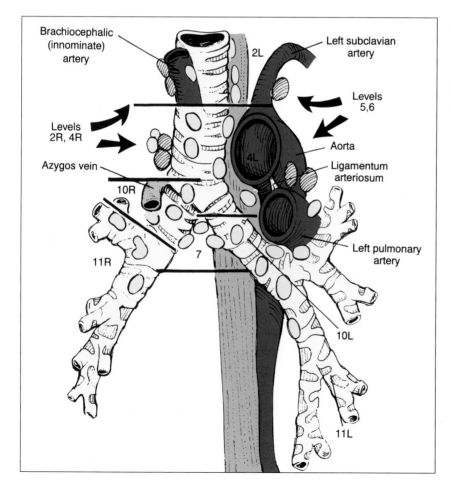

Figure 5. The American Thoracic Society's [28; with permission] classification of regional pulmonary lymph nodes. The thoracoscopic approaches to aorticopulmonary (Levels 5 and 6) and right paratracheal (Levels 2R and 4R) lymph nodes are shown.

tion of the hilar lymph nodes before the results of frozen section are available. Also, patients with right upper lobe tumors may have an involved azygos node that is not accessible by cervical mediastinoscopy but is readily seen at thoracoscopy.

Patients with left upper lobe masses provide another useful application of thoracoscopic nodal staging. Left upper lobe cancers preferentially metastasize to the aorticopulmonary (AP) window (levels 5 and 6). The conventional approach to diagnosing metastatic disease in the AP window is anterior mediastinoscopy (Chamberlain procedure). An incision is made in the second intercostal space, and the mediastinoscope is advanced into the subaortic mediastinal tissue. Anterior mediastinoscopy is usually performed without penetrating the mediastinal pleura. An advantage of an intact mediastinal pleura is that air or fluid does not enter the left chest. The mediastinoscopy can also be performed transpleurally, and the AP window can be biopsied from within the pleural space.

A more effective transpleural exposure of the AP window is obtained using thoracoscopic techniques. Patients for whom the computed tomography scan does not suggest nodal metastases are placed in the lateral thoracotomy position and prepared for surgery. The thoracoscopic ports are oriented to provide transpleural access to the AP window. Subaortic (level 5) lymph nodes are readily identified near the course of the phrenic and vagus nerves. In addition, lymph nodes at the base of the innominate artery (level 6) are also readily identified. Similar to the right-sided approach, the early stages of a video-assisted dissection of the upper lobe lymph nodes can be undertaken during processing of the frozen sections.

A disadvantage of a thoracoscopic approach is that it limits palpation of the lymph nodes. Palpation is helpful in identifying metastatic nodal disease. Also, thoracoscopic biopsies of the AP window and paratracheal lymph nodes require single-lung ventilation and the preoperative placement of a double-lumen endotracheal tube or bronchial blocker. This requirement is a minor consideration, however, in patients for whom an anatomic resection is anticipated.

POSTERIOR MEDIASTINUM

The thoracic surgical diseases of the posterior mediastinum are neurogenic tumors and lung cancers. Neurogenic tumors can be identified by plain chest radiographs (Fig. 6). The tumors are smooth walled and contiguous with the body of the vertebral column. The differential diagnosis of a patient presenting with a smooth-walled posterior mediastinal mass includes tumors of the pleura or lung, duplication cysts, and neurogenic tumors.

In patients without pleural adhesions or evidence of neural canal involvement, thoracoscopic surgery provides an excellent view of the pleural space. Visualization of the pleural space is useful in establishing the relationship of the tumor to vascular, neural, and bony structures. These relationships are critical in staging and assessing resectability.

Malignant tumors are typically identified by a characteristic retraction of overlying pleura or by invasion into adjacent structures. Direct assessment of the posterior mediastinum is particularly useful, as chest imaging has limited reliability in detecting invasion into vascular or bony structures. Thoracoscopic assessment of invasion can be performed with minimal morbidity and without complicating the subsequent resection. In cases of obvious malignancy, we also perform careful nodal staging at the time of thoracoscopic biopsy. This thoracoscopic staging has proved invaluable for the planning of subsequent resections.

Thoracoscopic resection of neurogenic tumors in the posterior mediastinum is performed with the patient in the semiprone position. An anterior access port is used to retract the lung, and two dissecting ports are used. In most cases, the tumors are easily visualized. The relationship of the tumor to surrounding vascular and neural structures can be defined. The parietal pleura is incised, and the tumor is retracted away from the vertebral body to expose the attachments of the tumor. We use vascular clips and avoid the use of cautery to minimize damage to associated neural tissue.

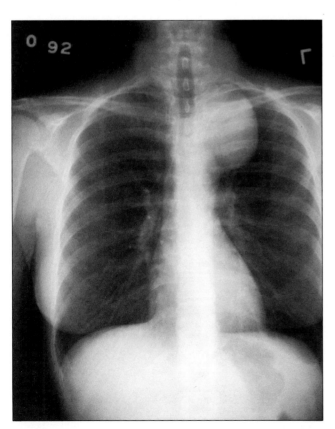

Figure 6. Chest radiograph of a patient with a posterior mediastinal mass. The neurogenic tumor (schwannoma) was thoracoscopically resected.

ESOPHAGEAL DISEASE

ACHALASIA

The most common motor disorder of the body of the esophagus is achalasia. Patients with achalasia typically present with obstructive symptoms. Medical management currently involves the use of endoscopic-guided pneumatic dilatation. Pneumatic dilatation provides effective palliation in the majority of patients. In approximately 20% of patients, however, pneumatic dilatation provides only temporary or minimal relief. These patients are usually referred for surgical treatment.

The obstructive symptoms of achalasia are the result of increased pressure in the lower esophageal sphincter and decreased effective peristaltic activity in the body of the esophagus. Surgical interventions have focused on the division of the lower esophageal sphincter muscle as a primary treatment of the obstructive symptoms. An extensive myotomy, however, may precipitate disabling gastroesophageal reflux. The gastroesophageal reflux can be exacerbated if the periesophageal tissue is ruptured during surgery and the lower esophagus migrates into the thorax.

The thoracoscope appears to be useful in performing an isolated lower esophageal sphincter myotomy. Experienced esophageal surgeons have promoted isolated myotomy in carefully selected patients; however, most surgeons believe that the myotomy must be performed with minimal disruption of the phrenoesophageal attachments to avoid gastroesophageal reflux.

An alternative to an isolated myotomy is the combination of myotomy and an antireflux operation. The addition of an antireflux operation permits the surgeon to fully mobilize the distal esophagus. Mobilization of the lower esophageal sphincter facilitates a careful examination and myotomy of the esophageal sphincter. We believe that in most cases of achalasia, failure of medical management and pneumatic dilatation requires a limited thoracotomy, myotomy, and antireflux operation.

BENIGN ESOPHAGEAL MASSES

Patients with benign masses in the esophagus usually present with mild obstructive symptoms. Barium esophagograms of these lesions typically demonstrate a smooth-contour obstructing lesion (Fig. 7), in contrast to the ulcerated "shelf-like" obstruction usually associated with esophageal malignancies. Most benign esophageal masses are leiomyomas.

Thoracoscopy provides a convenient approach to the resection of benign esophageal lesions. Our thoracoscopic approach to lesions in the distal 5 to 10 cm of the esophagus is through the left hemithorax. Lesions proximal to 30 to 35 cm are approached through the right hemithorax. The mediastinal pleura is incised and the mass is identified by inspection. A 42F Maloney bougie (Pilling Co., Fort Washington, PA) is inserted perorally to facilitate identification of the leiomyoma. After incision of the overlying muscular layer of the esophagus, the leiomyoma can be readily extracted from the esophageal wall. Almost all resections of leiomyomas can be performed without violating the mucosal integrity. In most cases, leiomyomas can be resected and the patient discharged after an overnight hospital stay.

ESOPHAGEAL CANCER

Many procedures have been advocated for the surgical therapy of esophageal cancer. These procedures include a partial esophageal resection with intrathoracic gastroesophageal anastomosis and an extended esophageal resection with cervical gastroesophageal anastomosis. The latter procedure can be performed with or without thoracotomy.

The extended esophagectomy with cervical anastomosis that is performed without thoracotomy is termed a *transhiatal esophagectomy*. Most of the dissection in a transhiatal esophagectomy is performed through the esophageal hiatus. Prolonged retraction of the crura provides adequate visualization of the esophagus up to the level of the subcarinal space. A second incision is made in the neck, and the dissection of the proximal esophagus is performed to the level of the azygos vein. This dissection can be aided with the use of a cervical mediastinoscope. Despite the efficacy of the cervical and

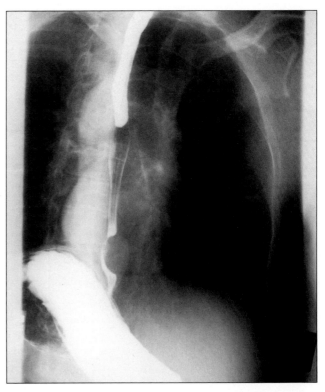

Figure 7. Barium esophagogram demonstrating the smooth-walled contour of a typical leiomyoma. The patient had mild obstructive symptoms, and the lesion was removed thoracoscopically.

abdominal approaches, there is a poorly visualized portion of the esophageal dissection in the region of the carina and azygos vein.

In selected patients, we have incorporated a video-assisted mobilization of the esophagus into the first stage of a transhiatal esophagectomy. A video-assisted approach provides an opportunity to visualize the distal airways and the azygos vein. In addition, video-assisted visualization of the midesophagus permits the resection of potentially involved lymph nodes. Another advantage of the video-assisted approach is that it provides an assessment of tumor invasion into mediastinal tissue. This visual assessment is a useful complement to transesophageal ultrasound (Fig. 8). Assessment of potential mediastinal invasion is particularly important when evaluating the need for open thoracotomy.

Video-assisted mobilization of the esophagus is performed with the patient positioned semiprone on the operating table. This position provides access to the posterior paravertebral recess and facilitates posterolateral thoracotomy if necessary (Fig. 9). With split-lung ventilation, the lung is retracted anteriorly and the mediastinal pleura is mobilized. We routinely transect the azygos vein with a vascular stapling device to permit visualization of the entire intrathoracic course of the esophagus.

The esophagus is initially mobilized at the level of the posterior pericardium. The dissection is carefully performed to avoid entering the contralateral pleural space. We routinely retract the phrenic nerves laterally to prevent an indirect traction injury to the recurrent nerves. Traction appears to be at least one potential cause of postoperative hoarseness. The esophagus is mobilized and encircled with at least one wide Penrose drain (Sherwood Medical, St. Louis, MO) for traction. The Penrose drains are circularized with a silk suture and positioned in the proximal or distal esophagus to facilitate dissection from the neck and abdomen. After video-assisted mobilization of the esophagus, the patient is turned to the supine position, and standard transhiatal esophagectomy is performed.

Whereas thoracoscopy is not used in many patients who require esophagectomy, video-assisted techniques do provide flexibility in the surgical approach to esophagectomy. In our experience, video-assisted techniques extend the indications for transhiatal esophagectomy to tumors in the proximal 30 cm of the esophagus and those with suspected mediastinal invasion.

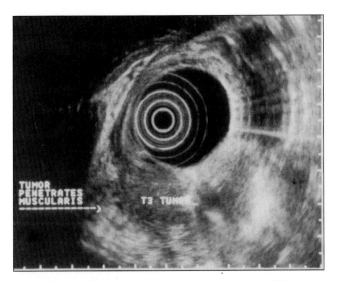

Figure 8. Esophageal ultrasound, demonstrating a T3 esophageal tumor that was thoracoscopically mobilized and resected using an abdominal and cervical incision.

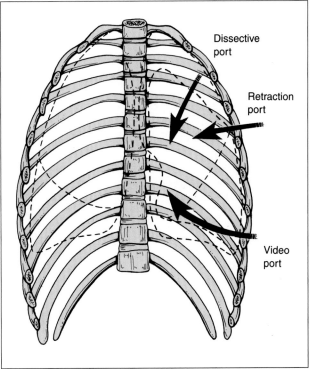

Figure 9. Schematic diagram of the access ports used in a right-sided thoracoscopic approach to the esophagus.

REFERENCES

Papers of particular interest, published within the period of review, have been highlighted as:
• Of special interest
•• Of outstanding interest

1. Jacobaeus HC: The Practical Importance of Thoracoscopy in Surgery of the Chest. *Surg Gynecol Obstet* 1922, 34:289–296.

2. Jacobaeus HC: The Cauterization of Adhesions in Pneumothorax Treatment of Tuberculosis. *Surg Gynecol Obstet* 1921, 33:493–500.

3.• McKneally MF, Lewis RJ, Anderson RJ, *et al*.: Statement of the AATS/STS Joint Committee on Thoracoscopy and Video Assisted Thoracic Surgery. *J Thorac Cardiovasc Surg* 1992, 104:1.

This is a statement of policy from the Committee. Thoracoscopy and video-assisted thoracic surgery should be done only by a trained and experienced thoracic surgeon who can do the procedure/s and manage the complications that might arise. The Committee advocates training for the techniques of thoracoscopy and VATS in approved thoracic residency and fellowship programs. It advocates training for current surgeons through courses which follow guidelines approved by the Committee.

4. Macha HN, Reichle G, von Zwehl D, *et al*.: The Role of Ultrasound Assisted Thoracoscopy in the Diagnosis of Pleural Disease. Clinical Experience in 687 Cases. *Eur J Cardiothorac Surg* 1993, 7:19–22.

5. Chen YN, Zhang DH: Application of Thoracoscopy in the Diagnosis of Pleuro-pulmonary Disease. *Chung Hua Chieh Ho Ho Hu Hsi Tsa Chih* 1990, 13:144–146, 190.

6. Raffenberg M, Mai J, Loddenkemper R: Results of Thoracoscopy in Localized Lung and Chest Wall Diseases. *Pneumologie* 1990, 44(1):182–183.

7. Faurschou P: Diagnostic Thoracoscopy in Pleuro-pulmonary Infiltrates Without Pleural Effusion. *Endoscopy* 1985, 17:21–25.

8. Kaiser LR: Diagnostic and Therapeutic Uses of Pleuroscopy (Thoracoscopy) in Lung Cancer. *Surg Clin North Am* 1987, 67:1081–1086.

9. Bagnato VJ, Ravo B: Modern Operative Thoracoscopy. *G Chir* 1992, 13:133–136.

10. Dotsenko AP, Potapenkov MA, Shipulin PP: Diagnostic and Therapeutic Thoracoscopy in Spontaneous and Traumatic Pneumothorax. *Vestn Khir* 1990, 144:14–17.

11. Hajbi O, Fico JL, Seitz B, *et al*.: The Value of Initial Thoracoscopy in the Treatment of Pneumothorax. *Rev Pneumol Clin* 1990, 46:14–18.

12. Inderbitzi R, Furrer M, Striffeler H: Surgical Thoracoscopy—Indications and Technique. Early Results in Spontaneous Pneumothorax. *Chirurg* 1992, 63:334–341.

13. Kabanov AN, Kozlov KK, Kabanov AA: The Use of a Plasma Scalpel During Thoracoscopy for the Treatment of Traumatic and Spontaneous Pneumothorax. *Grud Serdechnososudistaia Khir* 1990, 12:55–57.

14. Mouroux J, Benchimol D, Bernard JL, *et al*.: Surgical Treatment of Pneumothorax by Video-Thoracoscopy. *Presse Med* 1992, 21:1079–1082.

15. Oakes DD, Sherck JP, Brodsky JB, Mark JB: Therapeutic Thoracoscopy. *J Thorac Cardiovasc Surg* 1984, 87:269–273.

16. Rogers DA, Philippe PG, Lope TE, *et al*.: Thoracoscopy in Children: An Initial Experience With an Evolving Technique. *J Laparoendosc Surg* 1992, 2:7–14.

17. Torre M, Belloni P: Nd:YAG Laser Pleurodesis Through Thoracoscopy: New Curative Therapy in Spontaneous Pneumothorax. *Ann Thorac Surg* 1989, 47:887–889.

18. Wakabayashi A, Brenner M, Wilson AF, *et al*.: Thoracoscopic Treatment of Spontaneous Pneumothorax Using Carbon Dioxide Laser. *Ann Thorac Surg* 1990, 50:786–789.

19. Miller Jr JI: Therapeutic Thoracoscopy: New Horizons for an Established Procedure. *Ann Thorac Surg* 1991, 52:1036–1037.

20. Ginsberg RJ, Rubinstein L, for the Lung Cancer Study Group: Patients with T1 N0 Non-SCLC Lung Cancer. *Lung Cancer* 1991;7(suppl):83 (Abstract 304).

21. Menzies R, Charbonneau M: Thoracoscopy for the Diagnosis of Pleural Disease. *Ann Intern Med* 1991, 114:271–276.

22. Ladjimi S, M'Raihi ML, Djemel A: Pleural Talc Treatment Using Thoracoscopy in Lymphomatous Pleurisy. *Rev Mal Respir* 1991, 8:75–77.

23. Rusch VW, Mountain C: Thoracoscopy Under Regional Anesthesia for the Diagnosis and Management of Pleural Disease. *Am J Surg* 1987, 154:274–278.

24. Coltharp WH, Arnold JH, Alford WC Jr, *et al*.: Videothoracoscopy: Improved Technique and Expanded Indications. *Ann Thorac Surg* 1992, 53:776–778.

25. Landreneau RJ, Dowling RD, Castillo WM, Ferson PF: Thoracoscopic Resection of an Anterior Mediastinal Tumor. *Ann Thorac Surg* 1992, 54:142–144.

26. Goldstraw P: The Practice of Cardiothoracic Surgeons in the Perioperative Staging of Non-Small Cell Lung Cancer. *Thorax* 1992, 47:1–2.

27. Tsang GM, Watson DC: The Practice of Cardiothoracic Surgeons in the Perioperative Staging of Non-Small Cell Lung Cancer. *Thorax* 1992, 47:3–5.

28. Tisi GM, Friedman PJ, Peters RM, *et al*.: American Thoracic Society, Medical Section of the American Lung Association: Clinical Staging of Primary Lung Cancer. *Am Rev Respir Dis* 1983, 127:659–664.

INDEX

FREE POSTAGE! No stamp required if you live in the following countries:

AUSTRALIA, BELGIUM, BERMUDA, CYPRUS, DENMARK, FINLAND, FRANCE, GERMANY, HONG KONG, ICELAND, ISRAEL, ITALY, LUXEMBOURG, MONACO, THE NETHERLANDS, NEW ZEALAND, NORWAY, PORTUGAL, REPUBLIC OF IRELAND, SINGAPORE, SPAIN, SWEDEN, SWITZERLAND, THE UNITED ARAB EMIRATES, UNITED KINGDOM, UNITED STATES.

BUSINESS REPLY MAIL
FIRST CLASS MAIL PERMIT NO. 33925 PHILADELPHIA, PA

Postage Will Be Paid By Addressee

CURRENT SCIENCE
SUBSCRIPTIONS
20 N THIRD ST
PHILADELPHIA, PA 19106-9815

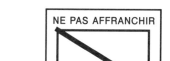

By air mail
Par avion

IBRS/CCRI NUMBER: PHQ-D/453/W

NE PAS AFFRANCHIR

NO STAMP REQUIRED

REPONSE PAYEE
GRANDE-BRETAGNE

CURRENT SCIENCE
34-42 CLEVELAND STREET
LONDON W1E 4QZ
GREAT BRITAIN

BUSINESS REPLY MAIL
FIRST CLASS PERMIT NO. 33925 PHILADELPHIA, PA

Postage Will Be Paid By Addressee

CURRENT SCIENCE
SUBSCRIPTIONS
20 N THIRD ST
PHILADELPHIA, PA 19106-9815

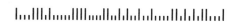

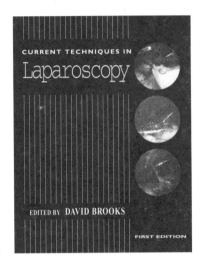